*Evaluating the
Impact of Nutrition and
Health Programs*

Evaluating the Impact of Nutrition and Health Programs

Edited by

Robert E. Klein
Pan American Health Organization/Institute of
Nutrition of Central America and Panama
Guatemala, Guatemala

Merrill S. Read
Pan American Health Organization
Washington, D.C.

Henry W. Riecken
University of Pennsylvania
Philadelphia, Pennsylvania

James A. Brown, Jr.
U.S. Agency for International Development
Washington, D.C.

Alberto Pradilla
Foundation for Higher Education
Cali, Colombia

and

Carlos H. Daza
Pan American Health Organization
Washington, D.C.

PLENUM PRESS · NEW YORK AND LONDON

Library of Congress Cataloging in Publication Data

Pan American Health Organization International Conference on the Assessment
of the Impact of Nutrition and Related Health Programs, Panama, 1977.
Evaluating the impact of nutrition and health programs.
Includes index.
1. Public health—Evaluation—Congresses. 2. Nutrition—Evaluation—Congresses. 3. Evaluation research (Social action programs)—Congresses. 4. Malnutrition—Latin America—Prevention—Congresses. I. Klein, Robert E. II. Pan American Health Organization. III. Title. IV. Title: Impact evaluation. [DNLM: 1.
Nutrition—Standards—Congresses. 2. Nutrition disorders—Congresses. 3. Evaluation studies—Congresses. 4. Public health America—Congresses.
QU145 C747p 1977]
RA427.P216 1977   614   79-11321

ISBN 978-1-4684-3491-0   ISBN 978-1-4684-3489-7 (eBook)
DOI 10.1007/978-1-4684-3489-7

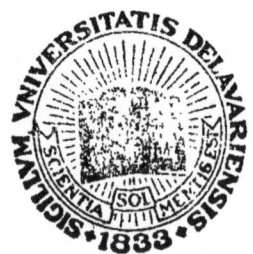

Based on the proceedings of the PAHO International Conference on the
Assessment of the Impact of Nutrition and Related Health Programs,
held in Isla Contadora, Panama, August 1—4, 1977

© 1979 Plenum Press, New York
Softcover reprint of the hardcover 1st edition 1979

A Division of Plenum Publishing Corporation
227 West 17th Street, New York, N.Y. 10011

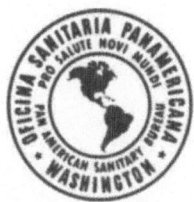 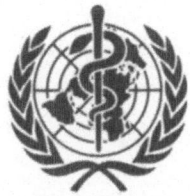

Preparation of this volume has been a joint effort of Plenum Press and the Pan American Health Organization, Regional Office of the World Health Organization. This volume also is to be published in Spanish for distribution through the Pan American Health Organization, Washington, D.C. 20037

Foreword

As is noted in the opening chapter of this volume, nutrition
and public health programs have been important throughout Latin
America and the Caribbean for many years. This is due to the special concerns of those responsible for setting national policies,
the program experience and leadership in public health developed
by the national governments, and the stimulus and cooperation of
the Pan American Health Organization (PAHO), including its twelve
associated centers which focus on research, training and program
development.

The need for a coordinated hemisphere-wide attack on malnutrition and other health problems was expressed clearly in the
"Ten Year Health Plan for the Americas" (1). This plan established
specific targets for reducing the prevalence of the major nutritional diseases and other health problems for the decade 1971-1980.
It was noted at that time that very few countries had formulated
adequate comprehensive national food and nutrition policies and
plans, nor had they developed strategies for combating the nutritional deficiencies known to affect large numbers of people throughout the Region. Following a review of the available data on a
country by country basis in 1975, the PAHO Directing Council endorsed recommendations for formulating the necessary national policies and strategies for the intersectorial execution of food, nutrition and health programs (2). This report also summarized the
available national data related to nutritional status, existing
programs such as food fortification, and the human resources available for services as well as for research and education.

The nutritional problems in the Americas are varied. The
most frequently encountered deficiency is protein-energy malnutrition (PEM). It affects the growth and health of large numbers of
young children and also contributes importantly to low birth
weight of infants born to inadequately nourished mothers. PEM is
seen most often among the rural populations and the marginal urban

poor in rapidly expanding cities. It is seen much less frequently in those areas and countries where health and community services have been extended to provide adequate coverage or in those areas where extremes of wealth or poverty are not great. In nearly all its forms under-nutrition is associated with higher incidence of gastroenteritis and other childhood diseases, either as a result of decreased food intake during illness or because malnutrition adversely affects the development of immunologic defense mechanisms. Therefore the development of appropriate national programs, and their evaluation, must be approached on a multisectorial and multi-disciplinary basis.

Several of the countries in the Western Hemisphere have developed extensive national food and nutrition plans. In these countries a variety of program activities have been projected or implemented. These include food stamps or food supplements for target populations, nutritional fortification of commonly eaten foods, extension of primary health care coupled with nutrition and health education, agricultural reform, and income maintenance.

Information systems, (i.e., health and nutritional surveillance) are being implemented in several countries to determine where problems lie, what services are being delivered, and what may be the impact of national programs as they are implemented (3,4). Frequently these efforts are centered in the health ministries (5). However, a multisectorial approach to impact evaluation will obviously be required if serious attention is to be given to the well-being of the needy populations. Papers in this volume make this point abundantly clear.

It is clear that evaluation of the impact of nutrition and health programs will become increasingly more important as countries throughout the world seek to provide services to meet the needs of their populations. We believe that this volume will stimulate new and innovative approaches to this end.

The Pan American Health Organization wishes to express its appreciation to the United States Agency for International Development for financial support of the conference and preparation of this volume.

Héctor R. Acuña
Director, Pan American
Health Organization

REFERENCES

1. Pan American Health Organization. *Ten Year Health Plan for the Americas*. PAHO Official Document No. 118, Washington 1973

2. Organiazción Panamericana de la Salud. *Políticas Nacionales de Alimentación y Nutrición*. Publ. Cientif. No. 328. Washington 1976.

3. Joint FAO/UNICEF/WHO Expert Committee. *Methodology of Nutritional Surveillance*, Technical Report Series #593. Geneva: World Health Organization 1976.

4. Coloquio sobre Sistemas de Vigilancia Epidemiológica Nutricional, IV Congreso Latino Americano de Nutrición, Caracas, Venezuela, November 1976. Published in *Arch. Latinoamer. Nutr.* 27 (2), Supplement, June 1977. (English translation: Pan American Health Organization 1978. In preparation).

5. Daza, C. H. and M. S. Read. Health-related Components of a Nutritional Surveillance System. Paper presented at Plenary Session of *IX International Congress on Nutrition*, Rio de Janeiro, August 1978.

Contents

V.   PRACTICE AND PROBLEMS OF IMPACT EVALUATION

RATIONALE FOR THE CONFERENCE AND

ORGANIZATION OF THE VOLUME

NEED FOR A CONFERENCE

Although health and nutrition services are expanding rapidly in Latin America and other low income regions around the world, surprisingly little is known about the various impacts of these services on the program recipients. Particularly, there is distressingly little information available on program benefits with which to design or redesign service delivery systems. Design decisions based on facts are increasingly important, however, both in terms of anticipating resource requirements and ultimately in terms of assuring that benefits accrue to target populations.

The impetus for a conference on methods for impact evaluation began during discussions in connection with the design of an integrated nutrition, health and social development program to be undertaken in Central America under the auspices of the Institute of Nutrition of Central America and Panama (INCAP), a specialized research center within the Pan American Health Organization (PAHO).

In the early planning for assessing the impact of this program, considerable literature was reviewed. This identified a number of useful references. It became clear, however, that the published literature was insufficient as the sole source for the design of new research projects. First, the literature is elusive in the sense that there are numerous journals that publish the results of intervention studies and it is simply impossible, without a massive effort, to locate all of them. Many monographs and journals carrying this information often are uncatalogued or unobtainable. Further, some of the most useful articles collected refer to completed or on-going studies with results reported in unpublished documents, while most of the very recent findings have yet to be published.

It was equally apparent that although attempts at assessment of large scale intervention programs in nutrition and health have increased markedly in recent years, a wide variety of outcome measures were being utilized in these studies. In fact, there appeared

1

to be little agreement even on the terminology for defining measures and outcomes. It was concluded that the use of common outcome measures would permit comparisons among projects, increasing
their utility as well as the generalizability of research findings
across various communities and countries.

Thus, the idea evolved for a conference which would draw upon
experts from various professions and disciplines, persons who could
contribute to a comprehensive review of the state-of-the-art in connection with the measurement of program impact. Because the United
States Agency for International Development shared the concern for
the refinement of outcome measures, they agreed to participate in
the planning and to provide major support for the conference.

The conference was designed to explore the conceptual difficulties of clarifying and ordering causal relationships among: (a)
the large number of health services; (b) an even larger variety of
social, economic, and environmental causal factors outside experimental control; and (c) a wide variety of program impacts. These
conceptual difficulties are matched by practical difficulties in
selecting and effecting concrete measurements in the field. Finally, there are social and organizational difficulties in starting,
controlling, and using impact evaluation.

ORGANIZATION OF THE VOLUME

This volume contains most but not all of the papers presented
during the conference, updated in greater detail than originally
drafted. In addition, two new sections have been added -- a final
overview of important themes and problems discussed during the
meeting, plus an integrated descriptive glossary of terms applicable
to evaluating the impact of nutrition and related health interventions. This glossary will be particularly helpful to those not
familiar with evaluation methodology; it also provides a useful
guide to different uses of similar terms among the various contributors.

The conference opened with a discussion of the multiple determinants of health and nutritional status prepared by Daly, Davis
and Robertson. This paper provides a general treatment of the impact of social and economic conditions on health and nutritional
status, providing a thoughtful introduction to the volume.

The remainder of the volume is divided into three major sections. The *first section* explores approaches to impact evaluation,
with the papers by Cook and McAnany, and by Townsend, Farrell and
Klein intended, respectively, to provide overviews of the conceptual
issues and of field data collection problems which are frequently
encountered.

The *second section* consists of four papers which discuss the impact of health and nutrition programs on health and nutritional status, and also on educational, social, and economic conditions of family life. This multi-criteria approach to the measurement of program impact reflects the belief that the development process is highly complex as it affects the individual and the family. We believe that social service programs modify the balance of the many factors that influence the family, and it is this overall balance that conditions the quality of life for the individual and family. Consequently, it is necessary to study the impact of health and nutrition programs not only in terms of explicit program objectives, but also in terms of the impact on other closely linked social and economic factors.

One may discuss the impact of health and nutrition programs on the individual, family, community, region, or nation. Each focus provides unique insights and requires specific measurements and approaches. Focusing on the individual tends to direct attention to the efficacy and utilization of medical treatment and nutrition interventions. Focusing on populations -- the community, region or nation -- emphasizes the social-structural and environmental setting of health and nutrition services. Emphasizing the family allows consideration of both the individual and the community. The family focus highlights the most important interpersonal interactions. It is in the family group that vital decisions are made regarding the distribution of food, the relative importance of various personal and familial objectives, and the behavior that will encourage health or change the vulnerability to disease.

The paper by Habicht and Butz discusses the impact of health and nutrition programs on health and nutritional status. In this area, we expect the clearest theoretical understanding of the relationship between program and objective, and the clearest demonstration of causality. Here is the acid test of programs; if impact on health and nutrition cannot be shown comparable to expenditures, health and nutrition programs will be severely criticized. Historically, the evaluation of health programs has been notoriously ineffective, and serious criticisms of health programs for lack of impact or for negative impact are current (1, 2). Consequently, this chapter presents the central theme of the volume.

The paper by Scrimshaw and Pelto focuses on family composition and structure as these relate to health and nutrition programs. It is obvious that the physical health of the family is a strong element in the socio-economic well-being of the family. The social pathology caused by the death of the head of a young family is a common historical theme. More generally, the history, existence, or high risk of disease and disability must influence family behavior in a variety of ways. An area of vigorous debate in this field is whether perceived high probability of death of children is a major cause of continued high fertility. In any case, evaluation of the impact of health and nutrition services on family structure and composition is a key element in holistic service evaluation, as well as a necessity in resolving major theoretical issues bearing on the value of health services.

The evaluation of the impact of health and nutrition programs on the household economy is treated in the paper by Chernichovsky. The theme is an extension of historically important work (3, 4, 5) in health economics relating to the investment value of health services, and to more recent work on nutrition and productivity (6). In the more modern treatment, however, it is recognized that the income redistribution and risk-sharing impacts of social services must be measured directly. Moreover, as health and nutrition programs are more fully integrated into a philosophy of generalized community development, changes in health and nutritional status may be indirect effects mediated through family economic changes. Finally, welfare must be estimated in terms of the family's own perception of its life condition. Without an appreciation of these conceptual issues and appropriate measurements of economic variables, we feel that evaluation of health and nutrition programs will be incomplete and, to some extent, misleading.

Finally, the impact of health and nutrition services on social competence is treated in the paper by Mushkin. Strong indications exist that severe malnutrition of young children causes irremediable reduction of mental capacity. More immediately, many health and nutrition projects are undertaken specifically to improve the performance of children in school. Moreover, health services are often described as non-formal education in that they educate traditional consumers as to the value of (governmental) services from the modern sector. In almost all cases, educational objectives of health and nutrition services postulate indirect causality. Educational objectives are important in the motivation for services, but difficult to evaluate in terms of service impact.

Each of the four papers of the second section is developed with discussion of (a) the conceptual framework linking health and nutrition programs with outcomes of concern, and (b) the indices and measurements required to measure the hypothesized impacts. This focus is fundamental to the approach to evaluation that the conference promulgated. Changes in the quality of life accrue from a number of sources: autonomous actions of individuals and families; direct and indirect impacts of private and public programs; changes in the environment beyond the control of man; and chance. In the evaluation of health and nutrition programs, it will not suffice to measure improvements in welfare that occur during the programs. Rather, it is necessary to deal conceptually with the causes of change, and to attribute to any program only those changes that it may reasonably be thought to have caused. For this purpose, a conceptual model of causality is fundamental. A model which allows the attribution of change to programmatic versus non-programmatic causal factors is as much a part of the evaluation method as is the measurement of the hypothesized causal factors and the measurement of impact variables.

The *third section* of the volume deals with social and organizational issues in impact evaluation. The paper by Emrey and Ugalde discusses the role of impact evaluation within an organizational and national framework. Evaluation programs will be meaningful and bureaucratically possible only if impact evaluation fits the perceived needs of decision makers and is facilitated by health and nutrition service providers. We perceive that the relative lack of success of impact measurement programs in the past was in major part due to failures in designing programs in terms of the political and organizational realities of their environments.

Finally, the paper by Stromberg deals with the diffusion of information. The literature on impact evaluation research is very small, in large part because information on the failures of projects and evaluation efforts is more often restricted than shared. The utilization of existing information available in the world for actual decision-making in public and private institutions is also of concern.

The scope of this volume is, therefore, (a) to acquaint the reader with a general overview of health and nutrition impact measurement; (b) to discuss in detail the conceptual and practical difficulties of measuring four types of impacts; and (c) to discuss the social problems of use of impact data.

REFERENCES

1. Cochrane, A. L. *Effectiveness and Efficiency: Random Reflections on Health Services*. Nuffield Provincial Hospitals Trust, 1972.

2. Illich, I. *Medical Nemesis: The Expropriation of Health*. New York: Pantheon Books, 1976.

3. Winslow, C. E. A. *The Cost of Sickness and the Price of Health*. Geneva: World Health Organization, 1951.

4. Rice, D. P. Estimating the Cost of Illness. *Health Economics No. 6*. U. S. Public Health Service Publication No. 947-6, Washington, D. C.: United States Government Printing Office, 1966.

5. Mushkin, S. J. Health as an investment. *J. Political Econ.* 70:129-157, 1962.

6. Viteri, F. E., B. Torún and M. D. C. Immink. Nutrition and productivity. Effect of energy (calories) intake and

supplementation on the productivity of agricultural la-
borers in Central America. In: *Proceedings of XIV
Meeting of the Advisory Committee on Medical Research,
PAHO, Washington, July, 1975.* Guatemala: Institute of
Nutrition of Central America and Panama, 1977.

DETERMINANTS OF HEALTH AND NUTRITIONAL STATUS

John A. Daly,
Joseph H. Davis *
     Agency for International Development
     Washington, D. C.

and

Robert Robertson
     Mt. Holyoke College
     South Hadley, Massachusetts

This volume stresses the impact of health and nutrition services on health and socio-economic well-being. In the breadth of focus, and in the explicit recognition of the mediating role of other socio-economic factors, we feel the approach is innovative.

This paper, however, complements the remainder by treating the impact of social and economic conditions on health and nutrition. Our intent is to go beyond the collection of intermediate and control variables described in other papers. We regard health as a fundamental indicator of the quality of life, and believe that health is affected by the human ecology and by complex social and economic policies of the society to an even greater extent than it is affected by health services *per se*. Consequently, in the following pages we sketch a model of the health and nutrition impacts of key public policies.

In practice, the great complexity of the interaction of health and nutrition programs with socio-economic development should lead us to great caution. The topic is among the most complex in modern society, and our theoretical understanding and measurement capac-

* Current address: Health Systems Planning Branch, Office of International Health, 3700 East-West Highway, Hyattsville, Maryland 20782

ity are frail indeed. Impact evaluation in these areas is of paramount importance, but should be approached with humility, and results interpreted with caution and restraint. We suggest that the
major benefit from improved evaluation programs will come as many
investigations contribute information to a growing worldwide understanding of health, nutrition, development, and social service programs.

At a minimum, professionals involved in evaluating the impact
of health and nutrition services should be aware of this larger context of public policy. Service evaluations should certainly keep
track of key policies affecting health, and should plan and modify
evaluation activities in the light of major socio-economic policy
shifts.

We look forward, however, to a future time in which health and
nutrition status will be among the key indices for the planning and
evaluation of public policy. If economic, agricultural, educational, and other major policies profoundly affect the survival and
health of the public, is it not reasonable to expect indicators such
as life expectancy to play as important a role in national planning
as does per capita income?

The following discussion is a very modest step in the direction of socio-economic planning for health. Figure I illustrates
the model that will be developed. Six major policy areas are discussed. For each, key elements that affect health and nutrition

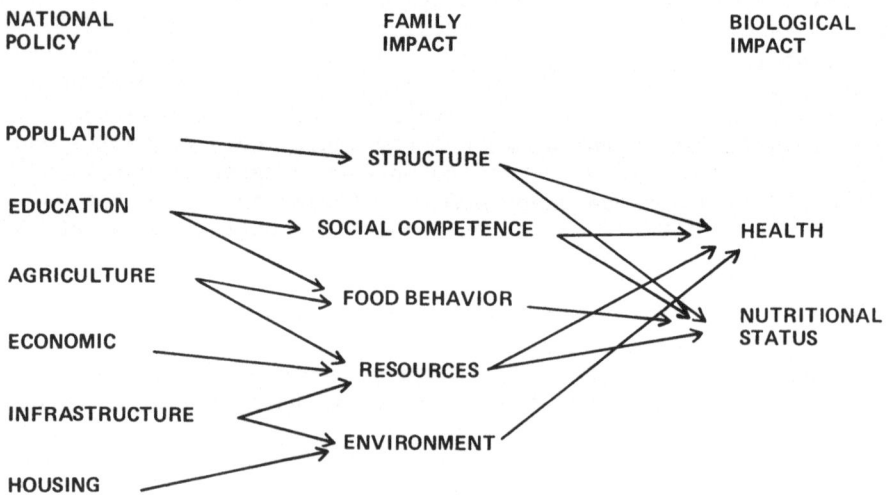

Fig. I. *Conceptual Linkage of National Policies (Other than Health)
and Health and Nutrition.*

are isolated, and causal paths are suggested by which the impact is made. The analysis deals with the structure of the family and the behavior, competence, resources, and environment of the family and individual.

In general, we believe in the following propositions. Development of food systems generally makes food more affordable and available, contributing to increased consumption, which at least early in the process of development reduces malnutrition and its sequelae. Demographic transition, specifically the lowering of birth rates accompanying development, results in women with high medical risk having fewer children. Fewer children per family in turn result in more family income and wealth being available for each member, in longer child spacing (allowing more attention per child), and finally in less interfamilial contact with communicable disease. Increasing personal and familial wealth and income allows purchase of a better diet, of more adequate clothing and shelter, and of services which contribute to health. Similarly, the infrastructure of aqueducts and sewage systems allows better personal hygiene, reducing the transmission of disease, and access to more potable water, reducing the incidence of water-borne disease. Education increases the individual's and the family's understanding of disease processes and thereby leads to increased capacity to prevent or treat illness. Finally, housing and urbanization alter the relationships among man, disease agents, and health services.

BIDIRECTIONAL CAUSAL SYSTEMS AND THEIR ANALYSIS

The major theme of this paper is that health and nutrition programs and improvements in health and nutrition have significant impacts on family economics, education, social competence, family size and structure, and other socio-economic factors. We also suggest in the following discussion that the latter factors strongly affect health and nutrition. The argument can obviously be generalized to the individual and community levels. Thus, the causal relationships between these socio-economic and biological variables are bidirectional.

The observations that the sick are often poor and the poor are often sick should not cause great surprise. The difficulty arrives when one tries to ascribe causality -- people are sick because they are poor or are poor because they are sick. Impact evaluation techniques must be chosen to answer these questions, or rather to identify the importance of each of the various causal processes which interact.

Simple models often incorporate unidirectional causality, whereby an outcome is determined by the influence of a number of controllable and non-controllable independent variables (1,2,3). We are postulating a more complex situation in which changes in each health and socio-economic variable tend to depend on all other variables (i.e., our model has few or no truly "independent" variables, and highly complex feedback situations exist). Data representing either a cross-section of communities or a history of one community will not be equivalent to the outcomes of independent experiments. Rather, they may be thought to represent a set of solutions to complex systems of social equations. In theory, this viewpoint suggests that two or three stage linear regressions are more appropriate than linear regressions (or to simple analysis of variance techniques comparable to linear regressions) (4).

We stress further the importance of this point. If economic conditions, educational and social behavior, demographic conditions and family structure, and health and nutrition are best analyzed as a set of simultaneously interacting causal systems, then the analysis will usually be complex, and data will generally be needed for collateral variables. Behavior of variables may often be non-intuitive or counter-intuitive. The task of assuring that communities or families are really comparable, and should be used as data for the same system, will not be trivial. Moreover, different hypothetical models may lead to serious divergencies in the estimation of the importance, or even the direction of key causal relations. In general, the explication of complex systems of bidirectional causal relations in social systems is extremely difficult in theory, and more difficult in practice. However, as the paper by Chernichovsky later in this volume observes, evaluators of nutrition and health programs and non-economist social scientists can learn a great deal about these matters from the theory and methods of econometrics.

THE IMPACT OF AGRICULTURAL AND FOOD POLICIES ON HEALTH AND NUTRITIONAL STATUS

In most developing countries, the primary problem of malnutrition is insufficient food consumption. To resolve problems of malnutrition, sufficient amounts of appropriate food must be available, local taboos or cultural practices must not prevent its consumption, and individuals and families must have the economic power to acquire that food. If there is insufficient food, or if people are too poor to buy an adequate diet, there will be malnutrition.

This simple statement has profound consequences in terms of nutrition planning. It suggests that an appropriate organization of major national socio-economic systems is required to assure food availability. In fact, macroeconomic planning for nutrition is being actively promulgated by international organizations (5, 6, 7).

The variable describing food as seen by the consumer, the major output indicators for agricultural and economic policy at the national level, are key variables for understanding nutrition. In principle, one would wish to monitor these national policies, their direct impacts on key intervening variables, and their further impacts on health and nutrition. Such a conceptual framework for evaluation would be useful for evaluating micro- or macro-programs. 1/ Some of the most important variables of this frame of reference are shown in Figure II.

Agricultural production policies are the most obvious ones determining food availability (8): Investments in land and water resources, improvements of technology, improvements of agricultural input and product markets, subsidies and taxes all modify the production of food. Policies implemented with sound agricultural bases, such as those directed toward improved balance of trade or maximization of agricultural income, may have profound negative impacts on food availability when farmland is devoted to high value, low nutrient crops such as coffee or tea. Alternatively, such policies may be nutritionally appropriate where comparative advantage favors purchase of food grains or other nutritionally appropriate foods with export earnings.

Food processing activities must also be considered. Increasing attention is being directed to the reduction of post-harvest food losses in developing countries. Such losses contribute significantly to reduction of availability of food grains and are very important for more perishable foods. Obviously, food storage and preservation is critically important in the case of seasonal food shortages. Similarly, fortification and the development of new foods offer significant potential for improving nutrient availability at low cost (8).

Food distribution systems also play key roles in determining food availability. Historically, famine has been a problem of local failure of food production rather than of global shortages. Crop failures in large geographical areas of the developing world can engender almost insuperable obstacles in moving adequate stocks of food. However, even in non-critical periods the food distribu-

---

1/ We define micro-program as one composed of direct medical or food services organized primarily for health or nutritional effects on individuals. A macro-program is one composed of macro-economic or socio-economic policy actions to achieve health and nutrition objectives for large groups of the society.

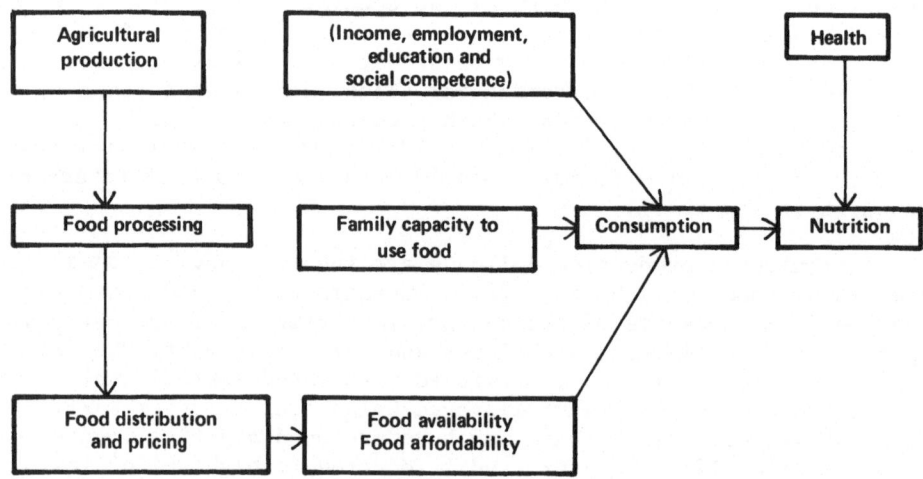

FIG. II. *Some Variables Involved in Food and Nutrition Policies.*

tion system involves relatively high costs, significant losses of
perishable foods, and invariably leads to geographical variation
in per capita amounts and prices of foods.

Food availability is defined as the amount available per person. It is normally measured by nutrient categories: calories,
proteins, vitamins, minerals, etc. As discussed in a following
paper by Habicht and Butz, per capita food requirements are subject to considerable uncertainty; nevertheless, it seems appropriate
to construct a standardized value of availability. In this respect,
demographic information on age structure and age-specific fertility
of the population would be needed.

Another major concern in evaluating food availability is the
degree of disaggregation of the data itself. We suggest that at
least three dimensions known to influence availability must be
used: geographic, temporal, and economic.

The affordability of food is determined by the price of food
relative to the income and wealth of the individual. Even in the
case of the subsistence farmer, the costs of food production must
be compared with the total resources he controls. When income for
the poor increases more rapidly than inflation, nutritional status
tends to improve (9). Thus, national policies that influence levels

of income and wealth are of key concern. Such policies as employment, income distribution, and land reform are obviously central to
Latin American concerns for food affordability.

The capacity of the family to use its economic resources appropriately to acquire a good diet must also be mentioned. Where
ignorance or superstition interfere with the family's ability to
acquire and prepare the most adequate diet available within its
economic means, there is considerable potential for malnutrition,
even in the presence of food availability and affordability. Education and modernization tend to overcome informational and cultural
barriers to good nutrition.

Obviously, health and nutrition are also closely interrelated.
Specific public health measures, particularly environmental sanitation, are often included in land and nutrition policies and programs. Poor health may reduce appetite, reduce absorption of food
consumed, and increase the food requirements of the individual.

It has been suggested that national, regional, and local policies that affect agricultural productivity, food processing, food
distribution, per capita income, education and modernization should
be monitored as they relate to food availability, affordability,
and consumption. These in turn can be related to changes in nutritional and health status. Practically, it appears unreasonable
to develop a comprehensive monitoring system for such variables,
except in the context of evaluation of exceptionally ambitious national, macro-economic, nutrition programs. However, in evaluation of a health or nutrition service, a record might be maintained
of important changes in food or income policy, and this record used
in interpreting control variables of food price, local food availability, and family income.

Food sanitation practices should also be monitored. Public
health practices normally include monitoring of quality of milk and
milk products, water, meat, and establishments which process or sell
these products. Obviously, as contaminated food causes disease,
and disease in turn influences nutritional status, strong direct
influences are possible. Often in Latin America, input data for
such analyses exist in health ministries but may not be centralized
nor regularly summarized in reports nor used in evaluations.

Lactation and weaning may be identified for special attention
because of the extreme vulnerability of the young child. Ideally,
child development in Latin America would involve an extended period
of breast feeding with an appropriately timed gradual transition
to high quality weaning foods. Breast feeding is advised for immunologic, food quality, and sanitary reasons. Food marketing

policies (10), public policies regulating advertising and nutrition education can all influence breast feeding and weaning behavior.

THE IMPACT OF POPULATION POLICIES ON HEALTH AND NUTRITIONAL STATUS

Population policy is an important consideration in designing social programs to affect health and nutritional status (11). Some of the more important relationships are shown in Figure III. For instance, effective population policies may be directed toward the provision of family planning services or motivational and educational programs, and may even extend to direct governmental incentives to the family to have additional children. Socio-economic programs are also generally conceded to indirectly influence demographic trends. These would include education and employment programs, especially those focusing on women and income redistribution. Generally, it is perceived that socio-economic interventions which increase the social competence and economic well-being of the poor (who have high birth rates) will result in smaller families (12).

The principal macro-economic rationale for reduced population growth have obvious repercussions on family health:

a.   Reduced population growth allows a higher rate of sustained growth in GNP, reflected in higher per capita production and income growth. This, in turn, should improve the poor families' socio-economic status, potentially facilitating improved health and nutrition.

b.   An increasing national ratio of wage earners to dependents would be a reflection of families where economic pressure from dependents on the wage earner should decrease and well-being should increase.

c.   As family size decreases, the number of persons in the average dwelling eating together and in close proximity should decrease. Since the highest rate of transmission of communicable disease is among proximate individuals, decreasing crowding of the household should decrease incidence and prevalence of disease.

d.   As the number of births is reduced, they may be confined more nearly to the optimal period in the life of the woman, and child spacing may be increased. These effects reduce biological strain and risk for both the mother and the child (13, 14, 15, 16). Specifically, the nutritional status of mothers and birth weights of offspring should

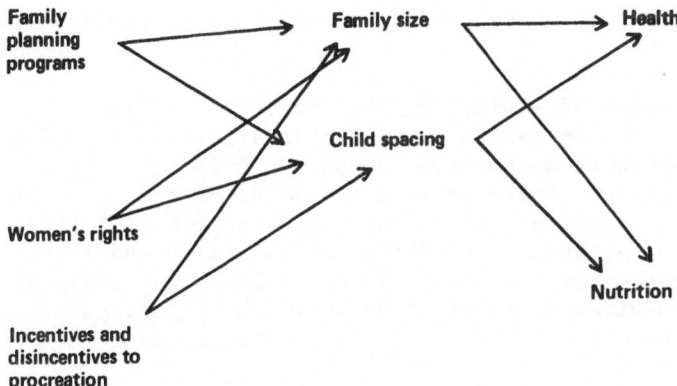

Fig. III. *Relationship Between Population Programs, Health and*
Nutritional Status.

increase and infant mortality rates and birth defects
should decrease (17).

In addition to these mechanisms, changing age, fertility, and
sex structures have profound impacts on health status indicators.
These demographic characteristics are very strong predictors of
morbidity. Specifically, as the population becomes older, the
relative importance of heart disease and tumors increases and that
of infectious diseases and diseases of childhood decrease. Consequently, changes in disease prevalence and use of medical services
must be considered in light of community demographic changes.

We postulate that family size is conditioned by a number of
socio-economic factors. These include such things as the prevailing
attitudes of the family concerning the most desirable number
of children, the availability of information and means for controlling fertility, the costs of raising children, and the economic
value of children to the family.

Many of these factors are related to the status and role of
women. Women's earning power increases with education and status.
Increased earning power both increases the opportunity costs of
bearing children and decreases incentives to early or repeated
marriages. Similarly, as social competence and income increase,
it may be postulated that couples have more opportunity and capacity to use health and family planning services, and are less
prone to fatalistic reasoning and behavior. On the other hand,
as economic incentives outside the home increase, there may be
a tendency to reduce child care. Reduced child care may in turn

cause nutritional problems and increase disease prevalence in children.

For purposes of evaluating the impact of population and socio-
economic policies on health and nutritional status as mediated
through demographic mechanisms, a number of indices are available
in many countries. These include estimates of the age of menarche,
initiation of sexual activity, marriage, and birth of first and
last children, as well as estimates of fertility and fecundity.
Often such estimates are available not only on the basis of census
data but from vital statistics and from sample surveys. Similarly,
marriage, divorce, legitimacy, and illegitimacy rates are often
available.

Indicators of the coverage and effectiveness of direct family
planning programs are well known. They include measures of attitudes, knowledge, and practice of family planning from field surveys, records of numbers of contacts, acceptors, and persons using
family planning services, and age-specific birth rates and estimates of births averted. Program statistics are also often available for education and motivation programs, for family planning
programs by type of contraceptive, and for key incentive or sanction activities.

In contrast, indicators of the indirect impact of socio-economic programs on health and nutritional status are often more difficult to obtain. There appears to be no single convincing indicator for women's status which would predict procreation. Nonetheless, employment, wages, literacy and educational attainment,
as well as differentials between men and women in these indices,
are commonly available and potentially useful.

Where national plans include a population policy, or where
population impact analyses of national plans have been prepared,
it may be possible to select and monitor key variables in the framework of health and nutrition program evaluations. But this will
normally not be the case, especially since it will be rare to find
control data available at the level of disaggregation needed for
health and nutrition project evaluation. In these situations,
either sample surveys or the addition of key population policy
indicators to existing instruments may be considered.

THE IMPACT OF INCOME AND EMPLOYMENT
ON HEALTH AND NUTRITIONAL STATUS

In this section we will deal with two principal sets of "household economy" variables: those relating to income .(or, more broadly, economic well-being) and to employment.

It is obvious that improved health and nutritional status may lead to higher levels of income through a more productive work force (18, 19, 20). The impact of expected illness or mortality on savings-investment decisions is not well understood (21). Theoretically, savings and investment should be reduced as the investor's expectation decreases that he will be alive and healthy to realize the returns from that investment. On the other hand, as survival increases through better health care, there are complex effects on saving and investment (22).

Hypotheses as to the ways increased incomes can benefit health and nutrition are found throughout this paper. Increased income should allow the family to buy a more adequate diet, to use health services more often and more appropriately, to improve the family environment by reducing crowding and improving sanitation, and to take advantage of educational opportunities, thereby to improve its competency to protect its health. Thus, in health as in other areas of human welfare, the advantages of increased income appear almost self-evident.

Since the initial computations of national accounts, the *per capita* values of national income, or closely associated magnitudes such as gross national product or gross domestic product, have been considered to be the principal indices of economic development. However, recently this point of view has been undergoing a change.

"There has been a growing realization in the development community as a whole that gross national product *per capita* alone is not an adequate measure of development and of its effect on human welfare" (23, p.24). A logical outcome of this realization for the World Bank and others has been increased attention to income distribution and to the social sectors (23). This focus includes a renewed concern with employment (discussed below). An important reason for this modification of view was the accumulation of evidence for the 1960's that "many countries experienced rising *per capita* incomes, but the lives of the people did not improve at all. Indeed, it seems to be the case that in the early stages of *per capita* income growth, the lot of the poor deteriorates". (24, as cited in 25, pp. 18-19).

Obviously, alternative economic measures are needed. One promising attempt is an indicator of the level and distribution of welfare based on a combination of current income and current net worth (assets minus liabilities), (26, pp. 13-15); with net worth being converted into an annual income stream by treating it like a lifetime annuity (27). Applying this measure to illustrative data for families in the United States, it was found that inequality increased when net worth was considered in contrast to income alone.

Whatever the exact selection of the indicators of economic and welfare status, the problem of analyzing the relationship between levels of income and of health and nutrition exists.

In the simplest terms, income and wealth are the vehicles whereby individuals and families implement their consumption decisions. Some changed consumption patterns directly influence health and nutrition, such as increased use of health services, purchase of a better diet, substitution of infant formulas for breast milk, or drug abuse. Other changed consumption patterns indirectly influence health, such as the health effects of improved water supplies or of a modified transportation system.

In general, those health conditions most characteristic of poor populations are the ones expected to change most with increasing levels of family income. Some of them are infant mortality, childhood mortality, malnutrition, diarrheal disease incidence, and infectious disease incidence.

To obtain a more precise idea of the relationships being studied, analysts might wish to attempt to identify the value of income of other economic level that denotes the cut-off points of ill health or malnutrition. Of course, such a value will depend upon one's notion of health or nutrition problems, and it probably will vary among populations. Still, the approximate "poverty line" for malnutrition, disease or death would have powerful appeal to many public decision makers. In principle, such a poverty line could be identified for ill health of one sort or another. In practice, there probably has been a closer approach to application of the concept as it relates to nutritional deficiencies.

Income elasticities of demand for health services, food and shelter could be used for more detailed analysis. Income elasticity of demand is the expression used to refer to the relationship between percentage change in income of the demanders in question and the corresponding percentage change in the quantity of product demanded, implying ability as well as willingness to buy. An elasticity coefficient greater than one would denote a greater than proportionate increase in demand as income rises. Elasticity is generally greater than one for "luxuries" and less than one for "necessities".

Thus, for poor populations in Latin America, food grains and pulses may be expected to have elasticities less than one. On the other hand, meat, as a relative luxury for the poor, may have an elasticity greater than one.

It is far easier to define the concept and to theorize on its values than it is to estimate it empirically, especially in poorer

countries with weaker data bases. There has been enough field research to indicate income elasticities for various foods, with important nutritional implications, but the values for health services are not well established. Among the reasons are the limitations of field survey instruments and the high random element in
health care utilization. A measurement problem that must be acknowledged is the likelihood that available demand data will be in
terms of monetary expenditures instead of product quantities, as
required technically for elasticities. In that case, price movements can confound apparent income-induced demand variations.

Among the diverse items of evidence regarding income elasticity values, two might be cited to point to additional work in the
health and nutrition fields:

a.   Working with data from 13 well-developed countries,
     Newhouse decided that "both cross-nation and time-series
     (within nation) data support the conclusion that the in-
     come elasticity of national medical care expenditure is
     greater than one" (27, p.16). The applicability to
     developing countries is open to serious question.

b.   A recent review of 1971 cross-sectional consumer expend-
     iture data in Colombia yielded no consistent income elas-
     ticities for urban or rural areas for a variety of pos-
     sible reasons (28, p.38; based on 29). More important
     findings of the project were the differences in patterns
     of health service utilization by different income classes
     in Colombia and in Santo Domingo, Dominican Republic (28,
     pp. 42-43).

The research of Swanberg and Shipley (30, pp. 111-125) contains
useful cautions for future investigators on the relationship between
income and health/nutrition. They obtained suggestive data from
two areas within the same rural region of Colombia. We cannot do
full justice to their experiment here, but their conclusions of
chief interest are:

a.   Incomes are probably not as important as other factors
     (perhaps, disease and unsanitary living conditions) in
     affecting overall health status (e.g., height and weight
     of preschoolers);

b.   "Protein and calorie intake were found to be more highly
     correlated with expenditure (and income) than were cal-
     cium, vitamin A or riboflavin" (30, pp. 123-124).

EMPLOYMENT AND OCCUPATIONAL HEALTH

There are many well-established indicators of employment or labor activity in a country, including the proportion of the adult population participating in the labor force, level of employment, and level or percentage of unemployment. Less settled but potentially important measures exist to estimate job vacancies and also the degree of underemployment or underuse of human resources.

This section will deal also with occupational health. Here too, there are fairly well accepted indices such as industrial accident rates and time lost from work due to health problems. Admittedly, data needs remain great, especially in obtaining broad-based information on population health status and in separating the effects of job-related problems from others. Most notable, besides the obviously positive effect of employment on income, is the perverse relationship, at least in the short run, between employment opportunities and health; increased chances for employment might worsen the health level of the affected population in the near run (e.g., several years).

There are two reasons for this strange situation. The first is that innovations creating employment may also create new health hazards. Thus, the development of new regions has led to a rise in certain diseases, like malaria. Development projects, such as dams, might have aggravated other threats, like schistosomiasis.

The second reason is exposure of more people to occupational health hazards. The nature of industrial accidents and of job-related sicknesses is well known (31). With or without good statistics on these problems, we can note their importance in poorer, as well as more highly developed, nations. Agriculture -- the backbone of a typical developing country's economy -- is notoriously unsafe, especially as mechanization increases. But the bodily threats multiply as industrialization proceeds. A body of information is accumulating through the efforts of agencies like the International Labor Organization and from case studies in developing countries (32, reviewed in 33; 34).

Health problems related to growing employment opportunities point to several needs for future work. One is to develop better data, such as data on industrial illnesses. Another is to devise programs or interventions to ameliorate the difficulties. By way of illustrating the challenge here, we point to the fruitful possibilities for combining market incentives (such as insurance contribution rates for companies) and governmental regulations to attack occupational health problems. The payoffs to such policies -- clarified by better data on health impacts -- can be great in the form of decreased absenteeism, increased productivity, lowered labor turnover, lessened disability and mortality, and reduced medical service requirements (35).

Health and nutritional status also have frequent impacts on the use of manpower resources (36). A malnourished or an ill labor force results in a different mix of factors of production than would be the case otherwise. This impact on labor force productivity is very difficult to measure, as it is subject to long-term adjustments in expected labor force productivity and levels of unemployment.

IMPACT OF INFRASTRUCTURE DEVELOPMENT POLICIES
ON HEALTH AND NUTRITION

In a simple model, disease may be considered the result of a biological, mechanical, or chemical toxic agent and a host -- for our purposes, man. The influences of the agents are specific to them, but their effects on the host are conditioned both by other factors in the host's environment and in the host himself.

The conditioning factors which can exist in the host-agent environment and confound the measurement of impact are almost limitless. The causal agents of diarrheal disease are only infrequently identified and include factors entirely unrelated to sanitation (37). The specific host-agent environmental changes produced by utilization of adequate amounts of potable water are almost never identified.

The most important host factors are physiological and dietary. Physiological conditioning factors include age, body size, immunological competence, level of nutrient intake, and presence of other debilitating factors. Among these, the most important factors to take into account appear to be those associated with the diarrheal-malnutrition complex, which will be discussed in other papers in this volume.

The impact measurement problems, therefore, appear to be inversely proportional to the directness of the contact between the host and the agent. In the case of waterborne epidemic disease or direct human contact with toxic materials, impact measurements are relatively simple. In the case, however, of sanitation measures that alter the environment of the host-agent contact, impact measurement and the specification of causality becomes enormously complex. Take the example of utilization of adequate amounts of potable water. Water can influence the environment of food preparation, personal cleanliness, and many other factors. We have little

knowledge concerning the impact of these factors on diarrheal disease; and all vary markedly with climate as well as social, cultural,
economic, and educational levels of households involved (38, 39, 40).

Different types of infrastructure mainly influence health, but
also may affect nutritional status, modifying the environment within
which the agent and the host interact. In a lesser number of instances, toxic agents are a direct by-product of development investments.

Two mechanisms for the influence of water supply can easily be
identified. Water can serve as a vehicle for bacteriological or
toxic substances which cause ill health upon ingestion of contaminated water. This was most vividly portrayed by John Snow's incrimination of the Broad Street pump as a source of cholera in 1951
(41). Despite the attention paid to such incidents, they are relatively infrequent when viewed from the perspective of total water-
related diarrheal case load. Although waterborne epidemics continue
to be identified (42, 43), currently the most frequent type of
health impact by ingestion of contaminated water supplies is that
due to metallic and chemical pollution of the water supply (44, p.
128).

The utilization of water as a cleansing and dilutional factor
to diminish contact between the host (man) and biological agents
is the mechanism whereby potable water has its greatest impact. Several studies have indicated that the major impact of potable water
depends upon its adequate utilization (45, 46, 47). The utilization
of greater amounts of water promotes more frequent bathing, washing
of hands, household cleanliness, cleaner eating utensils and so forth.

Industrialization and other types of infrastructure development
can also lead to air pollution, which in time can have a negative
effect on health. The variety of potentially detrimental air pol-
lutants is quite large, but the most important ones from the health
perspective are hydrocarbons, sulphur dioxide and carbon monoxide
(44, p. 228). Rather difficult measurement problems exist when
calculating the impact on the environment outside the industrial
plant due to the effect of climatic variation on pollutant density.

Investment in infrastructure for refuse disposal may be useful
for health. This includes investments for garbage disposal and
latrines, as well as disposal of toxic waste substances. By means
of these, a mechanical separation of disease agents and man is
achieved.

Configuration and components of the transportation system have
very important direct effects on health. In many societies they

form the largest single cause of death in the young adult population (48). Factors like seat belts, speed limits, public buses or
trains instead of private automobiles, and pedestrian overpasses in
urban areas, have significant impacts on accidental injury and death
rates (49).

A second area of potential impact of transportation infrastructure is the alteration of patterns of spread of infectious disease.
Improved transportation systems both increase the probability of
introduction by transportation of a large number of individuals into
a region from a wider source area outside the region and increase
the frequency of contact among individuals (50). The literature
cites many examples of the introduction of communicable diseases
into previously unexposed populations (51). These examples are
becoming less frequent, but they continue to occur in some instances, like the incidence of cutaneous leishmaniasis in workers
on the Trans-Amazonian highway (52). A more frequent occurrence at
the current time is the more constant reintroduction of common communicable diseases into the child population. This frequently implies higher mortality and complication rates than would otherwise
be the case.

Transportation and communication systems have major impacts on
relative prices for foods, health services and nutrient distribution
services. Occasionally, transportation of foodstuffs costs as much
as the food itself, with a resultant marked impact on family diets.
Also, travel costs measured both in real payment for transport and
in time lost due to slow or non-existent transport facilities, impacts on the frequency of utilization of health services. Reduction of real costs or travel time will be expected to have an impact
on demand for services as effective cost decreases. Although the
existent literature cites many examples of health problems influencing the construction of transport systems, this aspect presents fewer
problems today (53, 54).

IMPACT OF EDUCATION ON HEALTH AND NUTRITION

Next we will consider formal and non-formal education in terms
of their impacts on health and nutrition. While recognizing again
that causality is bidirectional, we wish to emphasize here the cases
in which health and nutrition are dependent variables.

The continued use of traditional (i.e., non-modern) health
services and foods in poor countries suggests serious cautions for
analysts in examining conventional variables and drawing policy
conclusions from their assessments.

It is often pointed out that education is positively correlated with health status. A simplified indication of this is the high (negative) coefficient of simple correlation between literacy and infant mortality from a world-wide, cross-sectional United Nations study (24, as cited in 25, pp. 18-19). While users of such results should be properly cautious about the interpretation of that correlation in the absence of control for other variables (with the knowledge that education and income are intercorrelated), they would be encouraged by research in the United States that seems to demonstrate "a strong positive correlation between health and length of schooling..... after allowing for the effects of such other variables as income, intelligence, and parents' schooling" (56, p. 46).

The natural question that follows such findings is: "Why?" Unfortunately, surprisingly little is known about the causal mechanisms behind these associations. Speculation over the reasons for the impact of formal education, via schooling and literacy, on health and nutrition has included at least the following: encouragement of better personal hygiene; improvement of child rearing; increase in safety practices; adoption of better diets and other living habits; modernization and proclivity to use modern health services; and ability to comprehend lessons from health education (23,25,55,56). Clearly, the subject is wide open for additional research.

Education, one may suggest, permits closer descriptions of health deficiencies, diagnoses of (certain) causes, and suggestions of (partial) remedies. Educational institutions can play roles besides schooling the population and developing (even supporting) researchers. In many countries, they fill the additional role of providing health services. School health programs including inoculation, screening and first aid are common in Latin America. Similarly, health personnel extend services as part of their training in many medical schools. More ambitiously, a medical school can operate its own community health and nutritional service programs (again linked to educational objectives). Out of the many examples which can be found, we might cite the widely-publicized experience of Universidad del Valle, Colombia, with its health center-hospital in Candelaria, along with other outreach activities (57,58,59).

Properly conceived, education extends to non-formal activities that potentially develop a wide range of economic and social skills. Their breadth is so great that analysis must be selective in order to use a few tractable independent and dependent variables for applied research. Customary manpower training programs and many systems of extension services resemble formal education in their possible effects on health and nutrition. They have potentialities for affecting human behavior -- as in the case of use of health services. They can offer external benefits in the form of direct service activities as part of the training or related processes. They can also affect the availability and perhaps deployment of specialized manpower, with important nutritional and health impacts (60,61,62).

Non-formal education forms a vital component for changing health and nutritional status, *particularly* for those aspects most subject to change by other sectors. Mass media, education by extension workers and multi-purpose information dissemination all become extremely important to the amelioration of problems determined by other sectors.

A rather different facet of non-formal education comes in the form of public campaigns to enlighten would-be users of services. "Health education" or "education of consumers in the use of health services" can have important effects on nutritional practices and on utilization of medical care and environmental and other public health services. It seems wise at this point to defer to health education specialists to explore the massive area. We close by noting that innovative delivery systems -- possibly integrating health, nutritional, and other services -- draw on the training programs mentioned above in order to obtain auxiliary health personnel of various skills (61,62,63).

IMPACT OF HOUSING AND URBANIZATION ON HEALTH AND NUTRITIONAL STATUS

For more than a century, there has been an active interest in and study of the relationships among health, urbanization, and housing. Historical perspective indicates that in early industrialized societies, increased communicable diseases resulted in a marked deterioration of health status (52). With advances during this century in the technology for prevention and treatment of communicable diseases, the magnitude of the health implications of urbanization and housing has markedly decreased. Still, there remains a significant problem related with urbanization in the least developed countries (64).

A variety of potential relationships exist through which housing and urbanization may influence health and nutrition. The three most important appear to be: 1) housing and urbanization as environmental factors in which the relationship between man and disease agents is altered; 2) the direct production of certain factors deleterious to health such as transportation, accidents and air pollution; and 3) health and nutrition factors which lead to increased urbanization due to increased accessibility to health and nutrition services (65,66).

The density and the quality of housing potentially influences health and nutritional status in a variety of ways. Density increases the probability of effective contact with communicable disease agents (67). Probably the two most important aspects of density are, (a) the larger size of the contact pool, and (b) crowding within the household, school, or neighborhood (68,69,70,71). There are data on animals and suggestive studies from prisons that crowding may also have psychosomatic effects on health and nutrition.

Housing, per se, has various aspects other than density of inhabitants which impacts on health and nutrition. General household sanitation, secondary to utilization of adequate amounts of potable water, was discussed in the previous section. Other aspects are related to safety, such as propensity for accidental falls (the most frequent accident-causing disability in most countries) and fire hazards. Other aspects relate to type of flooring and roofing materials, cooking and food preparation surfaces, and sanitary facilities.

Urbanization also results in breakdown of traditional cultural and familial factors. Some of these changes are beneficial to health but some are detrimental, such as increased alcoholism, drug abuse, and mental illness (72). The major causative factors are probably the breakdown in familial responsibility patterns and the increased likelihood of contact with a broader set of behavior patterns in urban areas. Urbanization is also associated with changes in fertility, which, in turn, has secondary effects on nutrition and disease (73).

Urban areas are frequently characterized by more readily available social services of all types. Specifically, health, nutrition, and water supply services are almost invariably more available to inhabitants of urban areas. This factor probably accounts for some of the improved health of urban populations and almost certainly accounts for some decisions by individuals or families to move to urban areas (50,64).

Lastly, the urban environment introduces new disease agents such as infant food alternatives for breast milk, air pollution, and new hazards from accidental injury or death such as occupational hazards or transportation accidents.

The two major impacts of all those outlined in this section appear to be those of the new health hazards characteristic of an urban environment and the tendency towards urbanization produced by the greater availability of health, nutrition, social, and environmental services.

Many measurement problems arise with regard to these two principal aspects. The health hazards of the urban environment can be measured directly and compared to hazards implicit in the rural en-

vironment. The extent to which the availability of health services
influences decisions of urban migration is very complex, however.
Many other determinants effect the urbanization decision, and multivariate analytical procedures are required to separate the health
and nutrition services impact.

CONCLUDING REMARKS

We have presented very quickly a complex view of a large number of national policy instruments and variables which interact
among themselves, and which are thought to impact on health and
nutrition through a wide variety of direct and indirect mechanisms.
An enormous quantity of literature deals with these hypotheses but,
given the complexity of the subject, it appears fragmented and
confusing (74,75). Not only are we not sure of all the mechanisms
to include in a conceptual framework, but we are uncertain of the
magnitude and even the direction of the major effects. In the face
of this complexity, we have tried to identify general references
which will provide the reader with a more extensive and useful understanding of the phenomena than is possible in this paper.

We have also tried to motivate the effort to begin evaluating
the impact of socio-economic policies on health and nutrition. The
effects are so strong and pervasive that they must be taken into
account in the evaluation of the impact of health services. More
important, health officials must more effectively monitor the health
impact of these national economic policies if they are to be able
to speak in national councils to protect the health of the public.
Finally, it would be most useful in the future for health officials,
armed with a quantitative knowledge of these interrelations, to
plan with leaders from other sectors for national development programs that would maximize the health of the people.

Underlying the concern for health and impact evaluation of social and economic policy instruments is our belief that there are
real differences among socio-economically similar policies in terms
of health impacts. Agricultural policy may find little to choose
between two crops in terms of employment generation, income, or
foreign earnings, but there may be major differences nonetheless in
terms of nutrients produced or occupational safety. Too often we
have seen agricultural policies stressing luxury export products
at the expense of domestic nutrition, or economic investment plans
leaving a legacy of greatly increased prevalence of tropical disease.

Finally, the socio-economic policies of a country have a very
large impact on health. Observers contrasting mortality rates
among developing countries with similar per capita gross national

products suggest health is most affected by the degree countries
attend to the basic human needs of their populations. That is,
health may be more affected by overall socio-economic policy than
by the availability of medical services.

In summary, we have tried to indicate the size and form of a
formidable intellectual problem, and simultaneously we have stressed
the benefits if solutions were available. The result should be a
fairly high degree of frustration. In the following paragraphs,
we will try to ameliorate that frustration.

This paper does not allow for an in-depth treatment of methods
which could be utilized for impact evaluation. However, some suggestions are presented below. A first step for a project or program evaluation could be simply the maintenance of a record of socio-
economic and other policies and events of potential major importance.
Thoughtful review of socio-economic events and possible health impacts could be done by an *ad hoc* committee. Simply relating such
events to trends of key health indicators through graphs may be
informative.

A more ambitious approach would involve the formalization of
the best judgments and intuition of knowledgeable observers of the
society and its health. It is suggested that a multidisciplinary
group of individuals knowledgeable in health, nutrition, and the
other particular sectors involved could be convened and charged
with the following tasks: 1) identification of potentially important intersectoral impacts; 2) development of impact measurement criteria; and 3) development of exogeneous group process techniques to specify the most important impacts to be measured. Subsequently, variables would have to be grouped.

Following the stage of variable specification in conjunction
with a health service impact measurement program, programs can be
established to measure complementary socio-economic variable impacts on health. Given the greater uncertainties of approaching
impact measurement in the way described above, it is preferable to
develop the measurement procedures such that they can be added to
and made more complex in the future if it proves feasible and useful to do so.

We suggest that one or more of the major international assistance agencies seriously begin to analyze the relation of socio-
economic policy to health and nutrition. A major study to define
the state-of-the-art and clarify the conceptual framework for future analysis is a necessary first step. Useful information for
this purpose is now accruing from a number of sources: evaluation
of the Colombian and other national nutrition programs; population

impact analyses of development programs, and environmental impact statements. Thereafter, a careful program of field studies might be considered. A few extensive studies in developing countries with relatively high socio-economic stability and good information would be advisable. Such countries should obviously be those with governments vitally interested in the topic.

The utility of information on the health and nutrition impact of socio-economic policy will increase with a greater understanding of their interrelationships, as well as with the authority of the user. A health official evaluating a relatively small health project will find such information most useful in determining how much of health status change he can attribute to his project's efforts. However, a national planning office, using an organized body of knowledge from many studies in several countries, might significantly improve national plans and programs. Thus, much of the benefit to be gained from such health impact studies will accrue not to the health project or researcher involved, but from the contribution to an international body of knowledge which may eventually be of great importance to a number of governments.

ACKNOWLEDGEMENT

The authors gratefully acknowledge the valuable comments and criticisms received from Dr. James Brown and Dr. Hector Correa during the preparation of this paper. Dr. James Levinson and Dr. George Poynor made several suggestions to the authors that have been incorporated in the paper, particularly with regard to nutrition impacts of various programs. Similarly, the authors wish to acknowledge the major influence that Dr. Lee Howard has had on their conceptualization of the interrelationship of health and development.

REFERENCES

1. Reinke, W. A. Alternative methods for determining resource requirements: the Chile example. *Int. J. Health Serv.*, 6:123-137, 1976.
2. Mertini, C. J., A. J. B. Allan, J. Davison, *et al.* Health indexes sensitive to medical care variation. *Int. J. Health Serv.*, 7: 293-309, 1977.
3. Brooks, C. H. Path analysis of socioeconomic correlates of country infant mortality rates. *Int. J. Health Serv.*, 5: 499-514, 1973.
4. Knowles, J. C. *The Economic Effects of Health and Disease in an Underdeveloped Country.* pp. 216-224. Madison: University of Wisconsin, 1970.

5. U.S. Agency for International Development, Office of Nutrition. *Planning National Nutrition Programs*. *1, 2.* Washington: U.S. Agency for International Development, 1973.

6. Johnston, B. F., and J. P. Graves. *Manual on Food and Nutrition Policy*. Nutrition Studies No. 22. Rome: FAO, 1969.

7. Cook, R., and Y. Yueh-Heng. National food and nutrition policy in the Commonwealth Caribbean. *Pan. Am. Health Org. Bull.*, 8: 133-142, 1974.

8. Berg, A. *The Nutrition Factor*. pp. 70-71, 108-118. Washington: The Brookings Institution, 1973.

9. Reutlinger, S., and M. Selowsky. The anatomy of hunger. *World Bank Occasional Paper No. 23*. Washington: The World Bank, 1976.

10. Jelliffe, D.B., and E. F. P. Jelliffe. The infant food industry and international child health. *Int. J. Health Serv.*, 7: 249-254, 1977.

11. King, T., *et al*. *Population Policies and Economic Development*. Baltimore: The Johns Hopkins University Press (for the World Bank), 1974.

12. McGreevey, W.P., N. Birdsall, *et al*. *The Policy Relevance of Recent Social Research on Fertility*. Washington: The Smithsonian Institution, Interdisciplinary Communication Program, 1974.

13. May, J. M. *Contribution of Family Planning to Health and Nutrition*. Washington: U.S. Agency for International Development, Office of Population, 1974.

14. Omran, A. R. Health benefits for mother and child. *World Health*.

15. Committee on Maternal Nutrition. *Maternal Nutrition and the Course of Pregnancy*. Washington: National Academy of Sciences, 1970.

16. Kessner, D. M., J. Singer, D. Kalk, *et al*. *Infant Death: An Analysis by Maternal Risk and Health Care*. Washington: National Academy of Sciences, Institute of Medicine, 1973.

17. Omran, A. J., C. C. Standley, *et al*. *Family Formation Patterns and Health*. Geneva: World Health Organization, 1976.

18. Weisbrod, B. A. *Disease and Economic Development: Parasitic Disease in St. Lucia*. Madison: University of Wisconsin, 1973.

19. Spurr, G. B., *et al*. Productivity and maximal oxygen consumption in sugar cane cutters. *Am. J. Clin. Nutr.*, 30: 316-321, 1977.

20. Barac-Nieto, M., *et al*. Aerobic work capacity in chronically undernourished adult males. *J. Appl. Physiol.*, 44: 209-215, 1978.

21. Barlow, R. The economic effects of malaria eradication. *Am. Econ. Rev.*, 57: 130, 1967.

22. Conly, G. *Impact of Malaria on Economic Development: A Case Study*. pp. 96-99. PAHO Scientific Publication 297.

Washington: Pan American Health Organization, 1975.

23. Sharpston, M. J. Health and the human environment. *Finance and Development*, 13: 24-27, 1976.

24. Adelman, I., and C. T. Morris. *Economic Growth and Social Equity in Developing Countries*. pp. 18-19, 26. Stanford, California: Stanford University Press, 1973.

25. U.S. Agency for International Development, Nicaragua Mission. *Health Sector Assessment for Nicaragua*. Managua: U.S. Agency for International Development, Nicaragua Mission, 1976.

26. Weisbrod, B. A., and W. L. Hansen. Measuring economic welfare. *Am. Econ. Rev.*, 58: 1315-1329, 1968.

27. Newhouse, J. P. *Income and Medical Care Expenditures across Countries*. p. 16. Rand Publication P-5608-1. Santa Monica: The Rand Corporation, 1976.

28. Zschock, D. K., R. L. Robertson, and J. A. Daly. *Health Sector Financing in Latin America: Conceptual Framework and Case Studies*. pp. 33, 42-43. Washington: U. S. Department of Health, Education, and Welfare, Office of International Health, 1976.

29. Heredia, R., *et al. Financiamiento y Destino de los Fondos del Sistema de Salud en Colombia*. Bogotá: CCRP, 1976.

30. Swanberg, K. G., and E. Shipley. *The Nutritional Status of the Rural Family in East Cundimarca*. pp. 111-125. Colombia: Unpublished paper.

31. Elling, R. H. Industrialization and occupational health in underdeveloped countries. *Int. J. Health Serv.*, 7: 209-235, 1977.

32. CIBA Foundation, (ed.). *Health and Industrial Growth*. New York: American Elsevier, 1975.

33. Baker, T. D. Review of health and industrial growth. *J. Econ. Lit.*, 15: 154-155, 1977.

34. Programa de Investigación y Desarrollo de Sistemas de Salud. Unpublished studies in Valle del Cauca, Colombia.

35. World Health Organization. *Interrelationships Between Health Programmes and Socioeconomic Development*. p. 40. WHO Public Health Paper 49. Geneva: World Health Organization, 1973.

36. World Health Organization. *Health Hazards of the Human Environment*. Geneva: World Health Organization, 1972.

37. WHO Expert Committee on Enteric Infections. *Enteric Infections*. pp. 7-14. WHO Technical Report 288. Geneva: World Health Organization, 1964.

38. The World Bank. *Village Water Supply*. Washington: The World Bank, 1976.

39. Saunders, R. J., and J. J. Warford. *Village Water Supply: Economics and Policy in the Developing World*. Baltimore: The Johns Hopkins University Press, 1976.

40. McGarry, M. G. Village water, health and a potential role for primary care. Unpublished paper, 1977.

41. Snow, J. *On the Mode of Communication of Cholera*. London:
       John Churchill, 1855.
42. Miller, A. P. *Water and Man's Health*. Washington: U. S.
       Agency for International Development, Office of Human
       Resources and Human Development, 1962.
43. Leach, C. O., and K. F. Maxey. The relative incidence of
       typhoid fever in cities, towns, and country districts of
       a southern state. *Pub. Health Reps.*, 41: 705-712, 1926.
44. Leh, F. K. V., and R. K. C. Lak. *Environment and Pollution:
       Sources, Health Effects, Monitoring and Control*. pp. 128,
       228. Springfield: Charles C. Thomas Publishing Company,
       1970.
45. Wagner, E. C., and J. N. Lanoix. *Water Supply for Rural Areas
       and Small Communities*. WHO Monograph Series No. 42.
       Geneva: World Health Organization, 1959.
46. Hollister, A. C. Jr., *et al*. Influence of water availability
       on shigella prevalence in children of farm labor families.
       Am. J. Pub. Health., 55: 354-362, 1955.
47. Stewart, W. H., *et al*. The relationship of certain environ-
       mental factors to the prevalence of shigella infection.
       Am. J. Trop. Med. Hyg., 4: 718-724, 1955.
48. Haddon, W., E. A. Suchman, and D. Klein. *Accident Research:
       Methods and Approaches*. p. 2. New York: Harper and Row,
       1964.
49. Reynolds, D. J. The cost of road accidents. *J. Roy. Stat.
       Soc.*, 119: 393, 1956.
50. Prothero, R. M. *Human Mobility – A Neglected Epidemiological
       Factor and a Restraint on Health in Sub-Saharan Africa*.
       Liverpool: University of Liverpool, Department of
       Geography, 1973.
51. Hughes, C. C., and J. M. Hunter. Disease and development in
       Africa. *Soc. Sci. Med.*, 3: 443-493, 1970.
52. Lenihan, J., and W. W. Fletcher (eds.). *Health and the Envi-
       ronment*. pp. 64-65. Glasgow and London: Blackie & Son,
       Ltd., 1976.
53. Heller, P. S. *An Analysis of the Structure, Equity and Effect-
       iveness of Public Sector Health Systems in Developing
       Countries: The Case of Tunisia, 1960-1972*. Discussion
       Paper No. 43. Ann Arbor: University of Michigan, Center
       for Research on Economic Development, 1975.
54. Heller, P. S. *A Model of the Demand for Medical and Health
       Services in West Malaysia*. Discussion Paper No. 62. Ann
       Arbor: University of Michigan, 1976.
55. Fuchs, V. R. *Who Shall Live?* p. 46. New York: Basic Books,
       1974.
56. Zschock, D. K. Economic aspects of health and development in
       Guatemala. Memorandum to E. C. Long, December 3, 1974.
57. Aguirre, A. Community medicine at the University of Valle.
       pp. 51-61. In: W. Latham and A. Newbury, (eds.). *Com-
       munity Medicine: Teaching, Research and Health Care*.

New York: Appleton-Century-Crofts, 1970.

58. Velasquez, G. Community medicine as an experiment in health
    care. pp. 121-131. In: W. Latham and N. Newbury, (eds).
    Community Medicine: Teaching, Research and Health Care.
    New York: Appleton-Century-Crofts, 1970.

59. Robertson, R. L., B. Barona, and R. Pabon. Hospital cost
    accounting and analysis: the case of Candelaria. *J. Com.
    Health., 3:* 61-79, 1977.

60. Butter, I., G. T. Moore, R. L. Robertson, *et al.* Effects of
    manpower utilization on cost and productivity of a neigh-
    borhood health center. *Mill. Mem. Fund Quart., 50:* 421-
    452, 1972.

61. Newell, K. W. (ed.). *Health by the People.* Geneva: World
    Health Organization, 1975.

62. Ronaghy, H. A., Y. Mousseau Gershman, and A. Dorozynsky. *Vil-
    lage Health Workers.* International Development Research
    Centre publication IDRC-074e. Ottowa: International Dev-
    elopment Research Centre, 1976.

63. Habicht, J-P., G. Guzmán, A. Lechtig, *et al. Community Control
    and Quality Control of Medical Primary Care Personnel.*
    Guatemala City: Institute of Nutrition of Central America
    and Panama, 1974.

64. Johnson, G. Z. Health conditions in rural and urban areas of
    developing countries. In: *Public Health and Urban Growth.*
    London: University College, Centre for Urban Studies,
    1964.

65. Andrzejewski, A., K. G. Berjusov, P. Genewatte, *et al. Housing
    Programmes: The Role of Public Health Agencies.* WHO
    Public Health Paper 25. Geneva: World Health Organiza-
    tion, 1964.

66. WHO Expert Committee on Environmental Health Aspects of Metro-
    politan Planning and Development. *Environmental Health
    Aspects of Metropolitan Planning and Development.* WHO
    Technical Report 297. Geneva: World Health Organization,
    1975.

67. Bailey, N. T. *The Mathematical Theory of Infectious Disease
    and Its Applications.* London: Charles Griffing & Co.,
    Ltd., 1975.

68. WHO Expert Committee on the Public Health Aspects of Housing.
    The Public Health Aspects of Housing. WHO Technical
    Report 225. Geneva: World Health Organization, 1961.

69. Britten, R. H. New light on the relations of housing to health.
    Am. J. Pub. Health, 32: 193-199, 1942.

70. Beck, M. D., J. A. Muñoz, and N. S. Scrimshaw. Studies on
    diarrheal diseases in Central America - 1. Preliminary
    findings on cultural surveys of normal population groups
    in Guatemala. *Am. J. Trop. Med. Hyg., 6:* 62, 1957.

71. Britten, R. H., J. E. Brown, and J. Altman. Certain character-
    istics of urban housing and their relation to illness and

accidents: summary of findings of the National Health
Survey. *Mill. Mem. Fund Quart.*, 14: 91-113, 1940.
72. Pasamanick, B., (ed.). *Epidemiology of Mental Disorder*.
Washington: American Association for the Advancement
of Science, 1959.
73. Smithsonian Institution, Interdisciplinary Communications
Program. *The Dynamics of Migration: Internal Migration
and Migration and Fertility*. Occasional Monograph Series, Vol 1, No. 5. Washington: Smithsonian Institution,
Interdisciplinary Communications Program, 1976.
74. Williams, K. N. *Health and Development: An Annotated, Indexed
Bibliography*. Baltimore: The Johns Hopkins University,
School of Hygiene and Public Health, 1972.
75. Howe, B., and J. E. Smith. *Health Care and Social Class: A
Selected Bibliography*. Ithaca: New York, Cornell University, Center for Urban Development, 1974.

COMMENTS

Héctor Correa, *University of Pittsburgh
Pittsburgh, Pennsylvania*

Daly, Davis, and Robertson deal with three topics: (a) the
environmental and social variables that influence the level of
health and nutrition in a population; (b) the problem of evaluating
the impacts of the specified variables on health and nutrition;
and (c) the bi-directionality of the relationships between environmental and social variables on the one hand, and health and nutritional status on the other.

The authors have managed to cover the main environmental and
social factors influencing health and nutrition, while dealing
with the influence of agricultural and population policies; changes
in the levels of income and employment; and development of infrastructure, education, and urbanization. In most cases they refer
to relevant research and point out some of its limitations. Despite
differences of emphasis or detail, I do not think much can be
added to their treatment of these topics.

As mentioned above, the authors, while dealing with problems
of evaluation, limit themselves to references about problems of
estimating the impacts of environmental and social variables on
health and nutritional status. However, the subject of the Conference is program evaluation for decision-making; this type of evaluation goes far beyond estimating parameters of some relationships
among variables.

A first point to consider in an evaluation for decision-making
is that the scale of the evaluation, and even whether it should

be performed at all, depends upon the benefits likely to be provided for the program being evaluated. Therefore, evaluations of
programs which are not likely to be modified as a result of evaluation are not worth the cost, whether the impossibility of modification results from political pressures or is because information that could be obtained from the evaluation does not substantially modify the information that already exists.

Also, evaluation for decision-making is likely to change with
the alternatives open for consideration. For instance, an evaluation to determine whether "education" or "nutrition" programs should
be implemented to improve nutritional conditions in a community is
likely to be quite different from an evaluation to select among
alternative "nutrition" programs.

The authors frequently remind us of the importance of considering the bi-directionality of the relationships between environmental
and social variables, on the one hand, and health and nutrition on
the other. They refer to the fact that the causal relationships
move in both directions, that is, from environmental and social
variables to health and nutrition, and vice versa.

Daly, Davis, and Robertson clearly state they are intentionally
leaving out discussion of causal relations that go from health and
nutrition to environmental and social conditions. Their choice, although regrettable, is understandable given the limitations of time
and space. However, they also give the impression that lack of
data and limitations in available methods make it unlikely that a
model integrating the bilateral relationships could be constructed
at the present time. For this reason it is worthwhile to mention
that an integrated model of the relationships among economic, educational, demographic, health and nutrition variables has been
constructed and applied to Mexico (1). In this application, the
model is used to choose among different types of investments in
the sectors previously mentioned in order to maximize the growth
rate of *per capita* income. According to the results obtained,
investments in population control seem to produce the highest
returns.

REFERENCES

1.   Correa, H. *Population, Health, Nutrition and Development.*
      Chapter 15. Lexington, Mass.: Lexington Books, 1975.

GENERAL DISCUSSION

Most of the discussion concerned the impact of overall food
availability upon health. The first speaker emphasized the influence

of food availability upon infant mortality and upon fecundity. He
and a later speaker stressed the similarity of human and animal
populations in this regard. He further noted that a few years ago,
a ten percent decrease in food availability had led to a ten percent increase in his country's infant mortality rate. Regarding
fecundity, he said that in a community he had studied, the provision
of adequate nutrition caused the average birth interval to drop
from 27 to 17 months, due to a shortened period of post-partum
amenorrhea. Two other speakers agreed that the direct *biological*
consequences of better nutrition would initially be higher population growth rates, but suggested that increased child survival
could eventually lead to lower fertility as a *behavioral* consequence.

It was also observed that global food shortages, evidenced by
the high prices of recent years, may have impacted more unfavorably
upon the urban poor than upon the rural poor in the Third World,
and that such effects deserve clinical consideration. A speaker
cited one study that showed adverse nutrition effects when farmers
switched production from locally consumed food to export crops in
response to improved export prices. It was also observed that
international development agencies may sometimes exacerbate nutritional problems by inducing subsistence farmers to adopt cash crops.

One speaker warned against generalizing about the situation in
a country on the basis of aggregate food availability data, since
not only will rural areas show different response patterns from
urban areas when food availability changes, but also there will be
differential responses (within the rural or urban sectors) depending
upon previous levels of program services in the various areas.
Several speakers stressed a need to look at the general orientation
of a nation's health policy and at the influence of overall social
and economic development policy upon health and nutritional status.

It was observed that even in cases where one can show adequate
food for each family, it is possible to document relatively high
levels of malnutrition among children due to maldistribution *within*
families. In fact, a survey in a Caribbean country showed a reduction in malnutrition of children in 1975, just after the large
increases in world prices of oil and food. The speaker suggested
the nutritional improvement in this case might have come from better household management, even though overall living costs were
increasing.

Citing the strong export performance of agriculture in many
poor countries, one speaker felt that food production for local
consumption also could be quite efficient and responsive if demand
were strong, i.e., if crop prices were competitive with prices for
export crops. This reasoning led him to conclude that nutrition
is especially affected by income distribution, particularly urban

income. Another speaker cautioned, however, about the likely conflict between interests of farmers, who need high prices in order
to produce abundantly, and poor urban consumers, who need cheap
food. The consequences of such a conflict may be that nutrition
frequently will become a serious political problem.

It was noted that many countries are seeking to establish
multi-sectorial food and nutrition plans that encompass some or
most of the variables cited by Daly, Davis, and Robertson. This
interest in impact evaluation is growing as governments attempt
to select the most appropriate interventions or programs while also
assessing which programs are achieving the desired goals. The ex-
ploration of food and nutritional surveillance systems is one part
of this effort. These range from fairly limited data gathering
and interpretation efforts tied to specific programs to more ambitious efforts to collate, analize, and interpret data regularly
gathered on a national basis by the many ministries and agencies
working in a given country. Regardless of the scale of each proposed surveillance system, it is recognized by all, that fairly
simple and reliable indicators are required for regular monitoring
of changes in health and nutritional status.

RECENT UNITED STATES EXPERIENCES IN EVALUATION RESEARCH WITH IMPLICATIONS FOR LATIN AMERICA

Thomas D. Cook
Northwestern University
Evanston, Illinois

and

Emile G. McAnany
Stanford University
Palo Alto, California

This chapter is intended to define and illustrate "evaluation" and to describe some lessons that have been learned over the last ten years by persons conducting evaluation research in the United States. Our hope is that these lessons will prove useful for those who commission or conduct evaluations of nutrition-related projects in lesser developed countries, especially Latin America. The lessons are relevant to:

a. Deciding which projects are or are not worth evaluating;

b. Determining who should ask the evaluation questions;

c. Deciding who should conduct the evaluations;

d. Determining whether random assignment to treatments is possible and where it is not possible;

c. Ascertaining which quasi-experimental or nonexperimental designs can be implemented;

f. Deciding upon the measures of project or program impact;

g. Measuring the extent to which a promised treatment has actually been delivered;

h.   Ascertaining the extent to which the findings from eval-
     uating a single project or program can be generalized to
     other settings, times, service providers, and service re-
     cipients; and

i.   Determining the relative emphasis to be given to "sum-
     mative" and "formative" goals.

AN ILLUSTRATIVE EVALUATION RESEARCH PROJECT

Before outlining each of these topics we need to define and illustrate what is meant by evaluation. By way of illustration, we
will describe a project carried out in Cali, Colombia (1). The
starting point for the project was the findings from nutrition research prior to 1971 that simply providing nutritional supplements
to economically disadvantaged preschoolers might not improve their
intellectual performance. The Cali researchers focused on two reasons why past research results appeared so pessimistic. The first
was that the nutritional supplements were provided for relatively
short periods of time, and the second was that nutritional supplements may not be as effective by themselves as when they are combined into a multidisciplinary intervention package which has both
nutritional, health, and educational components. The Cali investigators decided, therefore, that they would implement multidisciplinary treatments for a longer period than characterized past interventions.

To achieve this, they developed an intervention package in
which an average treatment day consisted of six hours of integrated
health, nutritional, and educational activities. Two-thirds of the
time was devoted to education and one-third to health and nutrition. The nutritional supplement was developed to provide at least
three-quarters of the recommended daily protein and calorie requirements. Low-cost foods were used together with vitamin and mineral
supplements. The health component consisted of constant observation of the children's symptoms, and prompt pediatric attention as
soon as symptoms were reported. The education component stressed
cognitive development and language, and was based both upon pilot
work undertaken in Cali by the same investigators and strategies
that had proven effective in the United States. This daily "dosage"
of six hours of treatment was provided to each child on an average
of 180 occasions during the year, and the treatment lasted one, two,
three, or four years for different groups of "experimental" children; and was not provided at all for the "no-treatment control
group".

The children selected for the study lived in poor sections of
Cali, and all met predetermined standards of malnourishment based
on ratios of height to weight. Eligible children had to have a

birthdate between June 1 and November 30, 1967, which meant that
they would be about to enter primary school in 1974, when the study
was scheduled to end. Seven hundred and thirty-three children met
the age requirement; 518 of them had parents who consented to the
initial anthropometric observations; 449 were identified as having
correct birthdates and no serious neurological or sensory deficiencies; and of these, the 333 children scoring lowest on indices of
nourishment, clinical signs, and economic status were selected for
the study proper. An additional 63 preschoolers of comparable age
were recruited from the more advantaged sections of the city. Their
intellectual growth was measured, but they received no treatment.
The purpose of this was to test to see how the intellectual performance of the economically disadvantaged children in the experimental groups compared to the performance of the more advantaged
children by the end of the study.

The experimental design involved six groups. Four were experimental, consisting of disadvantaged preschoolers who were in
the multidisciplinary project for either one, two, three, or four
years. The other groups were "no-treatment control groups" whose
intellectual performance was measured but who received no supplements. One was a group of economically disadvantaged children and
the other consisted of their more advantaged counterparts. Measurement of all groups took place five times before the study began,
and then at the end of each year, irrespective of whether a child
had received the treatment that year or not. Assignment of the
economically disadvantaged children to each of the treatment groups
was at random. This was accomplished by dividing the poor parts of
Cali into twenty sectors and then using a "lottery" to assign each
of the first five sectors to one of the five groups. Then, the
next five sectors were each assigned to one of the groups, and this
process was repeated a total of four times. From a technical viewpoint, districts of the city rather than children were randomly
assigned to treatments, but the result is the same. By giving each
child an equal chance of being in any treatment group, random assignment makes the average child in each treatment group comparable
before any intervention takes place. Consequently, when the sample
sizes are "large", and the process of random assignment is properly
carried out and is maintained during the total course of a study,
any group differences in intellectual performance that are apparent
by the end of a study are probably due to the different effects of
the treatments and are not likely to be due to different kinds of
children in each treatment group.

The measures used by the Cali researchers assessed each child's
performance in language usage, immediate memory, manual dexterity
and motor control, information and vocabulary, quantitative concepts,
spatial relations, and logical thinking. The tests called for responses that were about half verbal and half nonverbal. Because
any particular test is suitable for only a limited age range, dif-

ferent tests were empirically examined to assess their suitability.
The testers were nonprofessionals of both sexes who were supervised
by a professional psychologist.

The data from the study were analyzed in several stages. First,
the individual tests were combined into a general scale of cognitive development. Then, a multivariate analysis of variance was
conducted which showed that intellectual gains tended to be greater the longer a child had been treated. Finally, separate con-
trasts were performed which indicated that: (a) even one year of
the multidisciplinary treatment enhanced cognitive performance;
(b) but one year had a greater effect on younger than older children; and (c) the longer treated economically disadvantaged preschoolers tended to close the gap that separated their level of
intellectual performance from that of children from more advantaged
homes.

The Cali study is in many ways exemplary. But, like every
study, it raises some questions. For instance, one might wonder
about the financial cost of a multidisciplinary treatment that
lasts six hours per day, 180 days per year for four years. Unfortunately, no cost data have been presented in the reports we
have seen, but it should not be forgotten in this respect that cognitive gains appeared after only a year. One might also wonder
whether the evaluation of the Cali project should have been conducted by the same persons who designed the interventions. An
independent evaluation would have been more credible. One might
also question whether the dedication of the Cali staff can be
matched elsewhere and whether the same results would be obtained
if the intervention was implemented at other sites by other persons. One might also ask how the treatments affected individual
cognitive abilities, for the data analysis has thus far been restricted to a composite of all abilities. Finally, one might pon-
der whether teachers could have inadvertently taught the test items
to children so that their increased cognitive performance reflects
knowledge of a few specific items rather than of a whole domain of
knowledge of which the items are merely a representative sample.

Despite these questions, the Cali study is important because
it warns us against implementing puny interventions in the future
and it casts doubt on the argument that environmental interventions
cannot increase cognitive performance. If the Colombian group had
implemented their treatments *without evaluation,* or had implemented
them *but had used evaluative methods that result in more ambiguous
inferences about a treatment's causal impact,* then we would not be
in such a strong position (a) to oppose pessimists who think interventions will be ineffective, and (b) to call for treatments
that are of greater presumed power than has been the case in the
past. This is not to say we should give up looking for briefer,
cheaper treatments; it is merely to say that we should not over-

generalize from the pessimistic results of brief and puny treatments.

DIFFERENTIATING SOME TYPES OF EVALUATION

Evaluation is a vague concept. While it obviously entails placing a value on something, it does not by itself suggest either the criteria by which value is placed, nor the objects which are to be valued. Consequently, evaluation is used in quite different senses, and confusion often results in conversations where definitions are not offered. Indeed, one of the lessons that the present authors have learned over the years in the United States is to avoid the word "evaluation" unless it is modified in some way. Many modifiers have been proposed in order to enhance definitional fixity, and we shall present only the major ones here. However, little uniformity of definition exists among evaluators, and we want to warn the reader that not all the academic writings on evaluation contain definitions that are identical to those we shall offer. Indeed, our definitions are offered more in a spirit of illustrating working distinctions between types of evaluation than in a scholarly attempt to create identity-conferring boundaries around concepts.

Evaluations are undertaken to provide information about the extent to which projects or programs are meeting social needs. The hope is that the information generated from the evaluation will be valid, relevant to important decisions, and will be provided in comprehensible and timely fashion. By a program we understand an administrative thrust to meet a need, as when a national or international agency decides that efforts should be made to alleviate malnutrition in children and votes funds for this purpose. The money is likely to be spent in several different ways at different locations, and the efforts at the local level we shall call projects. The recent World Bank-funded efforts to increase the nutritional intake of Brazilians is an example of a program, and the many different types of endeavors to conquer malnutrition in the regions are examples of projects. In a sense, programs are administrative creations whose embodiment is local projects that directly touch the recipients of services. In contrast to programs, projects are usually characterized by more homogeneous activities, less geographic dispersion, fewer individuals delivering and receiving services, and a closer link between what is planned and what is delivered. *Program evaluation* is the name given to evaluating programs; *project evaluation* is the name given to evaluating local projects.

It is important to preserve a working distinction between programs and projects, since program evaluation is considerably more difficult than project evaluation. Logistics and coordination are

obviously greater problems with programs but so, too, is the design
of a framework for measuring consequences. Such a framework is
likely to be less sensitive for detecting effects with programs,
since they have many different local forms, than for detecting
effects of a single local project, which has a more fixed form.
Finally, program evaluation usually requires evaluating ongoing
activities, and so the evaluator is called in to study a program
after it has been implemented. This is also true of project evaluations in many instances, but with projects the evaluator is more
likely to be called in before a new project is set up and -- as we
shall see later -- evaluations are usually better if the evaluator
is involved in them from the very start. The major thrust in this
chapter will be on the evaluation of projects, but a strategy for
evaluating an ongoing heterogeneous program in one or more countries
is outlined in Cook, et al (2).

     A distinction is often made between *formative* and *summative*
evaluations. Normally, formative evaluation is intended to provide feedback to the implementers of a project so that its content,
execution, or management can be improved. Formative evaluations
are usually carried out either by staff members of the project being
studied or by persons hired by the project itself and, if there is
any conflict between rigor of method and ease of conducting the
evaluation, rigor tends to be sacrificed to ease. With summative
evaluations, the aim is to use social science methods to summarize
for funding agencies how a project or program has affected the
lives of the people who have been directly or indirectly touched by
it. The major thrust, of course, is towards determining whether
a project has had its intended impact on its intended target population. But good summative evaluations do not neglect secondary
issues concerning the unintended effects of a treatment on a target
group, and the intended and unintended effects on nontarget groups.
Typically, summative evaluations are conducted by persons who are
not employed by the project or program developers, and, if there
is any conflict between the demands of convenience and rigor, the
choice is not so easy as with formative evaluations. Since the ultimate goal of summative evaluations is to give funding agencies
valid information about causal consequences, and since invalid information can have widespread damaging consequences when used by
policy makers (3), most summative evaluators try to maintain the
maximal rigor and will accept only restrictions that are demonstrably unavoidable.

     Formative evaluations are in many ways akin to *process eval-*
uations and summative evaluations to *impact evaluations*. As the
word suggests, impact evaluations are concerned with the extent to
which a project has had causal consequences for an individual or
community (e.g., has a child's nutritional status improved; has his
health status improved; has his school attendance and performance
improved?). Process evaluations, on the other hand, deal with the

events that may have lead to a change (or no change) of state
(e.g., did parents learn of the nutritional campaign; did they
come to the local health center for supplements; did they use the
supplements as supplements or as substitutes?). Clearly, formative
evaluation -- with its emphasis on feedback useful to project personnel -- deals primarily but not exclusively with questions of process, while summative evaluation -- with emphasis on intended and
unintended changes of state -- deals primarily with questions of
impact.

It is important to differentiate the formative-process type
of evaluation from the summative-impact type.   There are well-
known cases in the United States of project developers and administrators who agreed to "evaluation" in the hope of gaining information about process but then saw the researchers begin a summative
evaluation. Since summative evaluations question the ultimate
value of a project, some of the developers became angry and did not
want to cooperate with the researcher. Their hope was for diagnostic feedback about how to improve rather than for evaluation
feedback about what they were accomplishing. Funding agencies,
on the other hand, tend to prefer summative information to formative, since information about accomplishment is one of the many
sources of knowledge on which decisions about funding levels and
new projects and programs are supposed to be based. There are
exceptions, though, to this preference for impact information,
the major ones being when (a) an agency is heavily invested, financially or politically, in a project and fears that a summative
evaluation will result in negative findings that may adversely
affect the agency's welfare, and (b) when the agency realizes that
a project is new and needs developing, so that it would be inappropriate to evaluate it by summative criteria. Another reason
for paying attention to the distinction between formative-process
and summative-impact is exemplified by some chapters in this book.
Unless the distinction is made it is not clear what kind of evaluation is being discussed, and differences between commentators
in the kind of evaluation to which they are referring (viz. impact
and process evaluation) inadvertently and falsely masquerade as
differences in opinion about the same object (viz. "evaluation").

Finally, we need to say something about a possible terminolo-
gical confusion over the very word "evaluation". For some readers,
"evaluation" may be equated with experts' views, site visits, or
other mostly qualitative methods. In some contemporary usage, however, "evaluation" designates procedures for gathering data directly from project participants according to a systematic research
design developed to yield causal influence about the impact of the
project. Typically, the design incorporates three principal features: (a) the division of participants into "experimental" and
"control" groups -- or some proxy such as difference in the length
of exposure to a treatment; (b) a framework for measuring possible

outcomes of the project; and (c) a statistical analysis of the quantitative data for the purpose of inferring the causal relationship
between project (treatment) and impact upon participants. Clearly,
such a procedure depends greatly on quantitative methods developed
for research in the social sciences. In fact, some authors have
deliberately used the term "evaluative *research*" to distinguish
evaluations based on more formal quantitative research procedures
from those based on more qualitative methods (4).

Our belief is that evaluation methods of a nonresearch character can sometimes be useful adjuncts to evaluation research, but
they are poor substitutes for it. This belief is based on two premises: the rarity with which nonresearch methods permit making a
strong case that change of any kind has taken place, and the rarity
with which any presumed change can be attributed to the treatment
rather than to forces extraneous to it.

Evaluation research on nutrition projects is not the same as
research on nutrition. Nutrition research is involved when one
tries to determine the efficacy of a supplement once ingested. It
would also be involved if one used quantitative methods to answer
questions such as: "When is a nutritional supplement for children
likely to be consumed by their parents?" or "Is a supplement more
likely to be used as a substitute than a supplement in large (as
opposed to small) families?" In each of these last cases, an important researchable question is asked that has implications for
the design of nutritional interventions, and so is relevant to
evaluation research in general. However, in neither instance is
there a sense of evaluating a particular nutritional project or
program.

The foregoing distinctions should help clarify the nature of
the Cali example given earlier. It was clearly summative, clearly
research, and clearly the evaluation of a single project. Hence,
summative evaluation research was used to evaluate a project. This
type of evaluation will be stressed throughout this chapter; and
less emphasis will be placed on formative and process evaluation
research. There will be no discussion of qualitative summative
evaluation methods or of general research on health and nutrition.

QUESTIONS ASKED AND METHODS USED IN SUMMATIVE EVALUATION RESEARCH

Summative evaluation questions are sometimes derived from a
careful analysis of the stated goals of a project. But in many
cases the goals are not stated explicitly. In other instances, the
goals cannot be readily translated into operational measures that
all would agree are suitable for assessing whether the project has
had its intended impact. And even if all the goals are well-stated,
they cannot exhaust the possible range of effects, planned or other-

wise, that a project may have. Given these realities, some evaluation researchers contend that summative evaluation research questions should be derived from a consideration of multiple factors,
especially: (a) project goals; (b) claims that responsible parties
have made about a project's possible effects; (c) a theory- or ex-
perience-based analysis of possible positive and negative side
effects of the project; and (d) a consideration of Suchman's (4)
major evaluation questions. Since the first three methods vary by
project, we shall present here a modified version of Suchman's evaluation questions which are outlined in Table I. The table also includes the techniques that are normally used to answer each question.

Suchman's first category -- effort -- involves asking how many
persons receive a treatment (a service or set of services) and who
they are. A host of subquestions are involved here, having to do
with: (a) the actual (as opposed to planned) availability of services; (b) the actual level of effort expended by service deliverers
to reach different kinds of persons in the target audience; (c) the
initial, and subsequent, levels of usage of the treatment by individuals in the target audience; and (d) an analysis of the types of
people who used the service most and of the possible consequences of
differences in usage patterns. Surveys of the target audience, and
subgroup analyses of the resulting data, provide the usual means of
answering these questions. Sometimes, although rarely, the questions
can be answered from the records that project operators keep for au-
diting purposes. The results of such surveys and audits are typically presented as percentages -- e.g., 30% of the target group of mothers come to the clinic within six weeks of their baby's birth; or,
among the mothers with three or more years of formal education 50%
attended the clinic, while among mothers with one to three years of
formal education 30% attended, and among mothers with no education,
the figure was 10%. Note that such results tell nothing about what
happened in the clinic or whether anyone benefited health-wise from
the visit. Nonetheless, the results are vital for assessing whether
the promised services were in fact delivered, and if they were, which
segment of the target population received or used more of the services in question.

Suchman's second set of questions has to do with whether statistically significant effects of the treatment are detected. This requires assessing whether the observed pattern of effects could have
occurred by chance and, if not, whether it was probably caused by
the intervention. Quantitative means for generating answers to causal questions are of two major kinds, and the means used in any one
summative evaluation depend on available data, cost, and disciplinary traditions, among other things. Most educators, psychologists,
and medical researchers lean towards the analysis of data collected
from randomized experiments or from quasi-experiments with both control groups and measurement before and after the intervention. Many

TABLE I.   SUCHMAN'S TYPOLOGY OF EVALUATION QUESTIONS

General Question	Research Questions	Means
Effort	a. How many persons ever receive the treatment?	Survey
	b. How many receive it for how long?	Audit
	c. What are the demographic correlates of availability and usage patterns?	
Effect	a. Does the treatment have statistically significant effect?	"Experiment" or "nonexperiment"
	b. On which subgroups is there an effect or a differential effect?	
Adequacy	a. To what extent does the magnitude of impact meet the need?	Impact analysis of the magnitude and generalizability of effects
	b. To what extent does the impact generalize and meet needs that are tangentially related to the target one (e.g., will improving motivational status improve academic achievement?)	
	c. To what extent does the impact of the treatment persist over time?	Long-term study
Process	a. What are the social factors that mediate impact or prevent it from being observed?	Questionnaire
		Interview
	b. What are the psychological factors that mediate or impede impact?	Observation
Cost-Benefit	a. What does the treatment cost per person per time unit?	Economic or audit
	b. In which ways might the costs for the project being evaluated be used more effectively within the project?	Analysis, always involving costs and sometimes
	c. What are the financial benefits of the project relative to its costs?	involving benefits

sociologists and economists, on the other hand, prefer regression
analyses of data collected before and after the intervention or only
after it if that is all that is available. Such analyses involve
correlating levels of exposure to the treatment with, say, health
status, and attempting to control statistically for all the confounding factors that might lead people with better (or worse)
health to make greater use of the treatment.

Suchman's third set of evaluation questions concerns whether
any observed effects of the treatment are likely to make a practical difference, for with large samples and measures of high reliability an effect of minuscule magnitude can be statistically
significant. The principal analytical tasks that help determine
whether an observed difference is likely to make a practical difference require estimating the magnitude, generality, and temporal
persistence of effects in relation to the magnitude of the human
need that led to mounting the intervention in the first place. For
example, is an average increase of 50 calories a day in a child's
diet a practically significant change? What about 10 calories?
The difficulties here are, first, obtaining widespread agreement
that a particular magnitude, generality, or duration of effect is
enough to make a practical difference; and second, obtaining agreement that questions about the magnitude and duration of effects
should even be asked. Some persons contend that Suchman's criteria
of practical significance imply higher standards than his criteria
of statistical significance, and that it is often unrealistic to
expect a project to have a socially significant impact. It is
likely that project developers and funders with a vested interest
in positive evaluation results are most likely to make this argument (5).

Suchman's fourth set of questions concerns the social and
psychological processes that might mediate or impede effects. A
crucial subquestion here concerns assessment of the content of the
treatment, for it can often differ quantitatively and qualitatively
from what was planned. As an example, it could have turned out
in the Cali experiment that children spent many of the six hours
per day, not experiencing the planned educational, health, or nutritional changes, but simply playing with each other or sitting
alone. It is one thing to measure Suchman's "effort" -- i.e.,
who receives the treatment -- and quite another thing to measure
the events that take place during the treatment period.

In studying process factors, questions other than about medi-
ators can be involved. For instance, it would often be useful to
know which aspects of a global treatment package are more effective than others. In the Cali case, this would involve asking
whether the nutrition component was more effective than the preventive health component. In a simple supplementary feeding project,

one might ask whether any observed changes are due to the supplement itself or to exhortations by the project personnel to induce
parents to change their family diets. If there were no observed
effects with the supplementary project, one might then want to
know whether the supplement had actually been used to increase
intake or whether it had served as a substitute for other foods.
Observational or interview techniques are used to measure process
variables, and measures are usually taken during the course of the
evaluation. Thus, observers might keep records on what happens
to each child, or observers might be sent into the home to inquire
about who actually ingests a supplement. Where resources do not
permit extensive interviews or questionnaires, one or the other
is frequently used at the end of the study and taps into retrospec-
tion about behavior rather than behavior that is ongoing or has
just happened.

The list of Suchman's questions has to do with costs. Usually three subquestions are involved here: first, what is the dollar
cost per time unit to reach each of the persons or communities in
the evaluation; second, what is the relative effectiveness of different ways of allocating the dollar costs within a given nutrition project; and, third, do the benefits of the project exceed
the costs when each is expressed in monetary terms. These three
questions are not equally easy to answer, and we have listed them
in increasing order of difficulty. Obtaining answers to these
types of questions lies within the scope of economists and account-
ants, but there are no well-articulated accounting conventions for
allocating the costs of the various components of health and nutrition programs; and estimating the dollar value of human or
social benefits has been very resistant to rational treatment. How
much is a human life worth? -- or even an avoided episode of diarrheal disease?

Suchman's typology of headings under which to note evaluation
questions has important implications. One is that his system of
comprehensive evaluation highlights the ultimate artificiality of
the distinction between summative and formative evaluations. For
any project, it would be useful for both project developers and
funders to know about both impact and process. Knowledge of impact would help developers realize to what extent they need to
make fundamental changes; while knowledge of process would help
funders begin to understand whether, say, the absence of impact
might be due to a puny treatment or a nondelivered treatment or
to some countervailing force in the local culture. A second implication is that comprehensive evaluation is necessarily interdisciplinary. Few individuals will have all of the necessary
skills at high levels, and team research is obviously required.
A third implication is perhaps the most important. It is desirable
in any evaluation to have answers to each of Suchman's five general

questions. Indeed, one can confidently predict that, when the evaluator presents answers to any subset of these questions, his audience will be curious to know answers to the remainder.

Unfortunately, the scarcity of evaluation resources often
makes it difficult to answer all five questions, and the crucial
issue then becomes: How should one choose priorities among the
questions? In the United States, questions about planned and unplanned effects and about financial cost have loomed largest in
evaluations of therapeutic interventions designed to improve health
practices, while delivery and cost concerns have loomed largest in
evaluating interventions designed to increase the coverage of services (e.g., medical care for the aged and the poor). In general,
process and adequacy criteria have played minor roles.

Suchman's questions primarily deal with the use of evaluation
research to throw light on whether specific interventions in, say,
nutrition or health change the nutritional or health status of
target populations. It is important to recognize at this point
that, like interventions, evaluations always incorporate assumptions about social values. However, we will not treat in any
significant way the underlying value assumptions about nutritional
or health status in Latin America, deferring this task to our
colleagues Ugalde and Emrey later in this volume, who argue very
strongly the political nature of the problem. It is also important
to recognize that explicit or implicit theories about nutrition
and health underlie hopes that certain interventions will prove
successful. For example, some persons' beliefs in the value of
supplementary feeding programs for preschool and primary children
rest on the theory that relieving the symptoms of protein-calorie
deficiency will by itself promote greater cognitive growth than
would otherwise have been possible. This may or may not be true.
Furthermore, the links in any argument justifying an intervention
will be stronger in proportion to the amount of empirical evidence
which has been accumulated in the past concerning the postulated
relationships.

We shall not concern ourselves in this paper with theoretical
issues about the postulated causal links between treatments and
outcomes. We shall instead content ourselves with pointing out
that the social desirability of any intervention is based on value
premises, and that its rationality depends upon the validity of
assumptions about the theoretical links between project actions
and expected impacts.

When is it Advisable to Evaluate or Not to Evaluate?

Some critics have argued that summative evaluation is often
used for slowing down social change, and that many policy-makers

invoke the need for it only when they see that the alternative to
evaluation is implementing some new practice which is ideologically,
financially, bureaucratically, or otherwise unattractive to them.
Evaluation, these critics argue, permits the appearance of sensitivity to needs and action to meet these needs without a practical
commitment to either. Thus, some have argued that INCAP in Guatemala has served to hold back pressure to implement large-scale
interventions for undernourished children while research on nutrition was being conducted and change strategies were being evaluated.

The most frequent response to this charge is to claim that in
many instances it is unclear whether a planned innovation will be
effective because no one has tried it before and the processes
that are presumed to lead to its effectiveness have not been well
tested in basic research. Lacking this knowledge, the argument
goes, resources can be poured into useless programs which give a
false appearance of being effective and create hopes that will
inevitably be disappointing. In addition, the argument continues,
it is difficult to phase out a program or project once it has been
funded on a broad scale, so that funds continue to be wasted on
ineffective programs and cannot be used to experiment with new
ways of alleviating the need to which the program was originally
addressed.

Both of these viewpoints have merit. It is important to take
them into account in order to abstract a general principle which
might suggest when the call for evaluation is likely to be a sin-
cere call to learn rather than a disguised call for inaction. Our
position is this: When it is known from prior studies, or from
a data-based *strong* theory, that an intervention is usually effective, then there is *generally* little purpose to evaluating the
innovation once again. Let us be concrete. In the nutritional
domain, years of research have shown which diet supplements can
reduce infant mortality and morbidity. Hence, to evaluate one of
the known supplements is generally wasteful if a crucial question
is whether the supplement improves health status. However, some
particular exceptions to our generalization have to be noted. First,
to know that a supplement is effective once ingested tells nothing
about whether the members of a particular target group will ingest
it. Second, to know that the supplement will be ingested tells
nothing about whether it will be used as a true supplement rather
than a substitute. Third, to know that a supplement (e.g., cow's
milk) is effective with one group of people in one part of the
world does not guarantee that it will be effective with all groups.
Finally, knowing that a supplement is effective provides no information about whether the resources or political atmosphere will
exist in a particular country for maintaining and capitalizing upon
any nutrition-related improvement in health that a supplement might

have conferred. When there are genuine doubts about any of these four issues, an evaluation should be carried out that is primarily targeted towards the issue in doubt.

Another circumstance where evaluation is not considered advisable by some is when individuals are in need and resources exist that are thought to meet the need. In this case, the argument goes: "Better provide resources that might be effective and forego the evaluation". Two very different responses can be made to this argument. One is to suggest that evaluation studies should be designed that permit distributing all available resources *and also* evaluating effectiveness. [For a list of such strategies, see (6, 7)]. The second and more philosophic response is to say: "While resources may be sufficient for everyone in a particular community, this does not mean they are sufficient for all the persons in need in a particular country (region, hemisphere, etc.). Would one not be doing a disservice to these other persons by implementing the treatment on a widespread *local* basis that precluded ascertaining its effectiveness?" In this context, imagine the gain to millions of children caused by *knowing from a few hundred children in no-treatment control groups* that polio vaccines were effective; and imagine the loss that would have occurred through giving the vaccine to all the children in the area and not learning with any reasonable level of confidence that the vaccine was effective.

One context where summative research is definitely not advisable is when a project has been in the field for a short time and so cannot have had a fair trial. All too often in the United States evaluations are conducted on new projects while operational mistakes are still being made and the project administrators are experiencing all the unexpected difficulties that inevitably accompany new projects. The time when it is appropriate to begin summative evaluation depends on many factors, most of which are project-related, and so it is difficult to give an estimate of when it is appropriate to conduct summative evaluation research. However, it is clear that fair evaluation requires a considerable project development period.

When is it most useful to conduct summative evaluations, particularly in circumstances where the resources for evaluation are scarce and so evaluable projects have to be chosen with special care? Our suggestion is that evaluation be done (a) after the project has passed through its initial shakedown period and (b) when the project holds promise for wider diffusion later. A pilot nutrition project, for example, whose effectiveness depends on the availability of an expensive food supplement will be useless for the poorest segment of a population who cannot afford the supplement. In this respect, it is questionable whether the expensive six-hour per day, 180 days per year Cali treatment is relevant to

many lesser developed countries. However, against this position
one has to note that, although evaluating projects which cannot be
easily implemented on a wide scale because of resource limitations
may do little for a *particular* country in the *short* term, it may
have other benefits. This is because information obtained in one
circumstance or country need not be used solely in that circumstance or country, and results that are obtained at one time may
have quite different relevance in the same country at a later date
if social and political conditions are different. Though we do
not dispute these possible benefits, we do not assign them as much
weight as we attach to using scarce evaluation resources for interventions that have an immediate national importance and generalizability.

Whose Questions Should be Answered?

Evaluations are political acts. At the broadest level, evaluation is political in that it implicitly assumes values of prag-
matism and a gradualist approach to social change, albeit gradual
within the social context chosen by a particular country. At a
narrower level, politics enters evaluation in influencing the research questions that are addressed. For instance, in the United
States most persons considered it appropriate to ask whether "Sesame
Street" raised the achievement level of economically disadvantaged
children. However, not everyone considered it appropriate to ask
whether the achievement gap between children from different social
classes widened or narrowed because of the show. Their fear was
that this distributive question might generate information suggesting that gaps were widening and that "Sesame Street" might be seen
as exacerbating a national educational problem.

One faces the same dilemma in the health area: Should one only
assess the impact of a health intervention, or should one also ask
about the differential consequences that might result because certain
social groups may or may not receive the new treatment, or because
groups do or do not benefit from it once they have received it?
The issue of distributive justice and its consequences might appear to be neatly side-stepped if an intervention is targeted exclusively at poor people. But even here the issue of distributive
justice may arise because -- as Rogers has suggested in the case of
agricultural development projects (8) -- the richer among the poor
may benefit most from the interventions and the new wealth they
have accumulated may help them acquire more land from their poorer
neighbors, consequently exacerbating local inequities. To choose
another example, the comparative issue has to be faced head-on
when one asks about the impact of professional services like nursing,
since such services may be more available to persons who need them
less, either because of where the nurses choose to live (viz., in

cities or large towns), or because they choose to work in locations to which only certain persons have access (e.g., hospitals as opposed to local health centers; or highly technical as opposed to less technical hospitals).

It would be wrong to think that the only possible evaluation questions with political/value overtones are distributional. For instance, all groups interested in agricultural development projects will ask evaluators to examine crop yields, but not all of them will ask the evaluators to examine how an intervention affects land tenancy, attitudes toward landholders, or the level or cooperation between farmers. Since these outcomes have very different political implications for different interested constituencies of the evaluation, "political" considerations obviously influence the choice of the evaluation questions that will be asked or not asked.

The crucial issue implied by the foregoing discussion is this: Which constituencies should have the opportunity to ask the major evaluation question? This is crucial since those who set the questions are most likely to have their interests fostered by the work. The opinion seems to be growing in the United States that, in the past, questions have come either (a) from evaluators' guesses about decision-makers' information needs or (b) from evaluators' interpretations of formal project goals. The growing fear is that little cognizance has been taken of what other interested constituencies might want to learn from an evaluation. For instance, in health matters, the questions are usually those of the project developers and do not include the questions that deliverers of health services at all levels might ask, or that would be asked by host country political figures or by representatives of the project recipients. In the United States, the concern with who asks the evaluation questions is made even more pointed by the growing realization, not only that it is unduly restrictive to exclusively ask decision-makers' questions, but also that it may not be useful to ask their questions. This is because their questions are not always analytically precise and unambiguous, because the rapid turnover of decision-makers sometimes renders their original questions obsolete, and because decision-makers are often not single persons or homogenous groups that can quickly come to a well-thought thorough consensus or hold an unconflicted view. Indeed, obfuscation and vague generalities are well-established political tools for managing the conflict that would arise if a decision-maker were pressed to come up with a restricted set of well-defined goals for anything, including an evaluation.

If one considers it important to ask a broad range of research questions reflecting the interests of several constituencies, a technical problem arises. How could one in practice perform a multi-constituency evaluation? Many obstacles to such work exist, including concerns of cost, time, and keeping the constituencies' expectations realistic. On the surface it would be appropriate to ask all the major questions of all the identified constituencies. However, assuming that cost is no issue, one still runs afoul of the fact that the more questions one asks in social research the lower will usually be the quality of the answers to any one question. The evaluator has therefore to select a subset of questions in such a way that each constituency feels it has some stake in the evaluation, and he can usually do this best by specifying new questions in terms of outcome variables to be added to the measurement framework as opposed to asking about additional possible causes, for in experimental research the latter sometimes requires new manipulable independent variables.

What is the significance of the political nature of evaluation? It means, we think, that everyone should ask certain things of actual and proposed evaluations: (a) Who decides what should and should not be evaluated, and are there inadvertent or deliberate biases in these choices -- e.g., are local self-help projects evaluated more often or more critically than nationally centralized ones? (b) Who poses the evaluation questions, and by what process are they arrived at -- is it the project developer, the funding sponsor, or the evaluator; and is the appropriateness of the major questions checked with groups that might have different interests in the program? (c) Who translates the general questions into specific research hypotheses -- who decides, for example, whether the general goal of stimulating the achievement of poor children in Mexico means narrowing educational gaps -- which implies a strategy targeted exclusively at poor children -- or raising their achievement in an absolute sense, irrespective of whether the means to do this raises the level of advantaged children more. [For the possibility of such an effect in Mexico, see (9)].

We do not know the answers to these questions for the majority of Latin American evaluations, nor are we sure whether the issue has the same salience there that it does in the United States. But we can feel sure that, sooner or later, political leaders, administrators, practitioners, and clients will ask:" In *whose* interests are evaluations in our country being conducted?" And this may boil down to: "Who decides now what should be evaluated?" and "Who decides now the actual form of the research questions?"

Sources of Bias in Evaluation: Personnel and Organization Factors

In the United States three related forces are suspected of contributing to biased evaluations. The first is where the evaluator works for the organization whose effectiveness is being evaluated, as would happen when the evaluator is a staff member of a community health center. The second is where the evaluator is not on the staff but is hired by the center and reports directly to powerful staff

members within it. The third is where the evaluator does not report
to the body being evaluated (e.g., the health center), but is hired
by the same office within the agency that is also funding the center.
This last relationship may mean that the office has a reputational or
budgetary interest in producing positive results. In all three of
these relationships, the evaluator is dependent upon the project
being evaluated or the funders of the project not only for access to
data, opportunity to observe operations, etc., but also for the con-
tinuation of his employment contract. Extrapolating from these three
situations, the preferred organizational structure would seem to be
where the evaluator is financially independent of the project being
evaluated and is funded by sources other than the organization sponsoring the project, or by an office within the sponsoring organization that is not responsible for the project under evaluation.

Is one of these organizational structures to be preferred? For
evaluations that are clearly formative in nature, it is extremely
useful if evaluators are members of the project being studied. When
they are, they know how it operates, have easy access, and enjoy a
local credibility that may facilitate utilization of any findings.
As for summative evaluations, it is desirable that they be truly independent, but we are not sure how many can be. The reason for this
is that there is in Latin America no "industry" of research firms
specializing in applied social research. Hence, there is no large
cadre of independent and easily available professionals. Most of
the Latin American evaluations cited in our references were conducted
by persons who were the developers of projects, or who were employed
by the developers of projects, or were persons who felt personally
committed to alleviating the target problem and often to the philosophy or concept behind the particular project being evaluated. Such
"passion" is not necessarily undesirable, but it has to be balanced
against a "dispassion" built into the interpersonal system of research in either of two major ways, or preferably both of them.
First, the potentially committed evaluator has to be closely monitored in critical fashion, which entails at a minimum the reviewing
of all he does at all major decision points. Second, it entails
placing greater stress on reviews of studies of comparable projects
rather than on the results from a single evaluation of a project,
always assuming, of course, that the same commitments are not inadvertently biasing all evaluators of a certain type of project. Since
we do not yet note either close external monitoring or frequent replications of evaluations, we have to conclude that the potential
for inadvertent bias may be more widespread in evaluations in Latin
America than in the United States.

How often this potential for bias translates itself into de-
monstrable bias is quite a different question. On the one hand,
we have been struck by the small number of Latin American studies
of which we are aware that found no differences between treated

groups and untreated controls. In this, experience is quite unlike
United States experience where "no difference" findings are typical.
On the other hand, there are cases of Latin American investigators
who in early studies found favorable results, but who reversed
themselves in later publications (9, 10, 11). It would be interesting, we think, for the agencies that fund evaluations in lesser
developed countries to try to estimate the prevalence of summative
evaluations by persons who are truly independent of the project
being reviewed, since it is clear from United States experience
that no-difference findings are more frequent when evaluations
are independent than when they are not (12). This is not to say
that external evaluation is a panacea. In some cases in the United
States, the outside evaluators have not taken their responsibilities
as seriously as they should and may not have had the same dedication as either employees of the project or external evaluators with
a philosophical commitment to the project. Nonetheless, dedicated
external evaluators give the best promise of uniting competence and
bias-free work, and the practical problem for Latin America is:
Where would such evaluators come from, given the currently restricted supply? If one or more independent evaluation agencies were
set up, how would they be structured, and which of the most crucial
evaluation projects should they undertake?

How Feasible is Randomization?

Most United States evaluators believe in the desirability of
randomization, but many doubt its feasibility. The skepticism
seems to be abating somewhat, largely perhaps because of the accumulating number of projects where random assignment was successfully implemented initially *and also* successfully maintained for
the course of the study. It is important here to be clear what
we are talking about, since randomization for group comparability
is often confused with randomization for representativeness. Only
the former is at issue here. It has to do with the process of
randomly assigning experimental units into different treatment
groups in order to create aggregates that are probabilistically
comparable to each other before the treatment is implemented.
Randomization for representativeness has to do with the process of
selecting a single group so that the chosen sample is representative
of the population from which it was selected within known limits
of sampling error. Random assignment for comparability is desirable because it rules out nearly all the threats to internal validity enumerated by Campbell and Stanley (13). However, it is no
panacea because, as Cook and Campbell have pointed out, random
assignment can be associated with other threats to internal validity -- systematic attrition, resentful demoralization of controls,
compensatory rivalry, and the like (7). But these restrictions
aside, randomization is the best single procedure we have for

facilitating inferences about the causal efficacy of a project or program.

The debate about the feasibility of randomization has, we think, been somewhat sidestepped, albeit temporarily, by altering the question. Now the focus is on conditions which maximize the probability of being able to randomize instead of on whether randomization is or is not feasible. Most scholars believe that randomization is most likely when new projects are under study rather than established ones; when the local demand for a service exceeds the supply; when several different treatments are to be compared; when individuals (or whatever unit is being used) cannot communicate easily with each other (as when different groups of people who do not know each other receive some service, say, job training); and when the persons or authorities granting access to respondents understand the need for randomization and are willing to endorse it. In the past, such conditions have led to randomly assigning whole villages to water treatments (14); intact nursery groups to Plaza Sesamo (9); households to birth control treatments in Taiwan (15); and sections of cities to multidisciplinary treatments in Colombia (1). Other examples of randomized experiments in lesser developed countries are outlined in Riecken and Boruch (6); their mere existence belies the contention that is often heard that randomized experiments cannot be carried out.

Since spatial isolation is usually important for preserving treatment groups intact, it is common to define the experimental unit at a higher level of aggregation than the individual -- e.g., villages or neighborhoods. In these cases, financial resources may be strained by having more than a few units in the experiment, and it is common to find, say, only two villages in some experimental group and two in the controls, as in the INCAP dietary supplementation experiment (16). In such cases, it is desirable to match the villages on variables that are thought to be most highly related to the outcome variable of greatest concern and *then* to randomly assign from within the match. This reduces the likelihood that the two best or worst villages might receive the same treatment. However, matching prior to randomization does not guarantee equivalence when so few units are available for assignment; but it does minimize pretest differences!

Since the cooperation of individuals who can control access to respondents helps in achieving random assignment, it is useful to anticipate their questions. In the United States, most of the questions and doubts of administrators relate to their discomfort at creating focused inequities between people who are deliberately treated differently. Many administrators are loath to allocate differentially unless there is a clear and socially approved justification based on individual differences in merit, need, seniority,

or the like. It is rare to distribute scarce and valued resources
by lottery, which is in essence what random assignment is.

Administrators seem most responsive to the following points
about randomization, especially if preceded by a brief and lucid
explanation of the basic function and importance of randomization
when compared to the alternatives: (a) Administrators of other
intervention programs have previously permitted randomization
without outward difficulties arising. (In this respect it might
be useful to cite from the previously mentioned lists of randomized
experiments). (b) The administrator can provide the treatment
to whichever persons or communities he deems particularly merito-
rious or needy, *and this need not preclude random assignment of
the remaining communities or individuals.* (c) If the treatment
proves effective, it will be made available to all the control
group members. The administrator should also be assured (d) that
steps have been taken to minimize contact between individuals in
different groups and (e) that the study has a low profile politically. None of these strategies guarantees success; but they
are said to increase the chance of it. Moreover, they are clearly
not appropriate where an ongoing project is being evaluated that
will not admit new clients. In such cases, the assignment process
has been implemented before the evaluators come on the scene.

The Desirability of Alternatives to Random Assignment

The two major empirical alternatives to random assignment are
some form of a quasi-experiment or a cross-sectional nonexperiment.
The major developer of quasi-experimental designs has been Donald
Campbell, who now publicly regrets the influence his work has had
(13). His argument is two-fold. First, the quality of causal
inferences from most quasi-experiments is lower than had been originally believed, based on the prevalence with which systematic
threats operate and/or the difficulty of controlling for them using
statistical adjustments. The exceptions to this general statement
are interrupted time-series designs, with their long baseline, and
designs like regression-discontinuity where the factors determining why some persons receive a treatment and others do not are
completely understood and, thus, not quantitatively expressible.
Unfortunately, interrupted time-series and regression-discontinuity
designs are rare in United States evaluation research, and they
are not likely to be found in any but a few Latin American settings.
Campbell's second concern is that the easy availability of quasi-
experimental designs may have caused applied social researchers
not to try to implement randomized experiments when they were
feasible. As a result he believes that some evaluators took the
line of least resistance, and sacrificed hard-headed causal inference for convenience. Campbell's position should not be taken

to mean a distaste for most quasi-experiments, *which are useful if
nothing better is available*. Rather, his position reflects a concern with settling for second best before it is clear that this is
all that can be achieved. He also is concerned with failure to
interpret the results of quasi-experiments more critically, clearly
expressing the assumptions that have to be accepted before the
stated research conclusions can be accepted.

The problems with quasi-experiments result, in Campbell's
opinion, because the average person in a treatment group is different from the average person in the untreated control group.
Consequently, the groups will differ on many measures even at the
pretest, and may be changing over time at different rates for reasons that have nothing to do with the treatment. Another source
of difficulties is the fact that most measures of social or cognitive behavior are unreliable, which can lead to statistical regression when matching takes place without subsequent random assignment or to underadjustment biases when multiple regression analyses
are conducted that attempt to control statistically for the initial
noncomparability that characterizes the different groups. These
same problems plague cross-sectional nonexperiments without a
pretest where differences in exposure to a treatment are measured
and then correlated with a dependent variable collected at the posttest. Unfortunately, the problems of causal inference are even
more tricky in this case than where there are pretest measures.

Ross and Cronbach have taken issue with Campbell (17). Their
position is that applied research is conducted to help make decisions, and so it is imperative that the information be available
when needed for such decisions. Often this means that randomized
experiments cannot be set up since it takes time to collect pretest measures, to implement the project, and then to collect posttest measures. Ross and Cronbach advocate powerful designs when
they are possible within the time-frame, but if they are not, then
they argue that one should conduct whatever data collection is
possible -- even if a correlational cross-sectional study or a
more qualitative study results, each of which has a greater risk
of bias leading to false causal conclusions.

This position implicitly assumes that some information on time
is better than no information at all or information that arrives
too late to enter into decision-making. Campbell, on the other
hand, argues that when rigor is sacrificed to timeliness, conclusions about cause may be wrong and may be used as part of the
justification for introducing new practices that are not effective
and for cutting back old practices that may be beneficial. In
this last regard, Campbell has cited the example of Head Start in
the United States, where he believes that positive results were
obscured by a statistical analysis which made the program look

misleadingly harmful. Of course, the likelihood of erroneous
causal conclusions is reduced if the results from a weak design
are intelligently interpreted and all the limitations and assumptions are listed. It is then up to the potential user to estimate
if he wants to use the information *despite its highly provisional
nature*. Unfortunately, results from weak designs are not always
wisely interpreted, and the sources of bias are often not made
explicit. Even when all the assumptions are expressly stated on
which accepting a conclusion depends, it is nonetheless frequently
the case that by the time results become part of the popular or
policy debate the qualifications to the conclusions have been forgotten or have been omitted from summary reports which are written
for general audiences (3).

Ross and Cronbach also argue that randomized experiments are
not useful for many of the more crucial evaluative tasks, which
they consider to be formative (17). One of their principal concerns is that treatments are often not delivered in anything like
the promised form, or are so heterogeneous as to be meaninglessly
classified under the single heading "treatment". For example,
they cite programs in which the treatment is to give administrative
entities funds which they are at liberty to spend as they want.
Some will spend them on diet supplements, others on nutrition-
oriented projects, others on media campaigns, and others even for
purposes that are irrelevant to nutrition. Given these concerns,
Ross and Cronbach want a major part of evaluative resources to be
devoted to formative and not summative tasks.

Even when a treatment is demonstrably somewhat homogenous and
is delivered in something approaching the promised form, Ross and
Cronbach would still argue that the random assignment is of low
priority. This is because random assignment helps in only one of
many research decisions -- viz., is there a *causal* relationship?
Ross and Cronbach doubt the importance to decision-makers of cause,
since they claim that causal information is most useful for making
funding decisions, and such decisions are less likely to be influenced by data than by political concerns. However, Ross and
Cronbach believe that decisions about the content of projects are
often influenced by data, and so they suggest that the most useful
kinds of evaluation data are formative. They also argue that,
even when causal information is needed for formative purposes, it
is usually wanted for managerial purposes that are local to the
project rather than for decisions about funding levels, and so they
suggest that the causal information required for formative purposes
need not be grounded in the degree of rigor associated with randomized experiments.

It is not yet clear to what extent information about impact
is or is not used to make or to justify decisions about projects

and programs. If it is not, then the argument of Ross and Cronbach
gains in strength. But if it is, their argument loses in cogency.
But even if impact information is not used to affect decisions
about politically impacted projects *today*, it could still be used
to affect decisions *tomorrow* -- decisions about whether a particular
project should be implemented elsewhere or whether a particular class
of similar-appearing projects looks so promising that a far-reaching
national or international program should be launched. Thus, the
issues to be decided are: when evaluations lead to weak or misleading causal inferences, how often does this have serious consequences for decisions about funding levels for projects and for
decisions about implementing a particular type of project elsewhere?

The current debate does not imply that evaluation is impossible
without random assignment. Rather, the moral is that the analysis
of quasi-experiments must recognize significant limitations on
causal inferences because multiple regression procedures to not
routinely adjust for all of the initial differences between nonequivalent groups in the absence of (a) an extremely plausible
model and valid measurement of the selection process or (b) near
perfect prediction of the dependent variable. In presenting causal
inferences drawn from quasi-experimental designs there should always
be a full and frank discussion of the assumptions on which causal
inference is dependent. We suggest that all evaluators should
resist all attempts to limit the qualifications they put on causal
conclusions and that they remain skeptical of their own findings
until they have been closely reviewed by knowledgeable persons who
try to point out the hidden assumptions and restrictions behind
them. [For an example of a critique of hidden assumptions in evaluation research, see (18)].

Measurement Issues

Most of this volume is devoted to measurement issues in evaluation research, particularly in lesser developed countries. Therefore, we shall deal briefly with only four issues that we consider
especially important.

The first revolves around a distinction between proximal and
distal measures of outcome. The former are measures close to the
treatment that is actually delivered in a project, whereas the
latter are more remote. For instance, if a nutritional program
is targeted toward improving the physical growth and mental development of children through increased consumption of home-grown
high-yield corn, the most proximal measure of outcome would be
whether the target families planted the seeds; a more distal measure
would be whether the children consumed the resulting crops; an even

more distal measure would be whether children became bigger and
heavier at a faster-than-expected rate; and an even more remote
measure would be whether children learned more and their life chances were significantly improved.

It should be clear from the foregoing example that the probability of obtaining any measured impact is greater the more
proximal the measure, but that the probability of obtaining an
impact of social significance is greater the more distal the measure. This relationship results because many steps usually intervene between an actual intervention and the responses indicating
solution of the target social problem, and extraneous forces other
than the intervention affect each of these steps and reduce the
strength of the relationship between the intervention and the most
desired impact. The distinction between proximal and distal measures is also important because project personnel want the project to be evaluated in terms of proximal measures, since these
are closely related to factors under their control (e.g., whether
the seed is planted and the food consumed). But policy-makers
and others ask about distal measures, since these are the indicators
of success in dealing with the social problem which justified the
project in the first place (e.g., morbidity and cognitive growth).

It is clearly advisable to measure both proximal and distal
variables, but since resources are finite, where should the stress
be? Our answer, once again, "depends". In particular it depends
on the longevity of the project being evaluated. To evaluate new
projects by distal criteria is premature, and formative feedback
about process and proximal measures is more appropriate. But even
established projects should not be evaluated by distal criteria
if the interval between pretests and post-tests is brief. Though
managerial problems are less with established projects than with
new ones, it should not be forgotten that, whatever the longevity
of the project, the passage of influence from proximal to distal
measures takes place in time. Consequently, "long" intervals between pretests and post-tests are appropriate if distal measures
are to be stressed.

A second measurement problem concerns side effects. We have
begun to learn in the United States that, for many social interventions, the unintended impacts are as important as the intended
ones. Think, for instance, of how the automobile has inadvertently
affected the residence pattern of North Americans and consider the
consequences of this. Think, also, of the side effects of a drug
such as thalidomide, or the side effects of many pesticides, or
the reputed detrimental side effects of bottle feeding babies by
working mothers in the urban areas of many developing countries --
effects that may be due to advertising campaigns by multinational
corporations which promote bottle feeding as more "modern" than
breast feeding (19, Ch. 7).

Since no one can hope to foresee and measure all side effects, the practical question is:" How can one increase the probability of measuring and detecting side effects?" Often, there may be a relevant theory about the intervention process, and this should be used. It can also be helpful to have frank discussions with persons who have had first-hand experience with treatments like the one to be evaluated. But ultimately the detection of side effects depends on a sophisticated on-site monitoring system that is not limited to a fixed set of measures. In this respect -- as we point out later -- we have been favorably impressed by some Latin American summative evaluation research (e.g., 1, 16). It is not clear, however, whether such monitoring is widespread, especially with smaller and less well-funded projects.

The third measurement problem we shall discuss relates to unfocused treatments. These are usually treatments aimed, not at alleviating a specific need, but rather at providing a general service. Nursing would be an example of this; the nurse might teach prospective nurses, lecture to community groups, clear up stagnant surface water in which mosquitoes could breed, treat cuts and bruises or diptheria and leprosy. By which criteria could one evaluate the nurse's services so as to be sensitive to the exact tasks that were carried out, and so as not to impose criteria that are appropriate to only a subset of the tasks that have actually been performed for perhaps only a smaller part of the nurse's time? The issue is also acute with satellite-controlled radio-telephone medical consulting services to remote areas in Alaska (20). In the Alaska study, it was difficult to show gains in health care, much less health status, though easier to show gains in the satisfaction of village health aides who could consult by telephone daily with a remote hospital staff. Given the host of things aides did, it would be difficult in any evaluation to show the relationship between their activities and any health gains in their target group of clients.

One way out of the measurement dilemma inherent in unfocused treatments is to throw up one's hands and say: "Such treatments cannot be evaluated. Let us use our evaluation resources elsewhere". A second response is to say: "Unfocused treatments can only be evaluated in terms of what is delivered and not in terms of effects -- in essence, rather like a process evaluation project that monitors the project activities". A third response is to say: "Unfocused treatments can be evaluated in terms of the satisfaction of the people reached"-- an evaluation based on "client satisfaction ratings". A fourth response is to say that unfocused treatments can be evaluated in restricted comparative terms, as when one asks whether nurses are more effective in disease control than, say, are paramedics. A final response is to say that," *given the passage of enough time,* unfocused treatments can be evaluated in terms of the

health status of individuals and families they have visited often."
In short, there are a host of *carefully phrased evaluation questions* that can be asked, but they all have to be sensitive to the
multitude of different tasks represented by unitary-appearing labels
such as nurse or paramedic.

The final measurement issue we shall mention is subject response bias. It is usually patently obvious to most persons in
treatment groups what the researchers would like to hear. This
means that certain kinds of responses (e.g., opinions and self-
reports of behavior) can be treatment-related and may masquerade
as treatment effects. This problem may be particularly acute in
some third world countries where respondents may have considerable
reason to want to please researchers who have higher status than
they and might be seen as representing formal authorities. Response bias may have been a problem with the radio-based nutrition
campaigns in Nicaragua, the Philippines, and Ecuador where effectiveness was measured by nutritional actions that were *reported*
to interviewers before, during, and after the campaigns (21, 22,
23). Since these studies did not have measures of overt nutrition-
related behavior, effects were not objectively assessed. To be
sure measures based on reported behavior are not always suspect,
and claims that, say, mothers' estimates of their children's height
and weight are reasonably valid are well worth investigating (24).

Well-kept statistics on morbidity and mortality might be an
answer to the problem of response bias, but in the radio-based
nutrition campaigns cited above a significant change in the behavior of people exposed to the nutritional messages would probably
not show up in national statistics because the target audience is
not a majority of the population. Archives are useful if statistics are well gathered and can be disaggregated by geographic area,
but this is rarely possible in much of the third world. Nonetheless, in some health projects there may be records from community
health centers, while in education there may be school records.
Careful scrutiny can determine whether such records are usable for
research purposes.

Recognition of the problems with subjective measures and national statistics had led some evaluators to espouse unobtrusive
measures, which are less susceptible to "compliance distortion" by
respondents. Such measures might include the amount of surface
water in which mosquitoes could breed, or the number of children
who are observed on the street to have certain symptoms. The major
problems with such measures are their validity, sensitivity, and
availability. Though unobtrusive measures have to be used with
considerable skepticism and background knowledge, they are probably
well worth searching for as an adjunct to other measures collected
in any evaluation.

The Need for Continuous Monitoring of Summative Evaluations

Time and again in the United States, evaluations have turned
out to be technically disappointing, if not an outright waste of
the taxpayers' money. Much of the disappointment resulted from
the implemented intervention being less powerful than the promised
intervention. But other sources of disappointment resulted from
the evaluation itself, as when testing was conducted in sloppy
fashion and reliabilities were low, or when sample sizes fell to
unacceptable levels because of the unwillingness to follow up hard-
to-reach individuals. (In some of these cases, the attrition was
systematic and led to differences in attrition rates across treatment groups.) The disheartening feature of most of these instances
is that the problems were either predictable or could have been
detected earlier than they were. The prediction and early detection of problems is important because each allows the evaluator
to modify procedures and so keep the study on track or "fall back"
to more feasible research techniques. The lesson we have learned
in the United States is that mechanisms are required for continuously monitoring evaluations in ways that are perceived by the
evaluators to be supportive. We are not speaking here of contract
monitoring; rather, technical monitoring is at issue. To be sure,
there is currently a job category in most federal agencies and
foundations called "Technical Monitor" or "Project Officer". But
too few of these persons have the necessary technical background
and field experience in evaluation to be able to detect evaluation
problems early and solve them. Consultants are often used to help
technical monitors in these tasks, but consultants tend to be used
once a problem is visibly serious or at fixed interim stages which
do not correspond to crisis points. Advisory boards are also used,
but these tend to be composed of luminaries who are so busy that
few of them can follow an evaluation in any close detail over time.
[For an extended discussion of these and related points, see (25)].

On-site monitoring has a second function in addition to the
early detection of the field problems that arise in implementing
an evaluation. All too often the treatment on paper does not correspond very well with the treatment actually delivered to individuals or communities. For instance, two evaluations of rural
primary school radio projects disclosed that at the time of site
visits a significant number of radios were not even in working
order. This meant that the "treatment" was not being delivered
to a large proportion of the target population and called into
question the results from an evaluation of the projects (26, 27).
Cases like these have made evaluators in the United States even
more aware than before of the need to measure directly how the
treatment is delivered and then to use these measures in the data
analysis. There is always a potential trap in doing this, for very
often more of the treatment is given to those in the worst health or

social circumstances. When this happens, most of the currently
used data analyses will inadvertently make the treatment seem harmful and relatively less progress will be apparent in the most disadvantaged groups (28). Nonetheless, most evaluators consider it
crucial to measure who receives the treatment (or various parts of
it) for how long.

     As we said before, we have been impressed by the care that is
put into monitoring treatments in Latin American evaluations, and
this may account for the relatively high technical quality and
ambition of some of them -- e.g., the Peru (11), Cali, Colombia (1),
and Guatemala (16) nutrition studies, or the Nicaragua mathematics
teaching experiment (29). But the intensive monitoring of either
the evaluation procedures or the delivery of the treatment costs
money, and this raises the issue of whether the growing demand for
monitoring in the United States is appropriate to Latin America at
this time. The basic question at issue is: "Is it advisable at
this time in Latin America to conduct summative, high-cost evaluations of a few projects, or coarser evaluations of more projects?"
Each strategy implies different research payoffs. In the first
case, one assumes that the project is promising and resources are
used to evaluate it as it is; in the other case one assumes that
the need is to pick out "successful instances", and so one makes
a gross cut from among many projects knowing that one may miss some
positive results that may be small in magnitude but will probably
detect most positive results of any magnitude. As we said, this
is a question about strategy, and we have no ready answers. But
the issue is an important one with grave consequences in light of
the restricted funds and personnel available for carrying out evaluation activities.

                        ISSUES OF GENERALIZABILITY

     There seems to be a growing realization in the United States
that the best formal procedures for ensuring generalizability are
the least feasible. Random sampling from a well-designated universe best ensures generalizability; yet how often does one see
respondents, settings, times, or measures being randomly selected?
Generalizability is next best ensured by sampling multiple instances
that are maximally different and then demonstrating that the same
cause-effect relationship holds across instances, as would be the
case if a nutrition program had similar effects in lowland and
highland settings in Guatemala at three different times and with
children of different racial backgrounds. Attempts to extend generalizability by this strategy of "purposive sampling by heterogeneity" require considerable resources but are technically more feasible than the random selection of persons, settings, and times.
The final means of extending generalizability is sampling to obtain

"impressionistically modal instances", as when one wants to conduct
a study with, say, poor inhabitants of villages and then goes out
to find convenient persons and villages that correspond to the
target profile. Obviously, this is a weak sampling procedure in
that (a) it does not readily permit generalizing *to* all instances
in the target population of villages, and (b) it certainly does
not permit generalizing *across* any other types of settings, persons, times, or measures.

The negative relationship between the desirability and feasibility of different means of assessing generalizability should
cause any person to hesitate who wants to use the results of a
single evaluation to justify widespread implementation. Because
of this, we detect in the United States a growing awareness that
the proper basis for implementation is the review of evaluations
on several similar projects or the review of several evaluations
of a single project, rather than the results of a single evaluation of a single project. As evidence of this awareness, we would
cite the many North American studies of prison rehabilitation,
negative income guarantees, and racial integration in the schools.

But not all reviews are useful. Ideally, one would like to
examine several studies which evaluated the same or similar projects in a variety of different settings with a variety of different kinds of persons at a variety of times, and one would like
studies that had different measures of what is presumed to be the
same outcome construct, and that were not subject to biases that
operated in the same causal direction. For example, an attempt
has been made to generalize results from evaluations of a number
of rural education projects using radio (30, 31). In this respect, it is heartening to note in Latin American research that
apparently successful projects are usually tested a second or third
time in different settings before decisions about wider implementation are made (viz., the projects on rural education by radio, or
nutritional supplements).

Consider the intensive on-site nutritional evaluations we
mentioned earlier. It is obvious that any results from these
studies cannot be generalized beyond the experimental settings.
It is more important to note that much of the intensive on-site
work, particularly attempts to recruit children, keep them in the
study, and keep up the high quality of the delivered treatment, is
carried out by persons in the development team, who are often motivated to make the project a success. One has to wonder whether
the same initiative and hard work would be manifested if the project became national policy *and so became part of an extensive
and routinized bureaucratic structure* instead of part of a smaller
team effort. In this respect it is worth noting that in the United
States several educational programs have appeared to have large

effects when they were evaluated by their developer, but had much
smaller effects -- or none at all -- when the projects were implemented elsewhere by persons without the same experience or dedication of the project developer.

    A kind of formative evaluation, often neglected but one that
could help toward the generalizability of evaluation results, is
the administrative history or case study. This kind of evaluation
focuses attention on qualitative elements of a project, like leadership, key administrative decisions and their consequences, or historical events that strongly affect the outcomes of intervention.
And it can help capture in a qualitative way the processes that
might facilitate or inhibit impact, thereby contributing to an
understanding of why a project is successful at one site, but a
similar project does not appear to be successful at another. This
kind of study is often conducted retrospectively, as a historical
document. There are few examples of administrative histories that
are written while services are still being delivered in a project
(cf. 32), but these latter have the advantages of working with
events as they occur, providing feedback about process to the project, and identifying special processes that might explain why
there appears to be a limited generalizability of results from one
setting to another.

    There is no way in any single evaluation that all questions
about generalizability will be answered. Indeed, when evaluation
results are explained to them, curious listeners often ask: "But
would the same results hold, do you think, for people of type X
rather than Y", where X is not the designated target group of the
evaluation. The evaluator can only admit his or her ignorance
about such matters, but he or she need not be defensive and should
stress: (a) that the major research thrust was towards the target
populations of persons, settings, and time to which decision-makers
wanted to generalize; (b) that he sampled to approximate these
populations even if it was only with "impressionistic modal
instances"; and (c) that the only non-target groups he was able to
measure with the evaluation resources at his disposal -- if any --
were those which theory or past experience led him to expect would be
indirectly affected by the intervention. If these last groups include the X's of the questioner, the evaluator is lucky. Often,
they will not.

            WHEN SHOULD EACH KIND OF EVALUATION BE CONDUCTED?

    As promised, we have emphasized summative evaluation research.
But we have referred frequently to other types of evaluation, and
it is appropriate to ask when each type of evaluation should be
employed. In a sense, the answer is simple. If the major evaluation

takes the form: "Are people receiving the nutritional supplement,
and are they using it as such?" then a process evaluation is all
that is required, even though it will be uninformative about the
health and social benefits caused by receiving the nutrition supplement. If the major question takes the form: "How can we make
the operation of our nutrition project more efficient?" then formative research is called for that concentrates on improving the
project's operation. However, if the major evaluation question
takes the form: "What are the health and other social consequences
of a particular nutritional project?" then the summative evaluation of a project is required. Deciding on the guiding research
questions is so important and determines the form of an evaluation
to such a considerable extent that we want to stress the necessity
for a careful appraisal of questions -- hopefully, an appraisal
undertaken with the interests of multiple parties in mind.

A decision is often required of agencies that fund evaluations
about whether they should place their priorities on one kind of
evaluation or another. In the best of possible worlds, there would
probably be no issue since one would call for the careful development of projects by means of formative evaluation, and one would
also call for the comprehensive evaluation of well-established
projects by summative criteria that include process (see Table I).
Unfortunately, this is not the best of possible worlds, and so a
difficult choice based on imperfect knowledge is required. If one
believes that, in general, current projects are not particularly
successful, then formative research is called for that stresses
developing the content of projects. If one believes that current
projects would be effective if only they were better implemented,
then process research is required which stresses internal project
management and outreach to the target community. If one believes
that many good projects (or programs) are currently being implemented, then one needs to stress summative evaluation. Finally,
if one believes that some good projects or programs are being
implemented, but one does not know which they might be, then summative research is called for in two stages: the first being to
gather data on many projects to find out which ones *might* be successful, and the second being to examine the projects that appear to
be successful in greater and more rigorous detail. When all is
said and done, the decision to stress one kind of evaluation over
another in the nutrition area depends on a necessarily underin-
formed judgment about the general quality of current nutrition
projects. Experience and informed guesses will have to be the
necessary guides.

If a decision is made to stress summative evaluation research,
then one has to ask "Evaluations *of what form*?" Should one aim
at the coarse-grained analysis of very many projects, or the finer-
grained analysis of a few projects of special promise and policy

relevance? Should one try to assign units to treatments at random
or allow systematic and probably biased social forces to perform
the assignment to treatments? Or should one randomize sometimes
(e.g., with experimental projects that are new) while not inter-
ferring with allocation on other occasions (e.g., when projects
are already ongoing). And if random assignment is not possible or
desirable, then one has to decide whether to rely on regression-
based quantitative means of analyzing information about a project's
causal impact, or to collect data of a more qualitative kind that
perhaps uses expert judgment or other non-statistical methods to
draw conclusions about impact. All of these are vital questions,
which we cannot answer for others. But we advise administrators
to ask themselves, in the context of each particular project:
(a) How important is it to ask causal -- as opposed to noncausal --
questions about this project?; (b) How serious will the consequences be if we receive the wrong answers to our causal questions?
The first of these questions determines whether one needs summative
evaluations, and the second whether one needs rigorous evaluation
research methods.

                               CONCLUSION

     The evaluation enterprise is many-faceted and the application
of its precepts will differ depending on the nature of the substantive area, the specific objectives of different programs and
projects in any area, and the social, political and professional
circumstances of the countries in which the evaluation takes place.
Given this, general statements about "evaluation" are hazardous
and worth treating with caution.

     We previously identified what we consider to be a strategic
question of great consequence for Latin American evaluation research -- whether it is advisable at this time to concentrate
scarce financial and personnel resources on intensive summative
evaluation research into a few projects, or to spend the resources
on less detailed evaluations of a larger number of projects in the
hope of detecting particularly successful ones. A danger in the
first approach is that one may invest most of one's resources in
a few projects that turn out to have no impact. Another danger is
that the impact detected by an intensive evaluation may have little
generalizability to other settings. The chief danger in the second approach is that when a large number of projects are examined,
there will probably be some "false positives" -- i.e., projects
that appear successful but are not, and "false negatives" -- projects that appear to have failed but in fact did not. The number
of false positives and negatives will depend primarily on how
intensive and precise the research is. Coarse-grained methods
which are speedier and cheaper in time and effort are likely to

yield more false conclusions. A compromise is to evaluate inten-
sively enough so that methodological sensitivity is not compromised and conclusions about causal impact lose credibility.

If time is not a problem, one can adopt a three-stage strategy
for evaluation research on nutrition projects. The first stage
would be to ask a heterogeneous group of informed persons about
the nutrition projects they *believe* are successful. Reputations
would therefore be used to define a pool of promising projects.
The second stage would be to conduct coarse-grained research on
all of the projects in the pool that meet criteria of policy relevance and logistical feasibility of conducting the research within
the budget. The purpose of this second stage would be to collect
data to determine which of the reputedly successful projects still
seem successful when data are used as a reality check on reputations. The third stage would be to conduct intensive evaluations
of the most promising of the projects from stage two, either studying these projects *in situ* or setting up projects like them elsewhere on a random assignment basis. This three-stage strategy takes
time, but if the purpose is to identify some successful projects
that have a high likelihood of being successful elsewhere, the
third and most time consuming stage can be dropped.

Identifying successful instances of nutrition projects is a
summative goal. However, it would be myopic to conduct only summative research, particularly once one has narrowed down the pool
of projects to those most likely to be successful. Impact information is most useful when it is *specified*. That is, when one can
relate the extent of impact to the quantity of the treatment delivered or the mix of the parts, when a global treatment package is
involved; or when the impact can be specified for different kinds
of persons or different settings. Indeed, once tasks of data-based
specification are accomplished, one should be close to having the
elements necessary for building a provisional theory of the conditions under which a particular intervention is successful. In
the total evaluation process which stresses multiple studies strate-
gically interrelated, there can be no substitute for detailed and
fine-grained research on some projects, and for the theory-like
statements that result from such work. The crucial issue is to
decide *when* such work is called for since it uses resources in-
tensively.

REFERENCES

1.   McKay, H., L. Sinisterra, A. McKay, *et al*. Improving cognitive
        ability in chronically deprived children. *Science* 200:
        270-278, 1978.

2.   Cook, T. D., B. R. Flay, R. A. Haag, *et al.* An evaluation
          model for assessing the effects of Peace Corps Programs
          in health and agriculture. Unpublished report prepared
          for ACTION by Practical Concepts, Inc., Washington, D. C.
          September, 1977.
3.   Cook, T. D., and W. E. Pollard. Guidelines: How to recognize
          and avoid some common problems of misutilization of eval-
          uation research findings. *Evaluation,* 4:161-164, 1977.
4.   Suchman, E. *Evaluative Research,* New York: Russell Sage
          Foundation, 1967.
5.   Cook, T. D. The potential and limitations of secondary eval-
          uation. In: M. W. Apple, M. J. Subkoviak and H. S.
          Lufler, Jr. (eds.). *Educational Evaluation: Analysis
          and Responsibility.* Berkeley: McCutchan, 1974.
6.   Riecken, H. W., and R. F. Boruch (eds.). *Social Experimenta-
          tion: A Method for Planning and Evaluating Social In-
          tervention.* New York: Academic Press, 1974.
7.   Cook, T. D. and D. T. Campbell. The design and conduct of
          quasi-experiments for field settings. In: M. D. Dunnette
          (ed.). *Handbook of Organizational and Industrial Psycho-
          logy.* Skokie, Illinois: Rand-McNally, 1976.
8.   Rogers, E. M. Communication and development: The passing of
          the dominant paradigm. *Communication Research,* 3:213-
          240, 1976.
9.   Diaz-Guerrero, R., I. Reyes-Lagunes, D. B. Wittke, and W. H.
          Hotzman. Plaza Sesamo in Mexico: an evaluation. *J. Com-
          munication,* 26:145-154, 1976.
10.   Baertl, J. M., E. Morales, G. Verastegui, and G. G. Graham.
          Diet supplementation for entire communities: growth and
          mortality of infants and children. *Am. J. Clin. Nutr.,*
          23:707-715, 1970.
11.   Graham, G. Feeding trials in children. pp. 358-364. In:
          *Proceedings of the Third International Congress of Food
          Science and Technology,* New York: Stuart and Wiley,
          1970.
12.   Gordon, G. and E. V. Morse. Evaluation research. pp. 339-361.
          In: *Annual Review of Sociology.* Vol. I. Palo Alto:
          Annual Reviews, Inc., 1975.
13.   Campbell, D. T. and J. Stanley. *Experimental and Quasi-
          Experimental Designs for Research.* Chicago: Rand-
          McNally, 1963.
14.   Dodd, S. *A Controlled Experiment on Rural Hygiene in Syria.*
          Social Science Series No. 7. Beirut: American University
          of Beirut, 1934.
15.   Freedman, R. and J. Y. Takeshita. *Family Planning in Taiwan.*
          Princeton: Princeton University Press, 1969.
16.   Freeman, H. E., R. E. Klein, J. Kagan, and C. Yarbrough.
          Relations between nutrition and cognition in rural Guate-
          mala. *Am. J. Publ. Health,* 67:233-239, 1977.

17. Ross, L. and L. Cronbach. Review essay evaluating the "Hand-
    book of Evaluation Research". In: G. Glass (ed.) *Eval-
    uation Studies Review Annual*. Beverly Hills: Sage Publi-
    cations, Inc., 1976.
18. Carnoy, M. and H. Levin. Evaluation of educational media:
    some issues. *Instructional Sci.*, 4:385-406, 1975.
19. Berg, A. *The Nutrition Factor*. Washington, D. C.: The
    Brookings Institution, 1973.
20. Kreimer, O. *Health Care and Satellite Radio Communications
    in Village Alaska: Final Report of the ATS-I Biomedical
    Satellite Experiment Evaluation*. Stanford: Institute
    for Communication Research, Stanford University, and The
    Lister Hill National Center for Biomedical Communication,
    June, 1974.
21. Manoff, R. K. *Mass Media Nutrition Education: Ecuador*.
    Washington, D. C.: Manoff International, Inc., 1975.
22. Manoff, R. K. *Mass Media Nutrition Education: Philippines*.
    Vol.I. Washington, D. C.: Manoff International, Inc.,
    1977.
23. Manoff, R. K. *Mass Media Nutrition Education: Nicaragua*.
    Vol.II. Washington, D. C.: Manoff International, Inc.,
    1977.
24. Freij, L., Y. Kidane, G. Sterky, and S. Wall. Exploring child
    health and its ecology: The Kirkos Study in Addis Ababa.
    Ethiopian J. Development Res., 11(2) Supplement: 1976.
25. Cook, T. D. and C. L. Gruder. Metaevaluation research. *Eval-
    uation Quarterly*, 2(1):5-51, 1978.
26. Schmelkes, S. The radio schools of the Tarahumara, Mexico:
    an evaluation. In: P. Spain, D. Jamison and E. McAnany
    (eds.). *Radio for Education and Development: Case
    Studies*. Working Paper No. 266 of the World Bank. Vol 2.
    Washington, D. C.: 1977.
27. Spain, P. The Mexican radio primaria project. In: P. Spain,
    D. Jamison and E. McAnany (eds.). *Radio for Education
    and Development: Case Studies*. Working Paper No. 266
    of the World Bank. Vol 2. Washington, D. C., 1977.
28. Campbell, D. T. and R. F. Boruch. Making the case for random-
    ized assignment to treatments by considering the alter-
    natives: six ways in which quasi-experimental evaluations
    in compensatory education tend to underestimate effects.
    In: C. A. Bennett and A. A. Lumsdaine (eds.) *Evalua-
    tion and Experiment: Some Critical Issues in Assessing
    Social Programs*. New York: Academic Press, 1975.
29. Searle, B., P. Suppes and J. Friend. Formal Evaluation of
    the Radio Mathematics Instructional Program: Nicaragua
    Grade I, 1976. pp. 651-672. In: T. D. Cook (ed.).
    Annual Review of Evaluation Studies, 3. Beverly Hills:
    Sage Publications, Inc., 1978.

30.   Jamison, D. and E. McAnany. *Radio for Education and Develop-*
          ment. Beverly Hills: Sage Publications, Inc., In press.
31.   Spain, P., D. T. Jamison and E. G. McAnany (eds.). *Radio for*
          Education and Development: Case Studies. Working Paper
          No. 266 of the World Bank. Vol. 2. Washington, D. C.,
          1977.
32.   Mayo, J. K. and J. A. Mayo. *An Administrative History of El*
          Salvador's Educational Reform. Stanford: Institute for
          Communication Research, Stanford University, 1971.

COMMENTS

Robinson G. Hollister, *Swarthmore College*
Swarthmore, Pennsylvania

INTRODUCTION

It is impossible to reduce recent United States experience
with evaluation to a few statements or guidelines. This is the
reason that Cook and McAnany quite often find themselves saying
"it all depends" when trying to come up with a recommendation.
The recent United States experience generates a multitude of particular problems in evaluation and various ways to deal with them
(or not to deal with them), through experiments, or non-experimental
designs. In a course that I teach at the University of Pennsylvania,
I spend a whole year trying to make students aware of the most
salient points of the United States experience and the syllabus for
that course seems to grow exponentially year to year. Thus, any
short discussion of what can be learned from the United States experience is bound to be highly selective and rather idiosyncratic
and my comments on Cook and McAnany will unfortunately be of that
sort.

At various points in the discussion below I will refer to one
or the other of several very large scale social sciences experiments in the United States. It would be most efficient, therefore,
if I give a very succinct description of each, at this point, and
some sources from which readers may obtain further references.

The Income Maintenance Studies (Table I) were a series of experiments the principal objective of which was to estimate the
effect of an income guarantee of the "negative income tax" type
on hours of work and earnings of low income families. Put suc-
cinctly, experimental families had a basic money grant, the size
of which declined as income increased. The size of the basic grant
and the rate at which it declined was different among several experimental subgroups.

Table I. INCOME MAINTENANCE EXPERIMENTS

Site	Duration of Treatment	Number of Experimental Subjects	Number of Control Subjects
Urban: New Jersey	3 years	725 families	632 families
Rural: North Carolina Iowa	3 years	374 families	435 families
Gary, Indiana	3 years	1,028 families	771 families
Seattle, Washington Denver, Colorado	Subgroups of 3,5,20 years	2,749 families	2,021 families

Note: For further information:
a.   Watts, D., et al (1).
b.   D. L. Bowden, Urban Institute, Washington, D. C.
c.   K. Kehrer, Mathematics Policy Research, New Jersey.
d.   R. Speigleman, Stanford Research Institute,
     Menlo Park, California

The objective of the Health Insurance Studies (Table II) is
to estimate the effect on demand for health care services (doctors
and hospitals) of different forms of health insurance coverage.
Experimental subgroups have different rates of co-payments (cost
sharing) and different limits on total out-of-pocket health costs.

The objective of the Housing Allowance Supply Study (Table
III) is to estimate the rate of increase of supply of housing in a
market area in response to a market-wide increase in housing demand
induced through housing costs subsidies (housing allowance) for low
income families.

In the Supported Work Studies (Table IV) employment is provided for up to eighteen months for workers drawn from among ex-
convicts, ex-addicts, women on welfare (AFDC), and youth who have
dropped out of school. The objectives are to estimate the effects
of the program on drug use, criminal behavior, and post-program
employment.

Table II. HEALTH INSURANCE STUDIES

Site	Duration of Treatment	Number of Experimental Subjects	Number of Control Subjects
Dayton, Ohio	Subgroups of 3, 5 years	390 families	0
Seattle, Washington	Subgroups of 3, 5 years	904 families	300 families
Charleston, South Carolina	Subgroups of 3, 5 years	153 families	526 families
Fitchburg, Massachu- setts	Subgroups of 3, 5 years	550 families	0

Note: For further information contact:
J. Newhouse, Rand Corporation, Santa Monica, California.

Table III. HOUSING ALLOWANCE STUDIES

Site	Duration of Treatment	Number of Experimental Subjects	Number of Control Subjects
Green Bay, Wisconsin	Subgroups of 5, 10 years	3,500 families	No control group
South Bend, Indiana	Subgroups of 5, 10 years	6,500 families	No control group

Note: For further information contact:
Ira Lowry, Rand Corporation, Santa Monica, California.

Table IV. SUPPORTED WORK STUDIES

Site	Duration of Treatment	Number of Experimental Subjects	Number of Control Subjects
Atlanta, Georgia	12 months	139 individuals	139 individuals
Chicago, Illinois	12 months	450 individuals	445 individuals
Hartford, Connecticut	18 months	452 individuals	646 individuals
Jersey City, New Jersey	12 months	484 individuals	486 individuals
Newark, New Jersey	18 months	361 individuals	386 individuals
New York, New York	18 (Youth) 12 (Other)	361 individuals	363 individuals
Oakland, California	12 months	389 individuals	390 individuals
Philadelphia, Pennsylvania	18 months	411 individuals	403 individuals
Fond du Lac, Wisconsin	18 months	16 individuals	16 individuals
San Francisco, California	12 months	131 individuals	128 individuals

Note: For further details contact:
R. Hollister, Mathematica Policy Research, Princeton, New Jersey.

THE ROLE OF EXPERIMENTS IN ALTERNATIVE MODES OF ANALYSIS

I want to begin with a discussion of Cook and McAnany's points
4 and 5, which they entitle "How Feasible is Randomization" and
"The Desirability of Alternatives to Random Assignment". The most
important point to be made on this issue is that experiments and
other modes of analysis are really not alternatives but complements.

The alternative modes referred to are statistical analyses of archival data (either existing program data or records from functional, usually governmental, units) of existing population or institutional surveys or of specially designed data collection efforts. There has been much too much discussion in the methodological literature in recent years which poses these alternative modes only as competitors with experimental methods; this is seriously misleading.

I want to mention just a few of the ways in which statistical analyses can be ·complementary with experimental methods. Statistical analyses of non-experimental data are virtually a prerequisite for design of any experiment. Before an experiment is undertaken it is necessary to have some prior estimate of the variance in the behavioral variable that is of interest so one can determine how large a sample will be necessary in order to have a reasonable chance of detecting the treatment effect. Data from large scale national surveys were used in this fashion in the planning of all of the major income maintenance experiments and in the health insurance experiment. However, for the housing allowance supply experiment, there were no such data available and the size of the experiment was determined by guessing at the sample variance.

Such survey data and analyses are also important in determining the location of sites for experiments and in some cases the location of subjects. In addition, such data have often been used to provide checks during the course of the experiment. For example, in the New Jersey Income Maintenance Experiment, it appeared at one time that sampling procedures had yielded a misrepresentative sample of the low income population because there was such a very low proportion of working wives. However, by simulating the eligibility criteria for the experiment on data from a national survey it was possible to determine that the sample was not misrepresentative but instead that the low proportion of working wives was a result of the income eligibility cut-off for the experiment. 1/

External, non-experimental data are also used during the course of an experiment to monitor changes in the environment in which the experiment is taking place. For example, in several of the experiments it was useful to know the conditions of the local labor market. The response to a manpower training program or

---

1/   Only families with incomes less than 1.5 times the poverty line were eligible to be included either as experimentals or controls. Families with wives working as well as husbands generally earned enough jointly to raise family income above the eligibility level. Therefore, the remaining sample of eligibles had a low percent of wives working.

income maintenance program may be very different when unemployment
is high than when it is low. Undoubtedly, knowing about changes
in food prices in regional markets may help in understanding about
fluctuations in responses to nutritional supplement programs.

The data from such surveys are of great importance in trying
to generalize the results from the experiment *ex post facto* to the
wider context of national policy (since as Cook and McAnany point
out, feasibility of taking representative population samples for
the experimental evaluation is often limited). In the case of the
income maintenance experiment the behavioral responses from the experiment have been built into simulation models for the population
as a whole using the population survey data in order to generalize
the results. The simulation model can also estimate responses to
alternative configurations of the income maintenance policy.

In a currently ongoing experiment, archival data are being
used to check for biases in responses of subjects to interview
questions. For example, checks of official arrest records show
underreporting of arrests, but equal underreporting by both experimentals and controls. Welfare records show errors in response
concerning receipt of welfare payments. Such information gathered
for a sub-sample can be used to correct estimates of responses for
the experiment as a whole. One experiment has been using archival
data to check on response biases from survey interview data.

Much of the literature discussing the advantages of experiments
in contrast to alternative procedures, has emphasized the use of
regression analysis or covariance analysis as a substitute for experimental, random assignment designs or as a corrective for design weaknesses. 2/ This argument has obscured the fact that the
experience with the major social experiments indicates that these
types of analyses *will inevitably be used with the experimental
data themselves.* First of all, these techniques will be used because they can increase power of the sample. That is to say, the
ability to detect a small but statistically significant response
to the treatment can be considerably enhanced by using regression
analysis to remove extraneous "noise" from the behavioral response
(i.e., to reduce the residual variance). In addition, it is in-

---

2/   The debate on this issue continues. I, personally, find the
arguments concerning the usefulness of regression analysis, except
in unusual cases, generally persuasive. That is, random assignment where feasible is preferred (except for some cases detailed
in the text below) but where not attained, all is not lost and
statistical control is useful. For a reasonably comprehensible
statement of the case, see G. Cain (2).

inevitably the case that investigators or decision-makers would like to know about the ways in which the response to the experimental treatment varies within the treatment group. Often the differentiations one would wish to make within the experimental group are based on characteristics which may themselves be affected by the treatment (i.e., are endogenous to the experimental system) (3). For example, the income maintenance experiments sought to discover how the experimental response varied according to the income levels of the families, but the income levels of the families during the experiment were affected by their response to the income maintenance treatments themselves. In order to try and deal with this problem one had to resort to rather sophisticated techniques of regression analysis.

To reiterate then, it is important to recognize that statistical analyses which use other non-experimental data or which are applied to the experimental data are complementary to rather than competitive with experimental procedures themselves. What future analysts really need is a better set of guidelines as to how to integrate these alternative modes.

As Cook and McAnany indicate in their section on generalizing results, the most convincing evidence for policy conclusions is a consistency of estimated effects across a number of different studies. In the case of income maintenance in the United States, there are now a number of studies based on econometric analyses of cross-sectional and time series data as well as of the income maintenance experiments. It is the consistency across these studies in estimates of labor supply responses to income maintenance treatment that provides the most convincing estimates of the likely response to a national program. The cross-sectional studies and the experimental studies reinforce one another.

However, recognizing all of the important complementarities outlined above, it remains true that at particular points in time evaluators or decision-makers do have to decide whether a particular set of resources will be devoted to an experimental study or a non-experimental study. At this point, these approaches remain competitive. Therefore, it is perhaps useful to list the limitations of each of these types of studies. I try to summarize the limitations of each type of study as I see them in the table below. I do not have the space here to discuss all of these limitations in detail, particularly as some of them are highly technical. However, I do want to comment on a few of them and try to explain the nature of the limitations of experiments.

Table V.   EXPERIMENTAL VERSUS NON-EXPERIMENTAL STUDIES

Limitations of Experiments
Inappropriate timing
Inability to simulate program context
Limited duration of treatment
Legal constraints
Difficulty of randomization
Interference from existing programs
Vulnerability to special local events
Inability to capture secondary effects

Limitations of Non-Experimental Studies
Unmeasured selection bias
Simultaneity problems
Non-existence of market observations of
  phenomenon of interest
Limited variability of independent variables
Conflicts in time series and cross-section
  estimates
Errors in measurement
Omitted variable bias
Sample selection bias (truncation, aggregation,
  limited small-area data)

LIMITATIONS OF EXPERIMENTS

Timing

Controlled experiments require a considerable amount of time from the starting period of design through the implementation state -- including the duration of the treatment which constitutes the experiment -- to the stage of analysis arriving at results. This matter of the time duration of controlled experiments means that such experiments will not be relevant for those policy decisions where a "fast fix" is called for. Experiments will not in general yield information in short time periods.

One must be somewhat careful, however, in using this limitation to define the role of experiments. It has been my experience that any policy objective toward which experiments might be directed is judged by some to be a policy issue that needs action today and

that is likely to be acted upon tomorrow. Subjective estimates
about the likelihood of a policy action in a particular arena are
notably unreliable. The field of income maintenance is a good
example. When the New Jersey Income Maintenance Experiment began
the experimenters expected that it would be at least five years
before the proposals for a negative income tax would be taken
seriously at the policy action level. Within a couple of years,
however, President Nixon had proposed the Family Assistance Plan,
and the subjective estimates seemed to be very wrong. Within
another two years, that plan had been defeated in Congress; today
the negative income tax appears at least a few years away, if not
longer. Every experiment that has been started has been faced with
people arguing that the policy being considered will have been
acted upon long before the results of the experiment begin to come
in and, therefore, there is no opportunity to experiment.

Inability to Simulate the National Context

There are certain issues for which, at first consideration,
controlled experimentation appears quite relevant. However, under
closer examination, it turns out that for certain types of behavioral responses, it is simply not possible to approximate the
national context in which such a policy would operate. I would
venture a couple of examples, though I am sure some would argue
with me as to whether in fact it is impossible to simulate the
national context even in these cases.

One example is with regard to the supply of health services.
There is already under way an experiment to deal with the demand
side of health services. It was recognized early by the designers
of that experiment that a very important consideration would be
the response on the part of suppliers to changes in conditions of
demand. It is a generally recognized characteristic peculiar to
health services that the consumers' decisions are greatly affected
by the suppliers' (i.e., the doctors') judgment as to what is
necessary and appropriate. Thus, an important element in decisions
about a national health insurance policy is the response of doctors
to a change in demand conditions. The way in which doctors respond
to changes in the cost constraints which result from national health
insurance is extremely difficult to simulate, however, since doctors' practices with regard to appropriate modes of treatment for
various illnesses are undoubtedly influenced by the flow of information through teaching hospitals, journals and professional
associations concerning desirable best practice techniques and
their cost feasibility. A small experiment will not simulate these
information flows as a national program would.

Another possible example of difficulty in simulating the national context arises with regard to public employment programs.

An important question in a national program with the government as
an "employer of last resort" is how many people would demand such
a public employment job at various wage levels. The factors which
influence secondary workers to apply for such jobs are not that
well understood (e.g., why the surge during the last few decades
in labor force participation of married women at all income levels?).   Whether the public employment is regarded by the general
public as stigmatizing ("just leaf-raking" or "leaning on a shovel")
can affect the demand for such jobs. I doubt whether these responses are likely to be well simulated in a limited experiment.

      Our state of theory and knowledge about the behavior of insti-
tutions (or large groups of people) rather than individual is,
in my opinion, pretty thin. For this reason, I remain skeptical
about our ability to design experiments which seek to estimate
responses of institutions to changes in policy. Sometimes "saturation" experiments, in which an entire neighborhood, city or
region is subjected to the "treatment", have been suggested to
estimate institutional or large group responses. Having joined
in several attempts to design such experiments, I am convinced
that a number of the very difficult problems which they present
remain unresolved. For similar reasons, I remain quite skeptical
about experiments where a few villages are matched and randomly
assigned, such as are described by Cook and McAnany in their fourth
point.

Limited Duration of Experiments

      One of the problems of experiments which has received the most
discussion concerns the limited duration of experiments and the
effect this has on the behavioral responses. Many decisions are
based on expectations of future patterns, (e.g., anticipated income
or expected rises in prices). How far people look into the future
when making a given decision is sometimes referred to as the time
horizon for that decision. The time horizon for buying an orange
is short; the time horizon for buying a house is long. If the time
horizon for decisions by individuals extends beyond the period en-
visioned for the experiment, it is likely that behavior will be
different under a limited duration experiment than it would be
under a continuing government policy. This topic has received some
specific technical attention by Metcalf and others (4). In addition, the design of several of the experiments has been shaped to
try to provide some insight on this issue. Most of the experimental group in the Denver and Seattle sites for the Income Maintenance Experiments will participate in the program for three years,
but part will continue on for five years, and a small sample will
be enrolled in an experiment that is to continue for twenty years.
The Health Insurance Experiment also has a five-year as well as a

three-year sample. Information from these experiments should at
least help to make clear how important this time horizon issue is
with regard to labor force and medical services decisions. The
extent to which these results will carry over to other behavioral
responses, of course, will have to be judged when these results
are available.

Legal Constraints

As we know from the recently issued Department of Health,
Education and Welfare regulations with regard to experimentation
on human subjects, there are legal constraints on experimentation
that must be observed. The issue of privacy and confidentiality
of data has come increasingly into the public discussion, and it
has received considerable attention from both a technical and legal
standpoint. 3/ As the number of experiments grows, the resistance
of potential subjects to enrollment in experiments and the willingness of researchers to carry them out may become increasingly
limited unless there is some clarification of the legal protection
of research data.

Since random assignment is at the center of controlled experimentation, there are some legal questions concerning the ability of governmental agencies to make available services on a random
basis for the purposes of experimentation. Thus far, the United
States courts appear to have sustained this privilege but, as I
understand it, the legal basis is not very solid and may be subject
to further challenge. The other side of the issue of randomly
assigning people to no treatment is, of course, the possibility of
compulsory participation in experiments.

Random Assignments and Controls

Aside from the legal issue regarding random assignment there
are some more practical operational issues concerning random assignment which may limit the applicability of controlled experiments
to policy questions. Random assignment is central in the experimental paradigm, but the ability of operators to actually maintain
the integrity of the random assignment process has sometimes been
open to question.

When the designers of the program and the operators are separated and the operators often have little appreciation of, or

_____

3/ Technical aspects of the confidentiality issue have been described in Boruch and Cecil (5).

tolerance for, research objectives, the palatability of a random
assignment procedure can be quite low. Rational arguments about
limited budgets and availability of positions in the treatment
program are of no avail in many cases. To many people, there is
something inherently repugnant about the random assignment process.
For example, in a major national experiment now in the middle stage,
involving a special employment program for ex-addicts and ex-
offenders, there was considerable complaint by operators of the
programs about hardships caused by random assignment. Only the
strongest insistence by the central funding agency allowed the
operator resistance to be overcome and random assignment completed.
In a similar smaller scale employment project run by the Vera
Institute, operators resented random assignment and managed to
partially subvert the creation of a control group.

In the large-scale social experiments to date, subversion of
randomization does not appear to have been a great problem. In
fact, the experience of the New Jersey Income Maintenance Experiment showed that the participants seemed to accept the idea that
assignment to treatment or control was like a lottery, preferring
it to the usual selection process which is related to some special
characteristic or knowing the right people. Undoubtedly, the ability to maintain the integrity of random assignment is related both
to the organizational structure and to the specific character of
the treatment.

Interference from Existing Programs

One lesson that emerged quite clearly from the experience of
the New Jersey Income Maintenance Experiment is that closely related programs operating in the context in which the experiment
is carried out can make it very difficult to control the treatments -- to know exactly what they are -- and therefore to carry
out the analysis. In New Jersey the creation of a welfare program
for male-headed families with benefits at a generous level, and
its eventual cutback a few years later, meant that the program with
which the Income Maintenance Experiment was, in effect, competing,
actually changed rather sharply through time. This makes it exceedingly difficult to tell what participants perceived as the net
gain to them from the experimental benefits, and thus difficult to
be very precise about the character of the experimental and control
conditions.

Similar problems arise with regard to the Health Insurance
Experiment, since many subjects already had available to them some
form of health insurance. An ingenious scheme was devised in this
instance to permit the experimental tests that were of interest
and, as I understand it, the experience to date with that scheme

seems to be fairly promising. (Essentially it is a matter of buying the people out of their existing health insurance program.) However, there remain the problems of whether, for example, in the case of the Health Insurance Experiment, people may not undermine the experimental treatment by buying additional special insurance to cover the deductions and co-insurance to which they are subject under the experimental treatment. In general, insuring that the integrity of the experimental treatment will be maintained and not interfered with by other programs is a problem that requires careful attention in every experiment.

Vulnerability to Special Local Events or to Changes Over Time

Closely related to the previous point is the possibility that in a given locality for an experiment, special events may occur that interfere with experimental treatment or interact with it in ways that are difficult to analyze. The already cited example of changes in welfare laws in New Jersey is one type of case. Changes in the labor-market conditions constitute another. In the Seattle Income Maintenance Experiment, changes in the level of employment in the aircraft industry had a great effect on employment opportunities of those in the experiment and may have swamped any experimental-control differences in labor-market behavior. In the Gary Income Maintenance Project, employment experience of the participants was also dominated by conditions in a single industry -- the steel mills.

Any experiment where the response is liable to be affected by external conditions that change over time is going to present problems for analysts. If, for example, the labor-supply response to income-maintenance programs is quite different when there is a recession than when there is an expansion, then one's ability to generalize from a given experiment may be limited. The existence of a control group always allows one to make inferences about pure effects of the treatment but they do not insulate one from conditions which affect both treatments and controls over time.

Inability to Capture Secondary Effects

One of the most frequent complaints of economists about experiments is that they do not permit estimates of secondary effects of the treatment transmitted through other markets and institutions. These effects may in some cases be substantial. For example, the income maintenance treatment caused changes both in the hours worked by low income workers and in their consumption patterns. These changes could in turn affect the price of goods produced by low-wage workers, the price and demand for goods consumed and,

thereby, have secondary effects on employment elsewhere. These
effects are often referred to as general equilibrium effects. 4/

LIMITATIONS OF NON-EXPERIMENTAL STUDIES

The idea of using non-experimental data to estimate likely
behavioral responses to policy is quite an old one. It is based
on the observation that the variability of institutional arrangements and social practices in society yield certain "natural experiments". One can try to use the existence of such variations
as a proxy for variation in policy parameters. To the extent these
proxies are adequate, one can try to draw inferences about the likely behavioral responses to proposed policy variations. A large
part of the training of economists has been devoted to developing
skills that use existing data to make inferences in just such a
fashion. Fortunately, there are now some very good discussions of
the usefulness of such non-experimental data which point out
limitations and contrast their usefulness with controlled experiments. 5/ Given these excellent detailed commentaries I will only
discuss a few of these limitations of non-experimental data to give
a flavor of the kinds of considerations.

Selection Bias

The most serious limitation of non-experimental data is the
possibility of selection bias. The problem arises from the fact
that, in a given population the treatment variable may be correlated
with some unmeasured variable which affects the behavior of interest. For example, in the case of health insurance, within the
United States, there obviously are differences in the characteristics of private health insurance which is available. It would
appear on the surface that these differences provide a good natural
experiment to study the effects of health insurance parameters on
the demand for health services. However, even if the problems of
gathering and coordinating such data could be overcome, there is
the underlying problem of adverse selection. It must be assumed
that people who buy health insurance have a better knowledge of
their likelihood of incurring large medical expenses than do the
companies who issue the policies. Therefore, those people who are

---

4/   See Golladay and Haveman (6) for an attempt to use simulation
models to trace such secondary effects.

5/   See Greenberg (7) and Cain and Watts (8) for a discussion in
context of labor supply response to income maintenance programs.

most likely to have high medical expenses will tend to buy those
policies which have the lowest co-insurance or co-payment requirements. There is adverse selection of risks; people who expect to
have high medical bills will select policies which require them to
pay a lower proportion of the total bill out of their pocket. If
adverse selection is extensive, then analysis of these data might
lead one to conclude that lower co-insurance or co-payment rate
leads to a higher use of medical services, but this would be an
incorrect inference. It is the result of the selection among existing policies and not a response to a change in the co-insurance
rate which leads to the correlation.

A sensitivity to the potential of selection bias is important,
but this sensitivity can be overdone. Some people with a distaste
for non-experimental studies tend to see selection bias everywhere
-- even in cases where there is no good reason to suspect it is a
problem. The controversy over this issue, however, has at least
made everyone aware that getting good information on how participants in a program are selected can be quite important and can
considerably enhance the usefulness of non-experimental program
data. Problems created by the absence of randomization can be
significantly reduced to the extent that good information is available on the procedures used for selection of participants in the
given program. Essentially, with good information on selection
processes, statistical techniques can be used to remove the biases
introduced by selection. These important points are explained
clearly by Cain (2).

Simultaneity Problems

In non-experimental data, the direction of causality often may
be open to question. Suppose we are interested in whether changing
the work opportunity of women is likely to encourage or discourage
marital breakup. If we look at non-experimental data and find unmarried women work more, we might conclude that improved work opportunities would increase family breakup. But, of course, the
causation may go the other way, or more likely, the decision about
how much the woman is willing to work and whether to change marital
status are simultaneously determined. Unless this simultaneity is
carefully untangled in estimating the likely response to improved
employment opportunity, seriously biased estimates may result.
Econometricians have gone a long way in trying to develop methods
for estimating the independent effects of variables within a simultaneous system. These methods have been used to provide a number
of policy relevant findings. However, anyone who has used these
methods realizes that there are many circumstances in which they
simply cannot overcome the confounding effects which exist in a
particular set of available data.

Selection bias and simultaneity problems are the major limitations of non-experimental data. The other limitations listed in
Table V are more technical in character and they would require much
more detailed explanation than there is space here.

Other Considerations

One other dimension in which experimental and non-experimental
methods are contrasted -- and which is mentioned by Cook and
McAnany -- is that of relative costs. It is apparent that to the
extent that survey data or archival data sources exist and provide
opportunity for analysis, the costs of estimating behavioral responses may be considerably lower than for an experiment and that
the results will be obtainable with greater speed. (Although here
experience should teach us that this is not always the case since
problems of data cleaning and data processing often are substantial).
In many cases, however, the choice is between an experiment and a
new non-experimental data collection effort. On the surface it
appears that the non-experimental data collection effort would be
both less expensive and faster than an experiment. But again,
experience in the United States has suggested that the cost and
speed advantages of the non-experimental method may be over-
estimated.

In closing this section I want to again emphasize that what
we need are not more conflicts over which is the appropriate method,
but rather a set of guidelines for timing and integration of both
methods. Certainly the experience in the United States has indicated that broad-based population surveys have tremendous value
as context for more detailed evaluations of programs, for generalizing the results of such evaluations and, in some cases, acting
as non-experimental substitutes for program evaluations. Thus,
over the last ten years, we have developed an impressive array of
annual cross-section population surveys and a number of large longitudinal studies of representative samples of the population. The
payoff in terms of policy insights from these surveys has been
phenomenal. It is important to realize that for certain questions
there are simply no substitutes for use of an experimental method
and experimental designs can give us more efficient estimates of
behavioral response. But the United States experience has shown
us that there can be many pitfalls in carrying out an experiment
and that there have been some rather serious misuses of substantial
resources to carry out experiments seemingly for the sake of experimentation or because it was the research style of the moment.
Once again, it seems to me that the most important question is to
develop research strategies which enhance the complementarity of
these methods.

DESIGN ISSUES

Basic Requirements of a Research Sample

An important lesson from United States experience is that the design of the research sample is of crucial importance. In my view, Cook and McAnany fail to stress this sufficiently.

First, it is useful to review the basic ingredients required for sample design. They are:

a.   The magnitude of the expected response to the treatment.

We need to know how big an effect we can expect in order to assure we will have a sample size with sufficent power to detect it.

b.   The degree of accuracy required (the confidence level).

We must decide what degree of uncertainty concerning any point estimate of effect we are willing to tolerate.

c.   The normal variance of the behavioral response variable (or more precisely, its residual variance, or error variance, after controlling for other measured characteristics).

This is a key measure of the amount of "noise" in the behavior which will make it difficult to detect the response to the treatment. The more "noise", the larger the sample size must be.

The degree to which some of these ingredients have been inadequately explored and specified in the design state of evaluation studies is rather distressing. In many cases the sample size has turned out to be too small to have a reasonable probability of detecting the level of response anticipated to be relevant to policy decision-making. In a few cases, the sample size has undoubtedly been larger than necessary and as a result resources have been wasted which could have been used to improve the quality of the data collection or analysis. I have already noted that the Housing Allowance Supply Study used guesses at the variance in supply when determining sample size and no one has any idea whether it will prove adequate to detect policy relevant responses.

There has been considerable progress in the last five years in developing techniques for relating the sample size decision to the relevant policy decisions so as to assure that the statistical

power of the sample is adequate for the policy issue posed (9).
Analysts have also developed sophisticated models for allocating
sample across treatments so as to maximize the information obtained
for a given cost (10).

While the theory for sequential experimental designs is well
developed and, I understand, applied in marketing and medical experiments, it has not been rigorously applied to social experiments.
Utilization of these designs probably should be encouraged.

Finally, with regard to design, the income maintenance experiments have shown the great value of long observation of subjects in the baseline period prior to entry into the program or
experiment. Such observations contribute greatly to reducing the
individual component of the overall behavioral variance and are
useful in avoiding the endogeneity problem in differentiating
responses among experimentals.

Non-Experimental Studies

It should be noted that all these sample design considerations *apply with equal force to non-experimental studies* which
involve creation of samples, even where sampling from existing
records. Very few non-experimental evaluations in the United
States in the 1960's were based upon carefully designed samples.

Secondary Data Gathering

In addition, the sample design criteria can and should be
applied to areas of investigation which are secondary in evaluation studies. In large studies there is a strong tendency to load
up the data collection instruments with supplementary questions
dealing with secondary hypotheses. For example, in the income
maintenance experiments we had numbers of questions on political
perceptions, organizational participation, etc. These were not
subject to the same design criteria as the central evaluation
hypotheses; yet they can impose great costs in terms of data collection, processing and analysis. The New Jersey Income Maintenance Experiment had a sample size of about 1,300 families.

In an ex-post study of some of the secondary hypotheses we
found several variables for which a sample size of 1,000,000 would
have been necessary to detect a reasonable response because the
variance in the variable was so large relative to expected response.

Specification of Treatment

Another important aspect of the design phase for an experiment which has sometimes been inadequately explored is the specification of the treatment. In particular, even the simplest treatments will be multidimensional and it will be impossible to experimentally vary and evaluate all the dimensions. Therefore, it is usually necessary to specifiy certain of the dimensions in a non-experimental fashion. In the income maintenance experiments these dimensions were called "rules of operation" and they dealt with such issues as: how income is defined; over what period is income averaged; how is the family unit defined; how often are payments determined and paid, etc.

In the design phase it began to become clear that these rules could produce a number of significant incentive effects. Defining these rules is important to assure that all contingencies are adequately anticipated and dealt with consistently. In addition, the analysis which goes into rule definition can anticipate many of the problems which those designing the eventual legislation creating such a program would have to deal with. In some ways, lessons learned from rule definition may have had greater impact on the structure of income maintenance programs in the United States than the central experimental findings.

Awareness of such rules is also important in trying to compare results of evaluations among different projects. For example, the various income maintenance experiments appeared to show rather different effects on family stability, but closer examination indicated that much of the difference was probably due to different family unit rules.

ORGANIZATIONAL ISSUES

In their discussion of organization factors conducive to bias, Cook and McAnany suggest the ideal situation is for the evaluator to be independent organizationally and financially from the program operators. These organizational issues are quite important and there have been a wide variety of configurations used in United States evaluations. But there are few systematic attempts to examine the effects of different organizational relationships on the quality of evaluation. For this reason, I think any generalization is hazardous and I would urge future evaluators to review some of the United States experiences in order to make their own judgments. I would like to make just a few observations which run somewhat counter to those of Cook and McAnany.

When to Initiate Evaluations

Cook and McAnany suggest evaluation should be undertaken only after the initial development phase when a program is likely to be implemented on a wider scale. This appears sensible but ignores the fact that it will be much harder to initiate an evaluation at this stage. Program operators are confident and set in their ways at this stage and, therefore, more likely and able to resist the interventions which are required for systematic evaluation. The framework for evaluation is best set up at the outset. Data can then be collected both at the development phase and in the mature stage. The evaluation may serve formative functions at the development stage and switch to summative at the later stage.

Randomization

Some further points on organizational aspects of randomization might be considered. The Supported Work Experiment turned up a major cost consideration in choosing the point at which randomization occurs. Subjects can come to a program through various referral filter mechanisms. The further back in the eligibility filter process the randomization occurs the greater the ability to generalize to the population universe but the greater the costs in following up ineligibles and dropouts. All ineligibles and dropouts *must* be followed or the resultant analysis may be seriously biased. It is hard to get funding agencies to accept the idea that for the evaluation it is important to spend significant resources in following ineligibles or early dropouts. Thus, a trade-off of costs and generalizability arises and must be dealt with.

In the Supported Work Experiment the sample accumulated over a period of three years. This created another set of randomization problems, for one must take steps to assure that controls from an early period are not recycled through the randomization process by operators hoping to get a second chance to get "desirable" subjects into the experimental group.

A strong organizational commitment by those with budget control is essential if randomization is to be maintained. Operator distrust of randomization is deep. I rather think that at base it is the explicit sense of loss of control in randomization which offends program operators. When you tell them there is nothing they can do to affect the odds, they balk, even though you make clear that those odds may be better than those they face with limited resources and other programs. Somehow, the perception that one may be able to "work with the angles" may be important to them.

Independence of the Evaluation Team

In an attempt to get unbiased evaluations, some people have gone so far as to suggest one team should gather the data and another independent group should evaluate. My experience leads me to believe this is completely unfeasible. A major problem in evaluations which are complex and take a long time is to maintain the morale of the research team. There is an awful lot of dirty work in the data collection effort. Yet if the data are to be of reasonable quality, these efforts must be closely directed by those with a thorough understanding of the analytic methods which will be applied to the data. One can only get that quality input in the dirty work by assuring the researchers that they will get the pay-off by being able to have first crack at the analysis.

Instrument Development and Data Processing

There are two other miscellaneous topics which deserve at least some mention. These are instrument development and data processing. Development of data collection instruments is an important, difficult, irritating, conflict-generating process. Evaluators should make greater efforts to capitalize on development work carried out in previous projects. In projects with repeat interviews it is tempting to alter questions to improve them. This is admirable but often creates terrible problems and associated costs in the data processing and analysis stages. More effort to thoroughly develop research instruments *before* the start of the evaluation process can have great long-term benefits.

Data processing problems have been the source of massive cost overruns and substantial delays in reporting results in every major evaluation -- experimental or non-experimental -- of which I am aware. I know of no simple rules for avoiding these problems, since I know of no case in which they have been avoided. I can suggest only a few tentative ideas -- and these I offer without much hope. In particular, on major projects, avoid data processing innovations. Every programmer has a radical new procedure to suggest which promises great advances on past systems. But data collection projects are not the place to introduce such innovations because any error in implementation generates big costs and delays. Try to force the data processors to use an established system of known capability. Each of the income maintenance experiments created their own unique data processing system and with it their own unique set of problems. There is plenty of relevant United States experience on how not to do it.

REFERENCES

1. Watts, H., D. Rees, D. Kershaw,and J. Fair. *New Jersey Income Maintenance Experiments,* Vol. I-III, New York: Academic Press, 1976-1977.

2. Cain, G. G. Regression and selection models to improve non-experimental comparisons. In: C. Bennet and A. Lumsdaine,(eds.). *Evaluation and Experiment: Some Critical Issues in Assessing Social Programs.* New York: Academic Press, 1975.

3. Hollister, R. G, and C. Metcalf. Family labor-supply responses of young adults in experimental families. In: H. Watts and A. Rees, (eds.). *The New Jersey Income-Maintenance Experiment.* New York: Academic Press, 1977.

4. Metcalf, C. Making inferences from controlled income maintenance experiments. *Am. Econ. Rev.,* 63(3):478-483, 1973.

5. Boruch, R. F.,and J. S. Cecil. *Assuring Privacy and Confidentiality in Social Research.* Philadelphia: University of Pennsylvania Press. (In press), 1979.

6. Golladay, F.,and R. Haveman. Regional and distributional effects of a negative income tax. *Am. Econ. Rev.,* 66: 629-641, 1976.

7. Greenberg, D. *Problems of Model Specification and Measurement: The Labor Supply.* Santa Monica: Rand Corporation, 1972.

8. Cain, G. G.,and H. Watts. *Income Maintenance and Labor Supply.* Chicago: Markham, 1973.

9. Conlisk, J. Choice of sample size in evaluating manpower programs: A comment. In: F. Bloch,(ed.). *Evaluating Manpower Training.* Greenwich, Connecticut: Johnson Associates, Inc. (In press), 1978.

10. Conlisk, J. and H. Watts. A model for optimizing experimental designs. *American Statistical Association - Proceedings of the Social Statistics Section,* pp. 150-156, 1969.

SPECIAL ISSUES FOR THE MEASUREMENT OF PROGRAM IMPACT IN DEVELOPING COUNTRIES

John W. Townsend
W. Timothy Farrell
Robert E. Klein
    Institute of Nutrition of Central America
    and Panama
    Guatemala City, Guatemala

The application of evaluation techniques in developing countries has expanded rapidly in recent years, although the absolute number of programs of social and economic development which explicitly contain evaluation components remains relatively small. Examples range from the evaluation of small non-formal education projects in rural Guatemala to wide ranging regional development programs in Brazil. Governments are not only concerned with assessing the benefits of long espoused development strategies (e.g., land reform or technical assistance) but also in improving methods for implementing existing as well as experimental projects (e.g., rural health care, community participation in development planning, etc.).

Undoubtedly this recent rapid expansion of evaluation research is due in part to the fact that funding agencies increasingly insist that the programs they support contain evaluation components. In addition, the present generation of politicians and program managers is generally more sophisticated and better trained than its predecessors, and more alert to the potential uses and benefits of program evaluation. They view evaluation as an integral part of the policy process, providing information to improve their decision making and planning capabilities. By employing evaluation in social programs, they are not only determining what are reasonable policies on paper but discovering the means for converting these policies into viable field operations and testing their program effects.

In our discussion of evaluation research, we employ three

terms which are widely used in the field (1). *Process Evaluation*
refers to the extent to which the program was implemented according
to its original design and stated guidelines. For example, did the
target group or groups receive the intervention as originally planned, and to the specified degree? Process evaluation is the prior
step to *Impact Evaluation*, or the measurement of the extent to which
the program or intervention resulted in a change in the situation
which the program was designed to produce. *Comprehensive Evaluation*
refers to studies which contain both process and impact evaluation
components.

In the succeeding sections of this paper we focus primarily on
some of the operational, technical, and ethical issues which are
important considerations in evaluation in developing countries.
Finally, we discuss some of the special opportunities and needs in
evaluation research in those countries.

STRATEGIC PROBLEMS ASSOCIATED WITH PROGRAM
IMPLEMENTATION IN DEVELOPING COUNTRIES

Two particular strategic problems stand out with respect to
program implementation in developing countries: timing of the intervention and the shortfall between plans and actual operations.
These implementation problems must be addressed in all projects regardless of their scope. What makes this particularly acute is that
social scientists have commonly limited their involvement in social
program evaluation to issues of experimental design and outcome
measures. [Recent exceptions in the United States include the Health
Insurance Experiment (2) and the Graduated Work Incentive Experiment (3)].

Recently some evaluation researchers (4) have argued the need
for a closer investigation of the process of program implementation.
Frequently, the implementation of intervention projects must be
planned according to the yearly cycle of the program participants.
This is particularly true in terms of expenditures, income, and
climatic conditions among rural populations in developing countries,
since these factors may fluctuate widely during the year. Funds
and foods are most available at the household level during and
shortly after harvest periods. If new material items or practices
come to the attention of villagers during this period, program recipients are more likely to invest money and time in the product or
service than when the post-harvest resources are nearly exhausted
and future expenditure decisions must await new harvest yields.
In addition, small farmers are much busier during some periods of
the year than at others and can undertake projects much more successfully during periods when they have more time available. Projects that are initiated too late in the agricultural cycle may

never be completed and may prejudice the recipients against attempting other projects in the future (5). Weather cycles may also affect the success of projects. For example, on-the-job training programs may be poorly attended during the rainy season due to difficult travel conditions and the increase of gastrointestinal and respiratory illnesses suffered by the rural poor during this period.

Another aspect of the issue of timing relates to the implementation of large-scale programs. Often, when a major program (e.g., an agricultural extension program) is introduced at the national or regional level, no appropriate comparison group is available. Time series analyses may be of some assistance in interpreting the results but only if two implementation conditions are met. First, the new program must be introduced abruptly, since a gradually implemented program may produce changes that often cannot be distinguished at the national level from long-term secular trends. It is only the relatively abrupt and coincident change in agricultural production, home diets, and health and nutritional status of small farm families that can provide some confidence in the causal inference that extension activities lead to improvements along these dimensions of change.

In addition, to avoid subtle regression effects, the implementation of the national or regional program should not immediately follow a major drop in development indicators. A quickly introduced corrective measure in response to an acute problem, while administratively attractive, may be very difficult to distinguish from the ordinary return to the normal trend exhibited by unstable indicators (6).

The second general problem in program implementation in developing countries is the shortfall between the interventions as planned and as implemented. Where program implementation is hampered by resource limitations, communication and transportation problems, or other logistical problems that hinder the delivery of the intervention, extra attention must be paid to monitoring the actual delivery of the treatment   (i.e., process evaluation). The rural development literature is filled with examples of "phantom" interventions (e.g., training classes not given, literature not delivered, equipment lost or stolen, etc.). In a recent evaluation of a radio nutrition program in Nicaragua, investigators discovered that the two-minute radio spots they had contracted stations to play were not being aired. Further, this lack of compliance was directly related to the power, technological sophistication, and location of the radio transmitter. Small rural stations simply did not comply with intervention plans (7).

It is obvious that for all types of evaluation it is imperative that the investigator be able to determine if interventions were

implemented as planned. Although interventions in developing countries are frequently relatively weak compared to the magnitude of
the problems, evaluations which focus on the strength and the timing
of the intervention may provide an important test of the policy
alternatives. Whenever the distribution, magnitude and timing of the
implemented intervention are crucial, the evaluation should include
a series of process measures. If variation in implementation is
independent of participant characteristics, valuable evidence on
the sensitivity of the intervention to variations in delivery may
result. For example, in projects that require community participation it is useful to know which local channels of influence are
more effective in spreading information and approval than others.
In one health project in India, workers were frustrated in implementing a vaccination plan until the community's religious leaders
provided their consent. Moreover, this type of information may
provide evidence for simple operational improvements rather than
basic policy changes.

   Another strategic problem often associated with evaluation
efforts is the differential attrition rates of program participants.
These differentials often occur between the intervention and control
groups due to differences in motivation or ability to continue in
the study (8) but also may be a direct result of the intervention
itself. The first type of attrition problem generally relates to
losses in the control group. For example, it may be easy to imagine
higher emigration rates due to rapid population increases and subsequent lack of land availablility and employment opportunities in
communities serving as controls for rural development programs.
Control families may move either because development benefits are
simply not available in their community or because access to benefits
not associated with a development program is limited. Although
having more subjects in control conditions may be relatively easy
as their participation is usually less costly, having larger control
groups will not generally solve the attrition problem because it is
the equivalence of groups during the experiment that strengthens
the control. If differential attrition results from differences
related to individual propensities to migrate from study sites, the
problem of attrition may also be viewed as a type of self-selection
and further threaten the generalizability of results.

   When the attrition is a result of the intervention itself the
situation becomes more complex. One result of most development projects is the introduction of novel ideas, marketable skills, and
problem solving strategies. This development of individual capacities along with the pull of urban life (e.g., economic gain, improved schools and medical facilities and higher standards of living)
may contribute to a "brain drain" from small rural communities. In
other words, those most likely to accept the innovations, those most
active in the change process also may be those most likely to leave.

In this case attrition takes on the character of a dependent variable. Follow-up of emigrants may be one solution but this also may pose problems. The major obstacle is the difficulty of locating people, particularly those from disadvantaged populations who may have highly mobile patterns of living. Biases due to attrition may be severe, since those emigrants who are easiest to locate are likely to appear more successful, both because of their apparent social stability and because those who have failed in the urban environment may be less cooperative in revealing their current status.

There are certainly no easy solutions to the attrition problem although a number have been proposed (6, 8, 9, 10), including paying for cooperation in interventions, making sure there are net gains to both intervention and control community, and improving the demand for labor within small towns to reduce emigration. Essentially, this means comparing two active treatments instead of comparing one treatment with a control. The most important point with respect to attrition is that comparability between intervention and control groups is ultimately more important than maintaining the absolute size of either group.

Still another technical obstacle to the development of evaluation capacity is the quality of data processing facilities available. The type of multivariate analytic problems evaluation researchers are faced with, and the pressures from program planners for quick feedback, require access to the latest in computer technology. However, severe limitations of trained programming personnel, availability of computer facilities, and availability of adequate software frequently force evaluation researchers to use data processing facilities outside the host country. Although often necessary, this may have unfortunate consequences. The exportation of the data for analyses further enforces the dependency of the host country on outside resources. It also divorces the administrative and program staff from the data analytic activities and precludes training of host country nationals in data analysis techniques.

OPERATIONAL CONSIDERATIONS IN PLANNING
AND IMPLEMENTING EVALUATION

In evaluation projects in developing countries, several operational issues demand particular attention. These are the problems of sample selection, language, cultural appropriateness, the relations between program staff and evaluation staff and the financing of evaluation research programs. Of course, other considerations such as the shortfall between social theory, program planning and implementation exist and are also important, but in the growing area of social program evaluation in developing countries the issues cited above appear in greatest need of examination.

Sample Selection

Perhaps the most important single criterion for sample selection is the generalizability of the experimental results (11). If the results obtained cannot be extended to other persons and settings in which a similar social program might be applied, little of immediate importance can be learned from the intervention. Because the nature of evaluation research implies immediate policy consequences, the importance of the representativeness of the sample and generalizability of the results cannot be overemphasized. Individuals or groups selected for participation in program evaluations should not have characteristics that make them inappropriate for the treatment or unable to use it. Thus, for example, small farmers whose agricultural practices are restricted by the type of land tenure (rental or tenant) would be a poor choice for participation in an evaluation of a long term pasture improvement program. Because farmers without land tend to change plots every few years, their responses to the intervention would most likely differ from those of the proposed target population (i.e., small farmers with long term interests in specific plots of land).

This is not to say that extreme cases should be restricted from participating in "non-research" development projects. On the contrary, one secondary benefit of the sample selection process in developing countries is the identification of individuals in particular need of assistance from service agencies.

A second general consideration is that sample participants should not be selected solely on the basis of their willingness to cooperate, availability, or previous experience with development program operations. The limitation of generalizability from volunteer samples is commonly referred to as the selection by treatment interaction (12) and occurs when the volunteer sample is more susceptible to social change, more inclined to cooperate with community change programs, or more able to take advantage of opportunity than the average target population member. This problem, however, may be unavoidable when experimental programs involve relatively high risks for program participation, when participation in the intervention itself runs counter to traditional cultural norms. For example, reliance on volunteers may be necessary in an experimental agricultural marketing program among marginal farmers. The reluctance of most marginal farmers to abandon traditional marketing strategies may not be an indication that they are not interested in the potential economic benefits of the program, but merely that in their perception the consequences of failure are too serious. In geographical areas where agricultural yields are low and subject to the vagaries of pests and weather, intervention strategies seeking to maximize generalizability should minimize additional risk associated with participation.

Minimization of risk could take several forms. These range from implementing the program in small steps so that the risks associated with any single harvest are relatively small, to budgeting sufficiently to protect the income of collaborators should unbearably low yields result.

Another consideration is that some subgroups may value innovation and change positively. For example, communities which have had extended contact with extension agents and have experienced the benefits of technical innovations are more likely to continue experimentation. The fact that a technique is new can be sufficient reason to experiment and perhaps adopt it. On the other hand, for individuals in rural areas of developing countries, innovation and change *per se* have less positive appeal. If an individual is conditioned to view new things with skepticism and caution because of cultural norms, he is unlikely to be cooperative (13, 14). In such settings, the sole use of volunteer samples would most likely reduce the generalizability of program results.

A somewhat different aspect of the volunteer problem is encountered in projects where community decision-making is an integral part of the development paradigm. Here, the community's selection of the intervention becomes the essence of the project. The evaluation literature offers little guidance in this area as intervention studies have generally involved the differential administration of public services rather than the more dramatic structural change implied in self-determination.

Ultimately, the sample selection problem comes down to balancing the need for logistical feasibility and local willingness to cooperate (10). In any case, evaluation researchers in developing countries must take care to identify the socio-cultural characteristics of their samples, and when representativeness is compromised for expediency, they should inform potential users of the sample's restrictive features.

The Problem of Language

When the evaluation staff comes from outside the cultural group being studied, they face problems common to all cross-cultural investigations. Among the most critical are the evaluator's ignorance of/or insensitivity to language and dialect differences, as well as cultural relevance and appropriateness of process and outcome measures used to assess program effectiveness. In the following discussion of these issues, we will present illustrations of how they may impede research efforts, and suggest some strategies for how such problems can be overcome.

The communication issue is complex for it is intertwined with other major cross-cultural research problems, and spans both verbal and non-verbal communications. This section deals principally with verbal communication, although some of the more critical non-verbal factors are mentioned (15, 16).

The basic problem is the mesh of the communication patterns of the evaluation staff, program personnel and the target population. Fluency in the national language of a country is not necessarily sufficient. Even a native speaker of Spanish may be unable to speak Indian languages, for example, and even in Spanish, differences in social class and regional dialect may produce communication problems. An evaluator must be prepared to cope with different kinds of language problems in dealing with various significant groups.

Evaluation researcher, the government and the scientific community. Although many scientists and government officials in developing countries are fluent in a number of languages, an evaluator should be reasonably fluent in the national language of the country in which he will work. Not to do so not only lays an unreasonable communication burden on the personnel of the host country, but also, depending on the language of reporting, reduces the probability of utilization of the evaluation results.

Researcher and the program and evaluation staff. When extensive survey interviewing is necessary to evaluate a program it must be conducted by interviewers who speak the "field language", that is, the everyday speech of the target population. The supervisors of interviewers may have to be bilingual in order to bridge the language gap between interviewers and the higher level evaluation staff who may be ignorant of the "field language". Since clear communication of tasks, data collection procedures, etc., are essential, it may be incumbent upon the evaluation staff to acquire a working knowledge of the language in which program operations and evaluation interviews are carried out, especially if bilingual supervisory personnel are unavailable.

Evaluation researcher and the language of the community. The language of the program recipients is a complex and important factor. Communication problems at the level of the community may arise not only due to distinct language groups, but also due to distinct dialects, colloquialisms and local pronunciation. Even when program participants claim to speak the national language it may be at a level that makes meaningful interviewing impossible. For example, in one study related to the concept of willingness to delay gratification for material goods, questions required the use of the present and future subjunctive. In pretests it was discovered that this was not a well understood verb form. So great was the misunderstanding that several informants felt they had been cheated since the researcher did not deliver on his "promise" of three cows within one year's time. In this situation, it was clear that even though the informants spoke the national language they did so at a level which was not adequate for complex interviewing. In this case it was necessary for the researcher to learn the appropriate field language and the particular phrases necessary to obtain data on concepts of this nature.

Although ideal, we must ask how realistic it is that evaluation researchers be fluent in the national language and have at least a working knowledge of the field language. In a society with multiple cultures and language groups, the target research population may include several such cultural and linguistic groups. What compromises can be made that maximize the quality of the research product while minimizing the time consuming and expensive process of mastering a series of languages and dialects? Minimally, the researcher should be fluent in the national language and a completely bilingual evaluation staff be engaged where appropriate. In a setting where the evaluator is unfamiliar with the field language it may be necessary to obtain the service of a good translator to facilitate communication.

Since spoken and written language is not the only means of communication, a word must be added regarding non-verbal communication. While it cannot be reasonably expected that researchers become multicultural, the meanings of certain kinds of non-verbal behavior should be appreciated. Some of the most critical of such behaviors in Latin America, for example, are proximity, eye contact, and tactile contact. Among Indian populations of highland Guatemala a penetrating "look-me-straight-in-the-eye" and a firm "masculine" handshake are a good way to terminate an interview before it begins. Such behavior connotes a marked lack of respect.

Cultural Appropriateness of Evaluation Measures

No less important than the language problem is the issue of the cultural appropriateness of evaluation process and outcome measures. If, for example, we wish to consider tilled land ownership as an outcome variable of a development program, it is incumbent upon the researcher to determine, through ethnographic investigation, the various aspects of land ownership relevant to a particular environment. If traditional tenancy practices are incompatible with tilled land ownership (i.e., non-formal communal tenancy patterns), the concept may not be an appropriate indicator of development. For example, in many developing countries rural residents are quick to resent the acquisition by their neighbors of personal property, because their traditional rules of sharing and reciprocity lead them to think that no one can prosper without taking something away from his neighbor (17).   Similarly, if the incidence of urinary infection in pregnant women is one concern of a rural health program, but cultural rules regarding modesty proscribe drawing a random sample of pregnant women for the appropriate tests, such a health indicator may have to be abandoned or the sample modified to focus on hospitalized patients with other gynecological complaints.

Measurement operations must be relevant to the target population. If the question involves the acceptability of a new cereal grain hybrid, then the dimensions along which the grain is appraised must be culturally relevant, especially with respect to descriptive and evaluative domains (e.g., corn must not only be palatable but also must have properties suitable for making tortillas).

Assessment of the acceptability of most program interventions should be done employing culturally appropriate instruments that measure acceptability along indigenous semantic domains. For example, preferences may be elicited using such tools as the Semantic Differential Technique (18), modified Thematic Apperception Tests (19) or Multidimensional Scaling Techniques (20). Such measures have the advantage of being understood relatively easily by informants and of having the characteristics of games, thus reducing informant boredom and fatigue (21). An accompanying disadvantage of such measures in developing countries, however, is that they require considerable interviewer sophistication, rigid standardization, and considerable statistical analytic skills.

The development of culturally appropriate measures frequently requires some ethnographic research prior to the design of evaluation measures in order to build an operational framework that fits with cultural reality. Such a framework often will need to be sufficiently sensitive to reflect variability over a number of communities. In some cases this will require that changes be made in operational categories without changing conceptual domains. For example, house construction materials may be used to index relative wealth within a community (22, 23, 24). Although this may appear to be a good surrogate of wealth in some communities it may also suffer from a lack of generalizability, that is, a low cost material in one community, for example wood, might be a higher cost item in another. A critical issue, then, is the search for conceptual equivalents in studies employing several communities or regions.

This may be relatively easy for material items where there are some physical referents. However, the question of conceptual equivalence of measures in the area of attitudes and beliefs is frequently much more complicated. In parts of Latin America, for example, some set of foods, appropriate in the treatment of an

illness, may be designated as "hot" and this category may be mutually exclusive of another set designated as "cold". Neighboring
communities, however, may have some food items that transcend the
"hot-cold" distinction or other food groups that are not relevant
in the first community. Responses to questions on appropriate
treatment based on the assumption of categorical equivalents would
then bias a summary score across several communities. The need for
equivalent measures should be determined for each intervention and
control group.

Generally, where social development theory exists, such theory
tends to be cast in abstract terms that are too imprecise to suggest specific variables that should be measured. While collecting
information on all variables of potential interest is clearly impossible, it is advisable to include supplementary observations
that will allow evaluation of alternative hypotheses about program
effects. For example, a study to test the impact of a family planning program on birth intervals must take into account corresponding
changes in religious beliefs, adherence to postpartum sex taboos,
and temporary migration patterns of spouses.

Issues such as these pose pragmatic problems for evaluation
researchers and for operational agencies. They also demonstrate
how evaluation research costs are increased in studies where extensive work must be done to insure the validity equivalence of the
outcome measures.

Although in many cases a uniform measure may be applied successfully in a cross-cultural setting, it is methodologically dan-
gerous to assume uniform comprehension of these measures in target
populations without substantiating data. Obviously, the cost involved in verifying the appropriateness of the outcome measures
must be balanced with other program needs.

Relations Between Program Staff and Evaluation Staff

A second major issue in the implementation of evaluation research is the relationship between program and evaluation staff.
Several writers on evaluation (25, 26) have considered the role
difficulties encountered by evaluation staff in a program environment. In developing countries this problem appears on at least two
levels.

The first level concerns the potential bias of an investigator
who is called upon to evaluate a program with which he is closely
affiliated. Ideally, an evaluator should have some technical expertise in the project area, and a level of familiarity with program
staff that allows for unrestricted communication and a detailed

knowledge of the process of program implementation. In developing
countries where technical expertise is less readily available, where
systematic record keeping on operation is less likely to occur, and
where a thorough review of daily operations would be available only
to on-site program staff, the advantages of using an evaluator who
is part of the program staff seems apparent. Gordon and Morse (27),
however, argue that there are hazards in such a strategy. From a
small survey of published evaluation studies in the United States,
they found that in 58% of the studies on which the evaluator was
affiliated with the sponsoring agency, the program was judged successful as compared with a success rate of 14% reported by outside
evaluators. If this bias can be generalized to conditions in developing countries, the use of program affiliated evaluators might
lead to the perpetuation of ineffective social programs and the
waste of already limited resources.

A second hazard is that affiliated evaluators often become
involved in the success of a program to the extent that they no
longer believe that the program needs to be evaluated (28). Their
role often becomes that of a project record keeper who is expected
to document the activities of program staff (e.g., number of literacy classes taught, pounds of seed distributed, etc.).

The evaluator without program affiliation, on the other hand,
may be viewed as a threat to the service role and continued employment of program staff. Rigorous research procedures may appear
hostile to program goals as they call into question the efficacy
of the skills and convictions of program staff. Improving the
quality of evaluation research by employing better methodological
techniques may exacerbate this problem by increasing the likelihood
of qualified or negative findings regarding program effectiveness.
Furthermore, the commitment of the evaluator to operating the project as a controlled experiment (i.e., providing services to some
randomly selected groups and not to others, etc.) may seem, from a
value perspective, incompatible with the general service goals of
program staff, particularly if the resources of the sponsoring
agency appear abundant. The term "evaluation" may itself present
problems. In the world of public service, where appointments are of
relatively short duration, a high degree of insecurity may exist in
the absence of a professionalized civil service. Evaluation by an
outsider may increase such insecurity unless the term is understood
clearly.

Several strategies have been suggested for reducing the perceived threat and suspicion of outside evaluation without comprising
the effectiveness of the evaluation staff. One is to cast the program evaluation in a larger perspective of program development and
by offering suggestions for improving program performance (e.g.,
improving procedures for identifying families in need of service,

or for strengthening the intervention). This is compatible with both evaluation and program staff interests in providing the strongest possible treatment and is consistent with demands of experimental design if it involves no major program changes during the course of the evaluation period. Another strategy is to design the experiment so that as the program's ability to accommodate clients increases, more members of the randomized control group are periodically assigned to the intervention group (11). Such a strategy is consistent with program development goals and does not reduce the power of the evaluation to detect program effects if the control group is large enough and transfers are selected randomly. Reicken, et al, (10), recommend that program staff be reassured that they will not be held responsible for the size nor direction of the intervention effects. The purpose of the program is to determine if the intervention has an effect and is worth replicating elsewhere rather than to provide a service at the research site. For example, the function of an experimental integrated health program is not simply to provide health care in the study communities but to test if such an intervention has an impact which is generalizable to a larger population. Placing the actual threat of evaluation research in perspective, Cain and Hollister (29) note that most social action programs are so complex in the variety of inputs and multiplicity of objectives that judgment to abandon programs is unlikely.

Generally, the purpose of evaluation projects is to rearrange the composition of intervention activities and to suggest marginal changes in the total scale of the program. The use of counterparts from the action agency as participants in the evaluation research activity can be extremely helpful, both in improving the quality of the intervention as well as increasing the utility of the evaluation results. Regardless of the strategy employed, the concensus of most evaluators is that the trust and cooperation of program staff are indispensable to an appropriate evaluation of social programs.

A second level of concern with staff relations is the community's perception of the roles and activities of both evaluation and program staff. In developing countries a majority of programs of planned change are carried out through government agencies. The mere fact that a program is sponsored by the government may lead some individuals to be reluctant participants. A general suspicion of the motives of government-sponsored projects grows from the demands of taxation, military conscription, and political affiliations of government representatives. In rural areas of developing countries not only may program personnel be handicapped by the fact that they are likely to be government employees, but also by the fact that they are outsiders whose motives and skills are unknown. Development specialists, regardless of their organizational ties, are suspect upon entering a community and it may take some time for villagers to be convinced that they are genuinely interested in the welfare of the community. For example, in a rural health project in a traditional highland Guatemalan village, suspicion of outsiders was expressed in terms of excessive land prices for a proposed clinic site as well as repeated demands in the community organization stage of the project for immediate material proof of program goals (e.g., supplies of medicines and an ambulance).

Thus, a major problem of program staff is to establish their role as a visiting advisor and advocate in communities that have traditionally known few or no such roles (13). A related problem of the evaluation staff is to distinguish itself from the program staff without losing its rapport with the community. For example, the identification of evaluation staff with the action team may cause difficulties if community members are reluctant to express negative attitudes toward the project due to cultural demands of courtesy, or the fear that negative evaluation will contribute to project withdrawal rather than improvement. However, over time, the separate roles become understood if staff project themselves consistently, and the program continues despite community criticism.

Financing of Evaluation Programs

The cost of maintaining social programs is enormous and presents a major financial burden for developing countries operating on constrained budgets. One way of maximizing the effect of these limited funds in the development of services is to systematically compare alternative methods for accomplishing development goals. For example, policy makers might contrast the benefits of investment in nutrition projects versus agricultural extension services in terms of reduction in the incidence of malnutrition. Traditionally, evaluation research has not concerned itself with the relative effects of such policy alternatives within a single target population.

Because of the preoccupation with detecting differences between intervention and control groups, until recently the question of whether differences in outcomes are socially significant given cost considerations has not received much attention (30). For example, a massive nutrition supplementation program may significantly reduce clinical malnutrition in a target population but the cost of the supplement, its preparation, and distribution may rule out such program as a public health strategy. The lower the cost of obtaining any particular development objective, the greater will be the contribution of the program toward achieving the goals of poorly financed action agencies. Thus, prototypical social programs in developing countries should be designed either to minimize costs given the desired impact or to produce revenues to support their operation in the event of adoption through, for example, progres-

sive taxes on increased agricultural production (particularly those
with large, more efficient production units) or sales of processed
foods made possible by increased production.

The high cost of evaluation research is also an issue of
considerable importance. Perloff, Perloff and Sussna (31) take
exception to the common guideline that 1% of a program's funds
should be allocated for the evaluation of that program. They note
that while 1% may be satisfactory for a large-scale programmatic
research, to devote 1% of funding to projects of modest size (e.g.,
less than one million dollars) would in fact, provide less than
$10,000 for evaluation. Such a figure would hardly suffice for the
comprehensive evaluation of low cost interventions in developing
countries when such research demands multidisciplinary professional
staff with adequate administrative and technical support.

Rather than a fixed percentage they recommend an amount
negotiable between the program sponsor and the evaluation researcher
on the basis of how much money is reasonably needed to implement an
evaluation research design capable of rendering at least minimally
acceptable evaluation results. The policy-maker always faces the
dilemma of running certain risks if he chooses to develop evaluation evidence with insufficient funds, and thereby waste funds on
useless programs, or even worse, run the risk of producing invalid
results, continuing ineffective programs, or sponsoring other program failures (32).

Developing countries may be interested in techniques for reducing the relatively high cost of evaluation research although
each technique presents potential problems as well as offering
savings. First, evaluation efforts might be tied to an existing
or modified government program. This may reduce the initial cost
of developing a model intervention and also allows a test of the
effect of the intervention in an atmosphere comparable to potential
adoption sites. The compromises of such a strategy realistically
include the high probability of relying on *post hoc* research designs and the lack of control over the implementation of the intervention. For example, an evaluation of a government water project
in Guatemala was hampered by the lack of opportunity to collect
pretest data and the operational failure of the government to
provide materials for the maintenance of the water system.

A second potential cost-saving technique is the use of program
participants to collect their own data. This method not only frees
funds normally used for hiring evaluation staff but also involves
the program staff and community in the process of program development. This technique has been used in Panama on community nutrition program evaluations, in a rural health program in Guatemala
(33) and in USAID-sponsored rural development projects in Africa

and Latin America (34). In numerous nutritional surveillance projects, participants have collected information on indicators of
malnutrition, the utilization of community services, cropping patterns, etc. On the other hand, problems associated with use of
program staff and recipients to collect data include the potential
unreliability of measurement techniques and procedures and it adds an
element of uncertainty to the estimations of effects. The inherent
competition between service and data collection activities often
leaves evaluation concerns with a lower priority. In addition,
there may be conscious or unconscious bias in favor of program
success. In spite of these potential biases and problems, these
techniques can be usefully employed if careful controls and safeguards are built in to avoid the biases described above.

A third method for reducing the cost of evaluation research
in developing countries is to undertake more short-term exploratory
research, including literature reviews, archival research, and
detailed pilot testing of possible interventions prior to large
investments in rigorous long-term summative evaluation projects.
Scriven (35) recommends that given the relatively weak nature of
many program interventions perhaps a wise investment of evaluation
funds would be in the formative phase of social programs. While
this strategy may be helpful for program developers, it offers
policy decision-makers little substantive information on probable
program effects.

One alternative would be separate funding for the intervention
program and for its evaluation. It could be argued that since the
governments of developing countries would expend funds for public
programs anyway, funds needed for the evaluation of these programs
could be sought in the private sector or from international agencies.
Several arguments favor such an approach. First, because comprehensive evaluation research requires a major organization with a large
multidisciplinary staff and a high level of administrative organization, one could hardly expect each developing country to maintain this kind of costly research capacity on a permanent basis.
Additional support for the argument of multiple funding of evaluation is that careful scrutiny of evaluation plans by national
governments and technical experts before funds are committed would
generally improve the quality of evaluation, thus minimizing the
risk that invalid evaluation results will be used in policy-making
or that sound results will be generalized beyond legitimate limits.

A number of drawbacks to this proposal are evident, however.
First, a program agency that is unwilling to commit funds and staff
to evaluation is probably unlikely to commit itself to preserving
the research design once the project is in the field, or to acting
upon its results. Second, the existing value difference between
program personnel and evaluation staff could only be increased if

evaluation were seen as essentially a foreign-sponsored and directed activity. Third, few international organizations would be
willing to provide funds if concomitant guarantees were not made
to insure some control or supervision of program content and implementation (e.g., maintenance of potable water systems). Finally,
international or private funding sources from more developed countries may not be politically acceptable to governments in developing countries.

Obviously, an ideal solution to these problems does not exist.
Researchers and program personnel interested in the implementation
of social programs in developing countries must balance the demand
for intervention funds with the necessity of evaluation efforts
to determine if those programs are indeed cost effective.

The point to keep in mind about cost-saving techniques in
evaluation research is that the real savings will occur in future
program operations. The documentation of the impact of replicable
low cost interventions made possible through quality evaluation
methods may ultimately be the greatest cost-saving technique.

POLITICAL AND ETHICAL CONSIDERATIONS ASSOCIATED WITH
EVALUATION RESEARCH IN DEVELOPING COUNTRIES

It is obvious from a review of the published literature that
political and ethical problems in evaluation research in developing
countries are of major concern since they occupy almost equal printed
space with the more technical problems associated with design and
sampling. We will discuss each in turn.

Politics and Evaluation

Carol Weiss (36) maintains that evaluation is a rational enter-
prise that takes place in a political context and the evaluator who
fails to recognize this is in for a series of shocks and frustra-
tions. Weiss identifies three major areas in which politics intrudes on the evaluative process (or in which evaluation intrudes
on the political process). First, social action programs are the
products of political process. They already have their proponents
and antagonists, and in implementation they remain politically
vulnerable. Second, evaluation is a political issue since its
primary rational goal is to assist in decision-making. Evaluation
competes for attention with other factors in the political process.
Finally, evaluation in and of itself is a political posture. It
critically examines program goals and strategies, and legitimizes
the role of social researchers in policy and program formation (36).

These issues are exacerbated in evaluations where the researcher, for reasons of expertise or the need for nonaffiliation, is not
a citizen of the country where the development program is operating.
In his own country the evaluator is a citizen as well as a scientist.
He votes, pays taxes, joins interest and pressure groups, and has
the right to participate in the social action process. In contrast,
a foreign evaluator enjoys none of these rights. Yet, if we accept
Weiss and others' definitions (6, 26, 37), every evaluator is in
the thick of the social action political process. His role, like
it or not, is to produce information which will influence public
policy. Since evaluation results are oriented toward decision-
making, and since decision-making is a political and administrative
process governed by power and compromise, the role of the evaluation researcher is potentially very complicated. Here it is obvious that reasonably precise definition of the goals of the operational program play an important role. If expectations for program
impact are unreasonably high, the evaluation researcher may encounter serious difficulties. Caro notes that when administrative
claims for development programs are usually unreasonably optimistic,
evaluative research results are almost inevitably disappointing
(38). Weiss agrees that among the many reasons for the negative
pall on evaluation results is that evaluators have accepted bloated
promises and political rhetoric as authentic program goals (36).
Given the complex nature of underdevelopment, intervention programs
should have more modest expectations and they should be evaluated
against more reasonable goals. Tripodi claims that useful social
program information is obtained only when the socio-political
climate is conducive to honest inquiry and where there is a commitment to the utilization of evaluation as a management tool for expanding knowledge and making decisions (39).

Thus, the evaluation researcher must contend with multiple credibility problems: the credibility of his own expertise in community
development; the credibility of the Government's policy goals; and
finally, the credibility questions involving the organization and
activities of the action agency (26, 36, 40).

Additionally, the evaluation researcher as member of a larger
scientific community is usually concerned with the publication of
evaluation results. The question of who has the right to publish
the data -- the Government, the sponsoring agency, or the researcher -- is potentially very sensitive. What are the implications of
an evaluation researcher submitting data on the outcomes of social
program to the public forum through scientific publications? Such
information may be politically sensitive and even potentially embar-
rassing to the host Government.

Viewed in this context, it becomes the responsibility of the
evaluation researcher to clarify publication policies at the outset
of, and perhaps as a precondition to engaging in a particular eval-

uation effort. Tripodi suggests that data rights and publication policy be part of the evaluation contract, thus eliminating
misunderstanding from the outset (39).

Ethics and Evaluation

Development program interventions typically supply some social
or economic service. Sometimes these are provided in response to
needs for assessment in target communities as advocated in the anthropological social change literature (14, 17, 41, 42). Currently,
more often that not, interventions are the products of national
planning programs and are imposed on the community, often without
regard for local perception of needs. Beyond this, evaluators attempting to make the best of a difficult situation should insist on
the closest possible approximation of an experimental research design, including a well-defined treatment, control groups, and random selection of program participants, if possible.

In developing countries most social action programs are aimed
at the poorest socio-economic strata. This means that nearly everyone targeted for the intervention has a pressing need for the service the program will provide. The question then is, how can one
justify the withholding of such service from one group of individuals however defined?

In contrast to medical research, social intervention research
participants can generally easily distinguish between placebos and
the real treatment. The concern of "net gains" for all is genuine
but difficult to realize if the efficacy of a particular intervention is to be evaluated. In some cases an experiment may test two
or more particular modes of intervention in order to determine the
best possible result. In this case some gain may accrue to all
participants. However, experimentation on distinct program modes
is not frequently done and usually a decision is made to test one
or another mode of intervention. In this context, Freeman (43)
laments that political pressures often determine the interventions
adopted in social programs.

Another problem of ethics in evaluation research involves that
of the privacy of the program participants and the confidentiality
of evaluation data. The focus of many program evaluations is the
individual. He is asked to divulge aspects of his personal life
to unknown and often impersonal interviewers. Since one common
characteristic of the poor in developing countries is lack of education, it is often difficult, if not impossible, to explain the
safeguards of confidentiality involved in the computer processing
of aggregated data. Beyond this, depending on his experience with
previous Government agencies (e.g., the census and tax collectors),

the informant may have reason to be suspicious or distrustful of the researcher's vows of protection of informants.

Finally, the evaluation researcher must decide who is the client. Is the client the Government and its action agency, the subjects of the intervention, or the organization that provides funds for the evaluation? This crucial question returns us to the issue of politics discussed earlier. To whom is the evaluation researcher ultimately responsible?

Many of the questions and issues raised in this section of the paper have not been satisfactorily answered. Serious debate that includes representatives from all sectors affected by the evaluation research process is necessary in order to determine some concrete guidelines. Through continuing debate, use of the evaluative research methods can contribute to the success of social action programs in developing countries.

OPPORTUNITIES AND NEEDS IN EVALUATION RESEARCH IN DEVELOPING COUNTRIES

Despite the technical, operational, and ethical problems discussed earlier in this paper, there is broad agreement that evaluation research strategies can contribute importantly to development programs. These contributions are several and range from encouraging the careful specification of policy and program goals, to the improvement of intervention strategies through the information provided by process and impact measures of program activities and effects. The general salutary effects of an evaluation component in a program can be seen at all administrative levels in improved planning, systematic record keeping on program activities, and in the healthy, and constructively critical orientation toward the program evidenced by program personnel.

There are three general factors which presently limit the wider use of evaluation research techniques as a tool in development strategy. The first is the availability of trained personnel. Only during the past five years have programs begun to appear in North American universities which are specifically designed to train professional evaluation research specialists. Most of the formally trained evaluation research specialists are presently from developed countries and thus the availability of trained personnel for participating in evaluation research activities in developing countries is severely limited. The training and organizing of evaluation research personnel from developing countries is clearly an important prerequisite for the expansion of these activities in the context of optimal development programs.

A second factor limiting the wider use of evaluation research techniques in development programs is the relative lack of an understanding and appreciation of the uses and advantages of evaluation research strategies by politicians and senior administrative staff in developing countries. Although evaluation is expanding in developing countries, it has been applied principally in the micro-level investigations of agricultural innovations, family planning, and a limited number of health and nutritional interventions. The transfer and adoption of this technology to a wide range of non - agricultural programs has been slow.

Although there have been positive and important changes in recent years, there is still a need to inform decision-makers of the role of evaluation and to disseminate existing evaluation research results broadly in a context which will promote awareness of the program benefits which can be derived from the systematic use of evaluation research techniques.

A third factor obviously related to the first two is the need for improvement in design, methods, outcome measures and analytical techniques in evaluation research. Here progress will be made as more experience is gained in defining the special needs of development evaluation and as more competent researchers participate in the evaluation of various components of national development programs. Advances in these technical aspects, and particularly in the development and use of comparable or uniform outcome measures, will allow the results of distinct interventions and delivery systems to be compared in terms of their impact and relative cost. Eventually a coherent body of published literature will evolve, building on the experiences of large scale programs in developed countries but making the greatest contribution in explaining the methodological and operational concerns of smaller scale programs suitable to the needs of developing countries. This will allow program designers and managers to select development strategies and design programs on a more rational basis than is now the case.

As we indicated in the introduction of this paper, there is a growing awareness, interest, and use of evaluation research as an important tool in development strategy. This trend could be accelerated by the development of a coordinated research and training network in Latin America. Such network could initially be set up in universities and research centers in several Latin American countries.

The principal activities of these centers would be training in the design and execution of evaluation research activities. However, centers could also serve as clearing houses for new evaluation data, centers for secondary analysis of existing development evaluation data, and as referral sources for program administrators seeking evaluation consultation.

The activities of such a research and training network would, by their very nature, address themselves to the three major limiting factors to the wider use of evaluation research identified above, and in this fashion promote and expand the application of evaluation research activities in the general area of social and economic development.

ACKNOWLEDGEMENT

The preparation of this paper was supported in part by the Agency for International Development (AID), Washington, D.C., (Contract AID-TA-C/1224); The National Institute of Child Health and Human Development, (NIH), Bethesda, Maryland (Contract No. N01/DH-5-0640); and the Ford Foundation, New York (Grant No. PN-801).

The opinions expressed are those of the authors and do not necessarily reflect those of the sponsoring institutions nor The Pan American Health Organization.

REFERENCES

1.   Bernstein, I., and H. Freeman. *Academic and Entrepreneurial Research*. New York: Russell Sage Foundation, 1975.
2.   Newhouse, J.P. *A Summary of the Experimental Portion of the Rand Health Insurance Study*. (Rev. ed.) Santa Monica: Rand Corporation, 1977.
3.   Watts, H., and A. Rees (eds.). *Final Report on The Graduate Work Incentive Experiment in New Jersey and Pennsylvania*. Madison: University of Wisconsin, Institute for Research on Poverty, 1974.
4.   Freeman, H.E. The present status of evaluation research. In: *Proceeding of UNESCO Evaluation Research Conference*. Washington, D.C., 1976.
5.   Batten, T.R. *Communities and their Development: an Introductory Study with Special Reference to the Tropics*. London: Oxford University Press, 1957.
6.   Campbell, D. Reform as Experiments. In: E.L. Struening and M. Guttentag (eds.). *Handbook of Evaluation Research*. Beverly Hills: Sage Publications, Inc., 1975.
7.   Manoff, R.K., and T.M. Cooke. *Changing Nutrition and Health Behaviors through the Mass Media: Nicaragua and Philippines*. New York: Manoff International, Inc., 1976.
8.   Kershaw, D. Administrative issues in income maintenance experimentation: administering experiments. In: L.L. Orr, R.G. Hollister, M. Lefcowitz and K. Hester (eds.). *In-*

come Maintenance: Interdisciplinary Approaches to Research. Chicago: Marham, 1971.

9.   Campbell, D., and J. Stanley. *Experimental and Quasi-Experimental Designs for Research.* Chicago: Rand-McNally & Co., 1963.

10. Riecken, H.W., and R.F. Boruch. *Social Experimentation: a Method for Planning and Evaluating Social Intervention.* New York: Academic Press, 1974.

11. Boruch, R. Coupling randomized experiments and approximations to experiments in social program evaluation. In: I. N. Bernstein (ed.). *Validity Issues in Evaluative Research.* Beverly Hills: Sage Publications, Inc., 1975.

12. Bracht, G.H., and G.V. Glass. The external validity of experiments. *Am. Educ. Res. J.* 5: 437-474, 1968.

13. Foster, G.M. *Traditional Societies and Technological Change.* New York: Harper & Row, 1973.

14. Spicer, E.H. *Human Problems in Technological Change.* New York: John Wiley & Sons, 1952.

15. Harrison, R. P. Non-verbal communication. In: I. de S. Pool and W. Schram (eds.). *Handbook of Communication.* Chicago: Rand-McNally, 1973.

16. Hall, E.T. *The Hidden Dimension.* Garden City, New York: Doubleday, 1966.

17. Foster, G. M. *Traditional Cultures and the Impact of Technological Change.* New York: Harper & Row, 1962.

18. Osgood, C. Semantic differential techniques in the comparative study of cultures. In: A. K. Rommey and R. D'Andrade (eds.). Transcultural studies in cognition. *American Anthropologist 66: Specific Issue 2, 1964.*

19. Rommey, A.K., R. N. Shepard, and S. B. Nerlove (eds.). *Multidimensional Scaling. Theory and Applications in the Behavioral Sciences.* Vol. II. New York: Seminar Press, 1972.

20. Pelto, P. *Anthropological Research: the Structure of Inquiry.* New York: Harper & Row, 1970.

21. Belcher, J. C. A cross-cultural household level-of-living scale. *Rural Sociology* 37(2): 208-220, 1972.

22. Farrel, W.T. *Community Development and Individual Modernization in San Lucas Toliman, Guatemala.* Unpublished Ph.D. dissertation, University of California at Los Angeles, 1977.

23. Klein, R. E., M. Irwin, P. L. Engle, and C. Yarbrough. Malnutrition and mental development in rural Guatemala: an applied cross-cultural research study pp. 91-119. In: N. Warren (ed.). *Advances in Cross-Cultural Psychology.* New York: Academic Press, 1977.

24. Rodman, H., and R. Kolodny. Organizational strains in the researcher-practitioner relationship. In: F.G.Caro (ed.).

Readings in Evaluation Research. New York: Russell Sage
Foundation, 1971.

25. Suchman, E. A. *Evaluative Research*. New York: Russell Sage
Foundation, 1967.

26. Gordon, G., and E. V. Morse. Evaluation research. pp. 339-361.
In: *Annual Review of Sociology*. Vol. I. Palo Alto:
Annual Reviews Inc., 1975.

27. Weiss, R. A., and M. Rein. Paper read at the conference on
The Evaluation of Social Action Programs sponsored by
the American Academy of Arts and Sciences, Washington,
D.C., 1969.

28. Cain, G. G., and R. G. Hollister. The methodology of evaluating social action programs. In: P. H. Rossi and W. Williams (eds.). *Evaluating Social Programs*. New York:
Seminar Press, 1972.

29. Levin, H. M. Cost-effectiveness analysis in evaluation re-
search. In: M. Guttentag and E. L. Struening (eds.).
Handbook of Evaluation on Research. Beverly Hills: Sage
Publications, Inc., 1975.

30. Perloff, R., E. Perloff, and E. Sussna. Program evaluation
pp. 569-594. In: M.R. Rosenzweig and L.W. Porter (eds.).
Annual Review of Psychology. Vol. 27. Palo Alto: Annual
Reviews Inc., 1976.

31. Rossi, P. H., and W. Williams. *Evaluating Social Programs*.
New York: Seminar Press, 1972.

32. Beghin, I. Improving nutrition at the local level. *Carnets
de l'Enfance Assignment Children,* No. 35 (UNICEF), 1976.

33. Morse, E. R., J. K. Hatch, D. R. Mickelwait, and C. F. Sweet.
Strategies for Small Farmer Development. Boulder: West-
view Press, 1976.

34. Scriven, M. The methodology of evaluation. In: R. W. Tyler,
R. M. Gagre and M. Scriven (eds.). *Area Monograph Se-
ries on Curriculum Evaluation*. No. 1. Chicago: Rand-
McNally, 1967.

35. Weiss, C. H. Evaluation research in the political context.
In: E. L. Struening and M. Guttentag (eds.). *Handbook
of Evaluation Research*. Beverly Hills: Sage Publications, Inc., 1975.

36. Rossi, P. Evaluating educational programs. pp. 97-99. In:
F. G. Caro (ed.). *Readings in Evaluation Research*. New
York: Russell Sage Foundation, 1971.

37. Caro, F. G. Evaluation research; an overview. pp.1-34. In:
F. G. Caro (ed.). *Readings in Evaluation Research*. New
York: Russell Sage Foundation, 1971.

38. Tripodi, T., P. Fellin, and I. Epstein. *Social Program Evaluation*. Ithaca: Peacock Publishers, 1971.

39. Davis, H. E., and S. Salasin. The utilization of evaluation.
In: E. L. Struening and M. Guttentag (eds.). *Handbook*

of Evaluation Research. Beverly Hills: Sage Publications Inc., 1975.
40. Goodenough, W. H. *Cooperation in Change.* New York: Russell Sage Foundation, 1963.
41. Arensberg, C., and A. Niehoff. *Introducing Social Change.* Chicago: Aldine, 1971.
42. Freeman, H. E. Foreword. pp. ix-xi. In: F. G. Caro (ed.). *Readings in Evaluation Research.* New York: Russell Sage Foundation, 1971.

COMMENTS

Guillermo Herrera, *Harvard School of Public Health*
Boston, Massachusetts

In their final statement the authors suggest that the severe shortage of trained personnel and the limitations of available consultants and part-time advisors are the principal constraints on evaluations of development programs. Recognizing these limitations as important, I would like to suggest that other constraints described by the authors comprise more significant barriers to sound evaluation today.

First, some action programs are planned and executed in a political context, not conducive to objective scientific assessment of program process or evaluation of impact. As pointed out by others, unreasonably high goals publicized for political reasons defy fulfillment and turn evaluation into a formal documentation of failure too costly to tolerate.

Secondly, most evaluation efforts thus far have been *post hoc*, rather than a planned component of the program in question. There are consequent difficulties in data retrieval and quality assurance as well as in selecting appropriate control or comparison groups. Related to this is the problem of the evaluator without program affiliation who may be viewed as a threat by program staff and even by those who contracted his services.

Third, the selection of instruments to assess impact, as emphasized by the authors, still poses methodological problems. Frequently because of difficulties in record keeping and data management, nation-wide indicators of health, nutritional status, family income, etc., are often unavailable or inaccurate. Moreover, as the authors point out, in many instances, culturally congruent outcome measures do not exist and must be evolved, modified, and standardized as part of the evaluation. Cultural appropriateness requires sensitivity as well as intimate acquaintance with the local milieu, qualities seldom found among foreigners. An example of

culturally inappropriate outcome measures is the widespread use of
I.Q. tests as sole measures of cognitive competence among dwellers
of rural areas and urban slums. The members of such communities
have adapted to an environment which places categorically different
demands upon them from those encountered among the middle class of
industrialized countries where the tests were developed. In contrast the authors are currently pursuing development of measures
of competence based on assessment by village members and designed
to quantify ability to adapt to the local environment.

Fourth, technical and design difficulties become almost in-
surmountable when assessing impact of multidimensional program
activities if the latter continuously change during the process
of implementation, as they often do. To control for other variables that may explain effects on outcome would necessitate the
design of a strictly-controlled, randomized trial, a task impossible
to achieve retrospectively.

Many of these problems could be minimized by casting evaluation in the perspective of program development as suggested by
Townsend, Farrell, and Klein. In order to achieve this goal, continued education of program planners and administrators needs to
be emphasized. Given the multiple demands made on the time of
public sector planners and executives, effective means must be developed to provide them with the necessary perspective and technical information locally and in their native language. Also important will be the improvement of communication between persons
confronting similar problems in different countries. A closer
liaison between institutions of learning and government, regional
workshops and conferences may partially fulfill this need. Training in evaluation methodology should receive emphasis in the education of public health planners and administrators. The curricula
of public health schools and regional health and nutrition insti-
tutes should include evaluation as a component of their training
programs in planning and administration.

I would now like to discuss two points mentioned by the authors
which deserve special emphasis. First, the need to conduct detailed
process evaluation and measurement of intervening variables, even if
the goal is to assess overall impact. Such measurements will yield
insights not yet available on the needs, priorities, and responses
to intervention among populations struggling under multiple material
and social deprivations. Let me illustrate this point with the following example.

Our experimental study currently under way in Bogotá, Colombia,
was designed in part to test the effects of prenatal supplementation on the outcome of pregnancy. It has been found that the distribution of food supplements in quantities sufficient to close the

calorie and protein gap resulted in only modest increments in actual
dietary intake among the pregnant women to whose families it was
given. The provision of 850 calories resulted in a mean increment
of only 135 calories above the baseline diet, largely because recipients reduced purchases of other food (1). The substitution
that occurred suggests that these families had needs more pressing
than insufficient food which they attempted to meet with the income
represented by the supplements. Identification of those needs will
be useful information in planning future intervention programs. In
the same study it was found that birth weight in the supplemented
group was significantly higher than in a control group randomly selected prior to the intervention. This apparently simple effect of
supplementation is actually a more complex phenomenon. Information
was obtained on dietary intake prior to and after supplementation.
The sample of mothers was stratified by the median into two halves
according to the pre-supplementation calorie intake (i.e., those
who consumed less than 1500 calories per 24 hours and those who
consumed more than 1500 calories per 24 hours). Surprisingly, only
the subset consuming 1500 calories or more prior to supplementation
showed a response to the program in terms of birth weight (2).
This finding, the result of process evaluation, suggests that birth
weight may not be a sensitive indicator of improved nutrition among
the most depressed sectors of the population.

Clearly, much remains to be learned concerning the interaction
of biological and environmental variables in the causation of poverty and malnutrition. Process evaluation and measurement of intervening variables carefully conducted as a component of intervention programs may yield this type of information at relatively
low cost.

In closing, I would like to refer to the authors' statement
that "prototypical social programs in developing countries should
be designed either to minimize costs or to produce revenues to support their operation in the event of adoption". This issue de-
serves emphasis and further discussion. I would like to suggest
that the degree to which a target population approaches self-
sufficiency as a result of an intervention must be considered when
judging program impact. Consider, for example, two rural health
and nutrition units with similar budgets which may match closely
in terms of number of patients attended, vaccinations applied, and
rations distributed to pregnant women and children under four years
of age. Yet in one unit the auxiliary nurse in charge is a native
of the village as was her predecessor, the community action committee donated the land to build the post, and they consider it one
of their accomplishments. Recurrent costs, although subsidized by
the national health service system, are defrayed in part by modest
charges for services rendered and contributions by the local association of coffee growers. In contrast, the second unit described
above was built on government land by the national health service,

is staffed, by auxiliary nurses from the provincial capital and is
financed entirely by the national health service. If evaluation
is limited to the quantification of services rendered and their
costs, the indigenization of services present in the first village
but not in the second would not be measured. This dimension is
almost certainly associated with the likelihood of the services
enduring into the future.

All too often social action programs are undertaken and soon
abandoned as external commitment falters. More often than not
target populations represent the politically disfranchised. Massive allocation of funds to the service of this sector of the
population is difficult to achieve or sustain. Only through effective community organization and incorporation into the economic
system will this subsector be able to compete effectively for services with organized labor and the middle class. Community participation and community organization are phrases that convey a
desirable objective but much needs to be done to give these terms
more precise meaning and to devise indicators to measure them.

REFERENCES

1.   Mora, J. O., L. de Navarro, J. Clement, *et al*. The effect of
         nutritional supplementation on its calorie and protein
         intake of pregnant women. *Nutrition Reports Interna-
         tional*. 17:217, 1978.
2.   Christiansen, N., J. O. Mora, L. de Navarro, and M. G. Herrera.
         Effects of nutritional supplementation during pregnancy
         upon birth weight: influence of pre-supplementation diet.
         Nutrition Reports International. 17:217, 1978.

GENERAL DISCUSSION FOR SECTION II: APPROACHES TO IMPACT EVALUATION

A lively debate centered on the question of how evaluations relate to the political process and, especially, to politically motivated program decisions. One participant argued that evaluation should not be tightly tied to political considerations, but that it was a good sign when bureaucrats request evaluation of programs. Such requests must be negotiated -- that is, the official may frame the evaluative question in one way, while the evaluator may consider a different question to be more appropriate. There was disagreement among the conferees as to whether the evaluator can really be free to answer the bureaucrat's question in a different framework. Some argued that one cannot avoid the question of independence of the evaluator from political purposes, but must recognize that evaluation must attract and hold the politician's interest even though the evaluator can have a totally different set of questions from the bureaucrats. Others took the position that it would be impossible to operate with two conflicting sets of questions and that evaluators must understand the politician's agenda and estimate whether his questions can actually be answered and whether the answers are likely to influence political decisions. Evaluation is not merely a technical matter. It should be relevant to policy, although not simply political in character. Unless an accommodation and an understanding of the political agenda is reached, evaluation will have no impact upon policy, even if it is technically perfect.

It is difficult to predict how an evaluation will influence the policy process. Sometimes the effect is long delayed, but one can have confidence that if a study focuses on central issues of lasting importance it will eventually affect policy.

Political constraints may not be as important as the limitations imposed by the state of the art of evaluation. For instance, we do not have much ability to take into account interactions between the intervention and the social reality in which it is embedded; we are not very good at measuring secondary effects. We need

127

to look inside our own shop and improve our methods rather than fretting over political constraints. Furthermore, we need to develop methods that are a compromise between the elegance of experiments and causal models on the one hand and the direct reflection of social reality on the other.

On the part of some Latin American participants, there was concern about the exportability of such technically complex methods of evaluation as social experimentation. No doubt the scientific methods of evaluation developed and applied with generous resources in the United States are powerful. Yet they depend not only upon large fiscal resources but also a reservoir of trained manpower for their success. Latin Americans must ask: "To what extent can these methods actually be applied in developing countries?" Perhaps they can be introduced gradually, but it may be difficult to stimulate explicit demands for evaluation from program administrators and planners, especially if they are approached with a formidable technical jargon coupled with expensive and sophisticated designs. A major need in developing countries is for appropriate methods of reaching marginal populations with health programs and social services. Perhaps evaluation can help to develop realistic approaches in health, education and nutritional status.

A question that may have to be asked prior to transferability is: What impact have these sophisticated evaluations had upon social programs in the developed countries, such as the U.S., which has had a number of large social experiments?

This was deemed not to be an easy question to answer. Social experiments do not always give complete answers to policy questions, and sometimes only confirm what lower cost cross-sectional surveys had found. Experiments may be appropriate for a few particular situations in the less developed countries; but less elegant, shorter-term evaluation strategies can provide useful information for decision-makers in many circumstances.

Evaluation has some unexpected side benefits. For example, in medicine, the recent emphasis on evaluation has made both doctors and patients more concerned about the real value of both well-accepted and innovative therapies.

At this point, the discussion was focused by a two-part question: "Was the discussion concerned only with evaluations that are designed to test experimental or pilot intervention programs, or was it to be concerned with the evaluation of inclusive, on-going national programs?" If the latter, does the evaluation necessarily include a control group, which would probably result in greater

methodological complications and possibly increased cost? The ensuing comments tended to focus on either the first part of this
question (issues of research policy) or the second (methodological
issues).

Comments on the methodological issues began with a suggestion
that it would be helpful to distinguish two kinds of research: one
kind is scientific research on outcomes of an intervention, which
could be called "effectiveness research". The other kind is "efficiency research". In a logical world one would proceed from the
scientific knowledge on effectiveness to design research on the
costs and benefits of various interventions to determine their efficiency. Presumably the most effective interventions would be
incorporated into pilot projects that would be evaluated for their
efficiency before going into inclusive national programs. Up to
that point, appropriate control or comparison groups are needed.
Once the program is in operation on a national level there is
little or no possibility of a comparison group because a national
program is presumably all inclusive. One must evaluate inclusive
national programs by observing changes over time in appropriate
indicators of health or nutritional status of the population.

Another participant pointed out that, whereas there might be
no possibility of defining a *random* control group in the context
of a national program, it was usually the case that some individuals
or communities in a national population did not receive or did not
use the services or material of the program because of differences
in distribution of goods and services over the country. Some areas
or groups are at least *under*served and these "hidden" comparison
groups may serve as "controls". Such groups are not randomly con-
stituted and hence cannot be considered true controls, but they may
help to estimate program effects.

Still another suggestion was to introduce national programs
gradually. There usually are not enough human, organizational or
material resources to install a national program everywhere at
once. · Accordingly, "staged introduction" is ethically justifiable
and allows one to estimate program effects by comparing regions
or sectors where the program was introduced early with those
where its appearance was delayed. This was the case with the family planning program in Taiwan. Program resources were dispersed
over the whole island in a way that was not truly random, but was
unsystematic enough to make it possible to carry out an analysis
of program effects.

One discussant argued that experiments are not an appropriate
way to evaluate nation-wide programs. Furthermore, it is important
to develop approaches that are less labor intensive and less costly,

given the personnel constraints and economic conditions that obtain
in Latin America. Causal modelling or "econometric" approaches
can sharpen insights and identify variables that must be controlled,
even if they cannot completely identify the causal structure of
intervention effects. Such approaches are, furthermore, useful
at the level of nation-wide programs. Finally, owing to recent
advances in statistical technique, the absence of randomization
in "econometric" approaches is not as serious a flaw as some critics seem to believe. Bias due to attrition can be measured.

Several participants emphasized the importance of a good
conceptual model of the intervention process that was to be
evaluated. Such a model directs attention to variables that can
have causal significance and a model can sometimes permit simulation of the process. Furthermore, conceptual models are inexpensive, although difficult. An adequate model for any process must
rest upon a basic scientific understanding of the relationships
among key variables.

Indeed, one participant took the position that experimental,
quasi-experimental and "causal modelling" were not mutually exclusive, alternative approaches to evaluation, but instead were
complementary. A causal model, in his view, is the indispensable
conceptual basis for an experimental design. Furthermore, once
one has such a conceptual basis, it actually means that *less* precision in measurement is necessary.

In connection with concern about the expensive cost of large
scale surveys and experiments, some participants argued that "bigger is not necessarily better". A small scale study of a sample
chosen to be representative of the population can yield useful
knowledge at lower cost. Furthermore, the evaluation of programs
need not be limited to surveys of impact upon recipients of services. Simpler and quicker approaches can handle certain types of
questions. For example, studies of feeding children school lunches
in the United States had two questions to confront: What proportion of the nutritional needs of school children were being met
by school lunches?, and What impact does the nutritional intervention have upon learning? A few quick "back-of-an-envelope" calculations based on existing statistics about participation in the program, dietary content and food wastage gave an answer to the first
question -- about 4% -- that was useful for policy purposes. Of
course, this result did not show how many children got their principal caloric intake from this source, nor did it answer the second
question about the impact of nutrition upon learning. That would
require a set of experimental studies.

Certain additional comments on method emphasized neglected aspects of evaluative research and fundamental principles. One par-

ticipant had commented that "external" evaluators, although presumably objective, might actually be the agents of program failure by
making a critical summative judgment of the intervention at a point
in its development when a more sympathetic understanding of its
weaknesses and feedback to help correct them could strengthen it.
A prematurely critical report lowers staff morale and staff give
up responsibility for improving the program, the sponsoring Ministry becomes concerned, and the program is deemed a failure. Another participant did not dissent from the criticism of prematurity,
but argued that it was essential to begin *planning for evaluation*
even before the very first steps of implementation are taken. If
evaluation is introduced early, that attests to the seriousness of
the program developers, attracts favorable attention from funding
agencies and policy-makers and gives orientation to the planning
itself. For instance, it makes program planners aware of how important it is to collect "baseline" data -- that is, measures of the
state of the problem and the situation prior to the beginning of
intervention. Since evaluation requires well defined objectives in
order to make appropriate outcome measures, the planning process is
further enlightened. So the early introduction of the idea of evaluation has many advantages, but, of course, the summative judgment
of the program should not be made prematurely.

Finally, this participant added, the Latin American countries
should begin with rather elementary evaluation procedures and sell
the idea of evaluation gradually, improving methods at the same
time. Another participant agreed, pointing out that even "elementary" steps had sometimes been omitted or carelessly carried out.
In the evaluation of one national program, he asserted, a well designed and rather expensive evaluation provided for collecting regular, continuing indicators of health and nutrition of the target
population. These data turned out to be almost useless because
they were so carelessly collected (e.g., obtaining the height and
weight of a child but omitting to record his age!). The biggest problem for Latin American evaluations may simply be to assure accurate
and careful execution in the field of the data collection requirements. Unless that is done, even the best designed studies are idle.

This last point provoked a further searching question: to what
extent can one actually initiate new programs which incorporate evaluation in countries where financial and trained human resources are
quite limited and where the possibility of getting valid results is
slim, given these limitations? Should countries like Bolivia and
Peru, for instance, try to do the kind of evaluations we have been
talking about at all?

Another discussant agreed that this question was appropriate,
but asserted that in Latin America new programs in health and nutrition were continually being developed and introduced but their
outcomes were unknown because they were not being evaluated. To be

sure, many Latin American countries lack the human resources and organizational infrastructure needed to make extensive evaluations.
Such studies are not easy to make. Even the more developed countries
began only ten to fifteen years ago to evaluate intervention programs.

Others argued that despite the admitted resource limitations it
was both timely and necessary to introduce evaluation into Latin
American social institutions. Evaluation methods, it was argued,
could be adapted to the special conditions of the country, the program, the situation. Specifically, one ought to do a rough cost-
benefit analysis to make sure that the evaluative research would not
increase the total costs of the program to more than the estimated
benefits of the intervention, since there is always the risk that an
enthusiastic investigator will spend all the available resources on
research! On the other hand, said a different participant, the allocation of funds to evaluation has a dual aspect: a large budget
will not only permit an evaluation to be well done but it signals
policy makers and bureaucrats that evaluation is important enough to
pay attention. Furthermore, if evaluation is to make a fundamental difference in health and nutrition programs, evaluation must
be located at a high level in the bureaucracy. If evaluation is
placed at a low level in the structure, it will have no prestige and
no one will pay attention to its results.

MEASUREMENT OF HEALTH AND NUTRITION EFFECTS OF LARGE-SCALE NUTRITION INTERVENTION PROJECTS

Jean-Pierre Habicht, *
   National Center for Health Statistics
   Hyattsville, Maryland

and

William P. Butz,
   Rand Corporation,
   Santa Monica, California

INTRODUCTION

Increasingly the nutritional impact of complex intervention packages is being sought. Typically these complex interventions include intentional changes in the economic, social and political environment as well as in medical and nutritional factors. We are concerned in this paper with the critical issues of the choice of indicators necessary to evaluate these complex interventions with multiple treatments.

We first will argue that large scale, complex interventions require knowledge about indicator variables that is likely to emerge only from careful evaluations of simple interventions. We then discuss a set of optimal properties for field indicators of nutrition and health. These properties have implications for the design and evaluation of interventions. In light of these implications we will review the few evaluations of nutrition interventions reported in the literature in order to assess the knowledge now available for structuring complex, large scale interventions. Finally, we will explore problems of design and measurement peculiar to interventions with multiple treatment.

*Current address: Division of Nutritional Sciences, Cornell University, Ithaca, N.Y.

OPERATIONAL DEFINITIONS OF HEALTH AND NUTRITION

The objectives of the program to be evaluated must be clearly defined and the evaluation must make the appropriate comparisons given these objectives. In the context of this volume, which focuses on very poor populations, good health may be defined as the absence of symptomatic illness, the absence of life-shortening processes and the absence of pathological constraints on performance. Although this definition is broader than that of the clinician, it is narrower than many definitions of health which cannot be translated operationally. More importantly, this definition concentrates mainly on the soundness of the body, little on the soundness of the mind, and not at all on the soundness of the soul. When conditions which threaten the integrity of the body have been obviated thanks to social and economic development, the fostering of the non-physiological components of health can receive a higher priority.

Also within the context of poor populations, good nutrition may be defined as food intake which is adequate enough so that neither health, performance, nor survival are impaired for lack or excess of food or of its components. Again, this definition is broader than that of classical nutrition, but is narrower than that of many nutrition demagogues. It may be considered a transient definition because other socially desirable components may come to be viewed as necessary as a population's physiological needs are met.

In the context of these operational definitions one should be able to infer from an improvement in indicators of health and nutrition that there is an associated improvement in performance, a decrease in overt illness, and/or longer survival. This requires previous demonstrations that these benefits are directly tied to improvements in the chosen indicators of health and nutrition. For instance, a reduction in infant mortality appears clearly to be a health benefit, while an increase in nutrient ingestion may or may not be. So much has been said about the interrelationships between nutrition and health that the interrelationships are presumed understood, at least at most practical levels. Unfortunately, this is only true in severe malnutrition and very poor health. Among those with moderate degrees of ill-health and malnutrition, characteristics of the vast majority of the poor, too few competent field studies have been done to establish the implications for performance, health and survival of changes in indicators of health and nutrition.

LEVELS OF EVALUATION OF FIELD STUDIES
AND PUBLIC HEALTH PROGRAMS

There is a logical sequence of evaluation studies depending

upon previous scientific and administrative knowledge (1). In general, these include field intervention studies, public health pilot projects, evaluations in conjunction with implementations of an intervention, and ultimately continuous monitoring of program impact. Each of these is discussed more fully in the paragraphs that follow. The knowledge resulting from each is not only important in deciding whether a given type of intervention is likely to be useful or not, but it also will indicate which experimental design to use and which variables to measure in an evaluation of new or ongoing nutrition and health interventions.

A.   Field Intervention Studies in Individuals

Some field intervention research is directed to identifying physiological and behavioral responses of individuals to public health intervention. It is not concerned with macrochanges at the level of the community. One might think that such individual responses could be done in a laboratory setting where conditions can be controlled. However, clinical and laboratory studies cannot substitute for a field study because the natural ecology of infections and nutritional stresses cannot be duplicated in metabolic wards.

An example of the value of such a field study is presented by Yarbrough and Habicht (2). Their population consisted of older preschool children whose dietary staple was maize, in whom they quantified the relative contribution to growth resulting from different doses of calories as contrasted to similar doses of calories combined with protein. Two unexpected results developed. The first was that a small increment in calories without added protein was as effective in improving growth as was a similar increment in calories with protein. The second was that even large improvements in protein-calorie nutrition could not improve growth rates to the levels seen in developed countries, in all probability because of recurrent and frequent diarrheal disease. These findings contradicted the inferences drawn from research in laboratory and clinical settings which could not take the village ecology into account (3).

This kind of prospective experimental epidemiological field study requires a large array of measures and a rigorous experimental design to assure the comparability of data from those individuals receiving the different kinds of interventions. Only by such careful control can the inferences be sufficiently strong and generalizable to individuals in other populations to be of use to scientists and clinicians in that they are assured of the effectiveness of the intervention for individuals.

B.   Community Field Intervention Studies

Field studies which show a benefit in individuals are not necessarily designed to show an effect at the community level. Yarbrough
and Habicht, for instance, reported a clear benefit to some individuals without any measurable impact in the entire population. Another
type of field research, which must be based on knowledge, such as
that acquired under the type of study discussed in (A) above, is
directed to evaluating community or a population response to an
intervention. Are there enough individuals who respond sufficiently
to the program so that one can identify a response from measurements
aggregated at the community level? This research is also expensive,
above all because it requires replication at the community level
and must have as rigorous an experimental design as in (A). A good
example is the group of fluoridation evaluation studies done by the
U.S. Public Health Service which examined many indices of fluoride
nutrition and many kinds of outcomes, including possible adverse side
effects (4). Collectively, these clearly demonstrated the effectiveness of water fluoridation to prevent caries in communities.

C.   Public Health Pilot Studies

Only when the results of field intervention studies have demonstrated effectiveness and thus promise a likely benefit from public
health programs, is it worth investigating the feasibility and the
cost-efficiency of large scale public health interventions. We call
these public health pilot studies. On the basis of the knowledge
gained from studies such as those described in A or B above, these
pilot studies can utilize the best and most sensitive measures of
mediating variables and of outcomes. Similarly, they only need to
measure the few confounding variables which have been shown in study
A or B to be important. However, they must also measure cost in
such a way that the three components of the intervention can be examined separately to permit cost-efficiency analyses. No such analyses
can be done without an experimental design which is at least as rigorous as in study (A) for cost-efficiency per individual benefited,
or as rigorous as in study (B) for cost-efficiency of community impacts.

D.   Evaluation During Implementation
            of Large-Scale Interventions

Once a pilot study has shown an intervention to be feasible,
effective, and efficient, it may be extended more widely. A well-
planned study needs to be conducted concurrently with this extension.
It must be intensive and rapid, measuring those variables which are
likely to change rapidly as the intervention is introduced. This
implementation evaluation compares baseline data with that obtained

later, or it compares geographic areas where the program has begun with those where it is about to begin.

The kinds of measurements are less numerous and more selective than those needed in the pilot study described in (C). The analysis of data should proceed quickly for each new geographic area benefiting from the introduction of the intervention to assure that the results correspond to those found in (C). If they do not correspond in spite of corrective action, either the chosen introduction is not feasible as a large scale public health activity, or the conditions which permitted the program to have an impact in study (C) do not hold at this large scale level.

E.   Evaluation Through Monitoring

Once a program is implemented on a large scale, the only concern is that it results in an improvement compared to past health and nutritional status and that these results persist. This requires the establishment of a monitoring system which must be functioning adequately before the initiation of the public health intervention program (5). It requires no rigorous control group and a minimum of crucial measurements.

CHOICE OF EVALUATION INDICATORS

The choice of an indicator depends upon whether the evaluation is directed towards change in individuals or in communities.

Indicator Sensitivity in Individuals

An indicator of nutritional or health status of individuals must be responsive to the improved health or nutrition for which the proposed intervention is designed. In other words, the indicator must be responsive over the range of improvement expected.

This requires that there is an abnormal value for the indicator in individuals before intervention. Furthermore, the abnormality must be due to that element of nutrition or health which is to be improved. Thus, for example, if the intervention only improves protein quality of the diet in a population which is stunted because of inadequate caloric intake, the intervention will not improve growth (6). Historically, the health and nutritional factors responsible for abnormal levels of indicators have often been incorrectly identified on the basis of descriptive studies which were not buttressed by intervention studies of the type described previously.

Even when an indicator's abnormal value is related to, or due to, the factor which the intervention is designed to improve, the indicator often may not be sensitive to improvement. This occurs because many indicators of health and nutritional status have been derived from comparisons between healthy, well-nourished individuals and clinically ill or malnourished patients. However, the majority of individuals in the usual target populations for large-scale interventions are not suffering extreme malnutrition or ill health.

The consequences of moderate malnutrition can often not be predicted from severe malnutrition. For example, the severe protein deficiency syndrome of kwashiorkor is accompanied by a deterioration of the body's defense mechanisms against infection and by impaired intestinal function, both of which result in diarrhea. However, protein deficiency sufficient to stunt growth does not result in increased diarrhea (7). Therefore, one may not presume that a strong effect on performance, health and survival, during severe malnutrition will necessarily lead to proportionately reduced indicator values under less severe malnutrition. In fact, trying to demonstrate the effectiveness of an intervention by using indicators demonstrated effective only under extreme conditions will usually fail.

Observations such as the above suggest that in many situations the dose-response curve may not be linear. Indeed, in those rare studies where one has looked for a dose-response on performance, health and survival, through improved nutrition in man, one finds a significantly lessened benefit as one improves nutritional state even at levels of nutrition universally accepted as inadequate (2,8). This means that for many indicators of performance, health and survival, one may not expect much improvement after intervention, unless the levels of the indicators in the malnourished population are quite different from normal levels in well-nourished regions (c.f. Figure 1).

Measured dose-response depends not only on the physiological response to dose consumed, but also, and sometimes importantly in field conditions, on the vagaries of measuring the intervention indicators and the response or outcome indicators. The larger and more frequent the errors of measurement of intervention and of outcome, the less sensitive will be the measured dose-response. For certain types of intervention (e.g., Vitamin A fortification of a food eaten occasionally by everybody) and for certain outcomes (e.g., an increase in fat folds) these vagaries in measurement can conceal any significant association between intervention and outcome. Where such errors are considerable, certain measurement strategies and statistical manipulations can help (19). It is much better to assure that the intervention and outcome variables chosen have little intrinsic variability and that the measurements are done carefully (10).

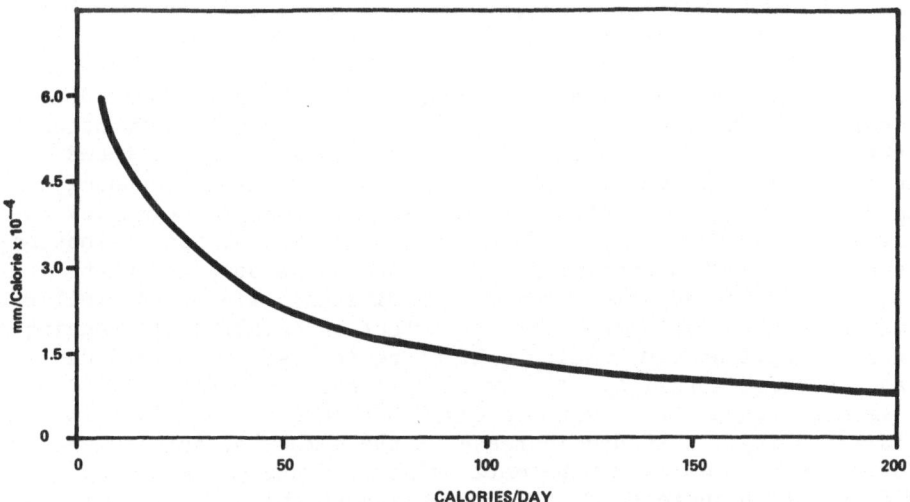

FIG. 1. Efficiency of calorie conversion to growth at different levels of calorie intake in young children. **Based on two year increments in growth at different levels of supplementation in one year old children (2).**

Indicator Sensitivity in Communities

So far we have discussed the effects of a health and nutrition intervention on indicators of performance, health and survival in individuals. Now we turn to problems which arise when one wishes to evaluate the results of an intervention on a population, rather than on individuals.

Evaluation of interventions in individuals usually depends upon sequential (longitudinal) measurements in the same individuals. The comparison is between improvement in those individuals who receive the intervention with the lack of improvement in those who do not. In contrast, the evaluation of interventions in populations often depends on sampling individuals at different points in time. Where the variability between individuals in some indicator is large compared to the expected response of that indicator to intervention, measuring different individuals each time instead of the same individuals longitudinally, will result in a marked decrease in the sensitivity of the indicator, similar to that which we noted will occur if the measurements are done poorly in individuals. The decision as to whether the improved sensitivity of evaluation acquired by longitudinally measuring the same individuals in populations is or is not worth the added cost and difficulty, as compared to sam-

pling different individuals each time, can and should be calculated
before intervention is started.

Usually, knowing the dose-response curve in individuals does
not permit predictions about the effectiveness of an intervention
in the community. One reason for this discrepancy can be found
when a certain critical reduction in disease or disease-causing
agents results in eradication of the disease from the community because a cause-effect chain is interrupted, as in malaria prevention
programs. In such a case, a greater response is obtained that
would be anticipated when looking at individuals alone. A similar
situation can be postulated for the effect on natality of reducing
infant and childhood mortality. If there is a sudden marked decrease in child mortality, it may be that the birth rate will decrease more rapidly than with an equal but more gradual fall in
child mortality. A sudden increase in the number of infants and
toddlers in the family may be more evident to the parents than
would be a slow increase in the proportion of children who survive.

A more general reason why individual response rates to a given
intervention do not predict population response rates to that same
intervention, lies in the fact that the population response depends
upon the characteristics of beneficiaries of the intervention compared to the rest of the population. Thus, one can expect different
dose-responses in similar populations depending on the way the intervention is distributed. For instance, nutrition supplementation
appears to be consumed in some nutrition programs inversely to the
individual's needs (11). The impact of such a supplement will be
negligible compared to a program with identical coverage which also
assures that maximum supplementation is ingested where it is most
needed.

For the above reason, many programs direct their interventions
to those most likely to benefit. Other programs may cover the whole
population but select for evaluation those who will most benefit.
This selection is done on the basis of indicators of probable benefit. For this purpose, one must not only choose an appropriate
"cut-off point" on that indicator which will permit the best selection (12). We call this characteristic the "selectivity of the
indicator's 'cut-off point'". 1/

_____

1/ Clinical pathologists with a concern for prognosis have
described the identical characteristic and called it "predictability". We have tried to use the term "predictability" in the context
of public health but found it so confusing that we have regretfully
retained "selectivity" for this presentation.

No variable is perfectly "selective". A child who is small for his age may be genetically stunted or he may be stunted for nutritional or health reasons. In the individual case one can ascribe a probability to the genetic and non-genetic possibilities if one knows two of the following three distributions: the distribution of growth of all children in the population of which the child is representative; the genetic distribution of sizes; or the distribution of stunted children. Figure 2 shows the probability of environmentally stunted growth at different heights among five-year-olds in a mixed population, half environmentally deprived (14) and half well-nourished (15). The smaller the child in this population, the greater the probability that the child's growth was stunted for non-genetic reasons.

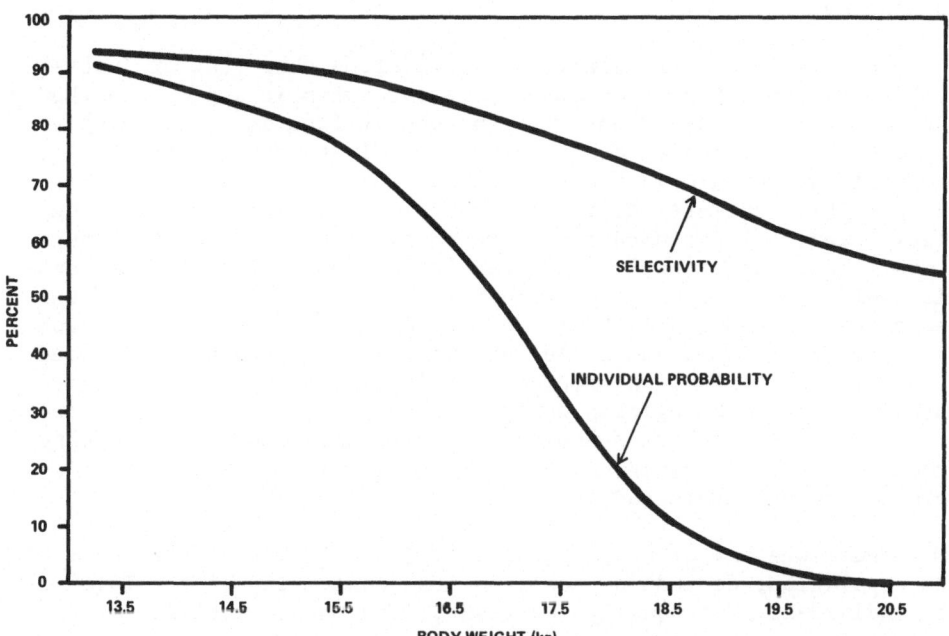

FIG. 2. *Individual probability as contrasted to selectivity of environment stunting.* Based on data for five-year-old boys of a mixed population with the same proportion of environmentally stunted boys (14) and well-nourished boys (15).

Selectivity of an indicator's "cut-off point" does not refer, however, to the individual's probability of being malnourished or ill, but refers to the number of individuals who fall below that "cut-off point" because they suffer from malnutrition or ill health rather than because of genetic factors. Figure 2 also shows how this selectivity changes with different "cut-off" points in this same population of five-year-olds. Selectivity depends upon three characteristics of a dichotomous diagnostic variable at a specified "cut-off point": the measured or true prevalence of the disease; the proportion of all correctly diagnosed as ill for this disease (sensitivity of diagnosis); and the proportion of non-ill persons correctly diagnosed as not ill with this disease (specific of diagnosis). Only one of these characteristics, the sensitivity of diagnosis, can be expected to remain constant under standardized conditions across different populations. It is obvious that the prevalence of disease can change. The specificity of diagnosis will also change with the changing prevalence of factors other than the disease or nutritional cause against which the intervention is addressed. Therefore, selectivity has to be estimated for each population.

Such estimates of selectivity will often show that an intervention can only have a modest impact even when it improves markedly the condition for all those who can benefit from it, because only a few of those selected can benefit. For instance, in the U.S.A., the official hemoglobin "cut-off point" for anemia is 12g. in Black women. This "cut-off" delivers a prevalence of 20% anemics among Black women, all presumed to be iron deficient based on the literature. In fact, probably less than 10% of those classified as anemic would benefit from iron therapy (16) -- the selectivity of this hemoglobin "cut-off point" is, therefore, only about 10%. If each of those Black women who could benefit from iron therapy responded to an iron fortification program by raising their hemoglobin 2g., this increase in hemoglobin would be diluted to a mean 0.2g. increase among those classified as anemic. Such results would not indicate iron therapy to be an effective intervention if the selectivity were not known beforehand.

Thus, whether or not an indicator is sensitive at the level of the population, depends not only on its sensitivity at the level of the individual, but equally important, upon the selectivity of the indicator.

It is clear from this discussion that, to ensure that evaluation does not result in spurious negative results, no large-scale intervention program should be evaluated unless certain facts about the intervention, the measurements, and the population's probable response to the program are known beforehand. The easiest and safest way to elucidate these facts is by conducting carefully designed and implemented intervention studies in similar populations beforehand. Tables I.a-e present the data reported in nine such intervention programs. The specifics of these tables are discussed in the next section.

Table Ia. EFFECT OF PROTEIN-CALORIE INTERVENTION IN PRESCHOOL CHILDREN ON TOTAL DIETARY INTAKE

Reference: Years Publication	Supplement	Supervised/ Measured Ingestion	Replacement Estimated	Age in Months	Intake Before Intervention or Compared to Control	Intake after Intervention	Change in Intake
(17)-1963	391 Kcal.* 13.4 g.	No	Yes	48-96	From previous study 1580Kcal. 37 g.	Not reported. Claim no substitution effect	?
(18)-1965	101-284 Kcal. 9.8-10.1 g.	No	No**	6-12	Not measured	Not measured	?
(19)-1967-9	Not specified	No	Yes	0-59	678 Kcal. 20 g.	1040 Kcal. 30 g.	+362 Kcal. +10 g.
(20)-1970	250 Kcal. 12.5 g.	No	Yes*	36-96	Not reported	Not reported	?
(11)-1970	300 Kcal. 10 g.	?	Yes	12-60	Not reported	Not reported. Claim no substitution effect	+300 Kcal.? +10 g.?
(21)-1970	?	Yes	Yes	35-59	486 Kcal. 13.7 g.	1181 Kcal. 35.3g.	+695 Kcal. +21.6 g.
(22)-1973	310 Kcal. 3 g.	Yes	Yes	12-60	700 Kcal. 18 g.	1010 Kcal. 21 g.	+319 Kcal. + 3 g.
(23)-1973	800-1300kJ. 6.7-11.8 g.	?	Yes	24-72	3700 kJ.	Not reported. Claim no substitution effect	+800-1300kJ.? +6.7-11.8g.?
(2)-1977	200 Kcal 14 g.	Yes	Yes	12-36	78% of recommended energy intake	Claim 10% substitution effect	+180 Kcal. +13.5 g.

Legend: * = Energy intake/day and Protein intake/day
    ** = Cause for doubting author's inferences
    ? = Uncertain

Table Ib. *EFFECT OF PROTEIN-CALORIE INTERVENTION IN PRESCHOOL CHILDREN ON HEIGHT*

Reference: Year Publication	Type of Height	Age in Months	Best-Worst = R **	Before Intervention or Compared to Control		After Intervention		Change in		Statist. Signif. (p<.05)
				Level	% of R	Level	% of R	Level	% of R	
(17)-1963	1 year increment in cm/year	48-96 Boys Girls	6.0-5.6=0.4 6.0-5.3=0.7	4.3* 3.7*	0% 0%	4.4* 4.1*	0% 0%	0.1 0.4	– –	No No
(18)-1965	6 month increment in cm/year	6-12	14-6.0 =8.0	7.4- 7.6	18- 20%	6.9- 7.9	11- 24%	-0.1	-1%	No
(19)-1967-9	3 year increment in cm/3 year	0-11 12-48	41-20=21.0 30-17.5=12.5	17.6* 19.9	<0% 19%	16.7* 22.0	<0% 36%	-0.9 2.1	– 17%	No Yes
(20)-1970	Attained developmental age	36-96	1.0-0.5=0.5	0.7	40%	0.7	40%	0.0	0%	No
(11)-1970	Attained height cm after two years supplementation	24-35 36-47 48-59 60-71	90-75= 15.0 99-81= 18.0 106-88=18.0 113-95=18.0	77.1 82.0 91.0 97.4	14% 6% 17% 14%	78.3 84.6 90.9 98.7	22% 20% 16% 21%	1.2 2.6 -.1 1.3	8% 14% -1% 7%	No No No No
(21)-1970	6 month increment in cm/6 month	35-59	3.5-2.9= 0.6	1.94*	<0%	2.7	33%	0.8	133%	Yes
(22)-1973	14 month increment cm/14 month	12-23 24-35 36-47 48-60	12.5-6.8=5.7 9.5-6.8= 2.7 8.5-6.8= 1.7 7.5-6.8= 0.7	6.5* 7.8 7.4 7.3	<0% 37% •35% 71%	9.3 9.5 9.1 8.4	44% 100% 135% 229%	2.8 1.7 2.0 1.1	49% 63% 118% 157%	Yes Yes Yes Yes
(23)-1973	6 month increment in cm/6 month	24-72	3.5-2.9= 0.6	2.0*	<0%	3.2	50%	1.2	200%	Yes
(2)-1977	2 year increment in cm/2 year	12	20-12= 8.0	15.7	46%	18.3	79%	2.6	33%	Yes

Legend: * This growth rate is lower than the lowest extrapolated from the most stunted population reported in the literature (24).
         ** R = Physiological Range (see text, page 155).

Table Ic. EFFECT OF PROTEIN-CALORIE INTERVENTION IN PRESCHOOL CHILDREN ON WEIGHT

Reference: Year Publication	Type of Weight	Age in Months	Best-Worst = R *	Before Intervention or Compared to Control Level	% of R	After Intervention Level	% of R	Change in Level	% of R	Statist. Signif. (p < .05)
(17)-1963	1 yr. increment as kg/year	48-96 Boys Girls	2.0-1.6=0.4 1.4=0.6	1.6 1.3	0% <0%	2.1 2.6	125% 200%	0.5 1.3	125% 217%	No Yes
(18)-1965	6 month increment presented as kg/yr	6-12	4.0-1.5=2.5	2.2-2.3	29-32%	2.2-2.5	26-35%	.04	1%	No
(19)-1967-9	Regression Coefficient (kg/year)	0-11	6.0-3.5=2.5	3.6	4%	3.9	16%	0.3	12%	No
	Regression Coefficient (kg/3 yrs)	12-48	6.0-4.5=1.5	5.2	47%	5.7	80%	0.5	33%	Yes
(20)-1970	Attained Developmental Age	36-96	1.0-0.5=0.5	0.68	36%	0.68	36%	0.0	0%	No
(11)-1970	Attained weight after two yrs. supplementation (kg)	24-35 36-47 48-59 60-71	14.5-8.0 =6.5 15.5-9.0 =6.5 17.5-11.0=6.5 19.5-13.0=6.5	8.8 10.1 12.0 13.3	12% 17% 15% 5%	9.2 10.9 12.0 14.0	18% 29% 15% 15%	0.4 0.8 0.0 0.7	6% 12% 0% 11%	No Yes No Yes
(21)-1970	6 months increment (kg/1/2 yr)	35-59	1.0-0.7=0.3	1.23		2.28		1.0	350%	Yes
(22)-1973	14 month increment (kg/14 months)	12-23 24-35 36-47 48-71	2.6-1.7=0.9 2.3-1.7=0.6 2.3-1.7=0.6 2.3-1.7=0.6	1.74 1.71 1.58 1.38	4% 1% <0% <0%	2.35 2.34 2.04 1.86	72% 71% 38% 18%	0.61 0.63 0.46 0.48	68% 70% 51% 53%	Yes Yes Yes Yes
(23)-1973	6 month increment (Kg/1/2 year)	24-71	1.0-0.7=0.3	0.2	<0%	1.5		1.3	433%	Yes
(2)-1977	2 yr increment (kg/2 yr)	12	4.0-3.0=1.0	3.67	67%	4.50	150%	0.83	83%	Yes

Legend: * R = Physiological Range (see text, page 155)

Table Id. EFFECT OF PROTEIN-CALORIE INTERVENTION IN PRESCHOOL CHILDREN ON MORBIDITY

Reference Year Publication	Type of Morbidity	Age in Months	Before Intervention or Compared to Control (Level)	After Intervention (Level)	Change in Level	Statist. Signif. (p< .05)
(18) 1965	Illness score based on effect of illness on growth rate	6-12	0.5 - 0.6	0.6 - 1.2	-0.3 Better	No
(19) 1967-9	Average days ill per year	0-59				
		No Intervention	13	22	+9 Worse	*
		Medical Interv.	71	48	-25 Better	-
		Nutrition "	10	46	+36 Worse	-
(11) 1970	% children with symptoms of protein-calorie malnutrition	12-60	23.0	11.3	-11.7 Better	Yes
			17.0	5.6	-11.4 Better	Yes
Legend: * No statistical significance testing done						

Table Ie. EFFECT OF PROTEIN-CALORIE INTERVENTION IN PRESCHOOL CHILDREN ON MORTALITY

Reference Year Publication	Type of Mortality	Age in Months	Best-Worst R = *	Before Intervention or Compared to Control Level	% of R	After Intervention Level	% of R	Change in Level	% of R	Statist. Signif. (p <0.5)
(19) 1967-9	Infant (deaths/ yr/1000 births)	0-11 No Intervention	16-200=184	186	8%	191	4%	-5	Worse	No
		Medical Intervention		136	35%	88	60%	46	25%	No
		Nutrition Intervention		182	10%	146	29%	36	20%	No
	Preschool (deaths/ 1000 children)	12-48 No Intervention	0.3-90=89.7	81-9	10%	50-40	45%	31	35%	Yes
		Medical Intervention		50-40	45%	35-55	61%	15	17%	No
		Nutrition Intervention		56-34	38%	24-66	74%	32	36%	Yes
(20) 1970	Infant (deaths/ yr/1000 births)	0-11	16-200=184	135	34%	48	83%	87	47%	Yes
	Preschool (deaths/ 1000 children)	12-48	0.3-90=89.7	40	56%	22	76%	18	76%	No
Legend: * R = Physiological Range (see text, page 155)										

These Tables present the results of nutritional interventions in populations of preschool children with malnutrition and they reveal that growth in height is the most sensitive indicator, increments in weight are less sensitive, and improvements in health and post-infant survival are so insensitive that they cannot be used as indicators of nutritional status or to measure the effect of nutritional interventions in populations.

We do not review here the results of nutrition intervention studies in pregnant women because we reviewed this literature previously (25) and concluded that birthweight and duration of pregnancy probably were not related to nutrition of the mother except in severe maternal deprivation. We have since persuaded ourselves otherwise, at least as far as birth weight is concerned (26,27). We will try to justify our conversion at the end of the next section. We hope soon for a similar justification in the literature for thinking that infant mortality is sensitive to maternal and infant nutrition -- but that is not yet available.

This evidence about the sensitivity of indicators can only come about from careful, well-designed intervention studies such as those described previously.

Intervention, Outcome and Intermediary Indicators

Later we will review the evidence for the sensitivity of outcome (impact) indicators which reflect cellular responses to improved nutrition because these indicators alone provide evidence of physiological benefit from a public health intervention. No evaluation study can, however, rely on such outcome indicators alone. These outcome indicators must be complemented by indicators which measure the intervention itself and its intermediary results. In field intervention studies the intermediary results are crucial for substantiating that the intervention caused the outcome. For this purpose the intermediary variables chosen will be those which biology indicates should change together, and they will be analyzed for such congruity of response. This analysis is imperative to substantiate causality between an intervention and a coincidental outcome.

The evaluation of all intervention studies is greatly facilitated if one knows how much intervention various members of the population receives relative to their needs. To achieve this, the intervention indicators should be as unambiguously tied to the intervention as possible. For instance, including in food supplements a tracer that can be measured in the urine permits one to ascertain who is consuming the food supplements. This and similar

strategies for evaluating interventions are particularly essential
when an intervention does not succeed in improving health, performance or survival. In such circumstances, one must differentiate
between the question, "Was the failure because the intervention
failed to reach those who needed it?" as contrasted to the question,
"Was the intervention itself inappropriately chosen?".

EVIDENCE THAT CONVENTIONAL HEALTH AND NUTRITION INDICATORS ARE SENSITIVE TO NUTRITION INTERVENTION

Establishing the Specificity of Indicator Response

To document the sensitivity of an indicator of nutritional
status requires nutrition intervention studies, which demonstrate
that the indicator responds to improved nutrition. Demonstration
of such a response includes exclusion of the probability that the
response was caused by non-nutritional factors. This exclusion,
which assures the specificity of response to the nutrition intervention, can only be achieved by carefully designed and implemented
intervention studies.

This section presents the criteria necessary to judge whether
a response in an indicator was likely to be due to nutrition, in
which case the indicator is sensitive to changes in nutrition, or
whether the change could have been due above all to non-nutritional
influences. In the context of testing the sensitivity of an indicator, these non-nutritional influences are "confounding" factors
in statistical parlance.

The need to control for confounding factors is of course as
important in evaluating the success of an intervention as in identifying sensitive indicators. Therefore the considerations reviewed
in this section are important for designing all evaluations. This
is especially true where the biological response to an intervention
is under investigation as in Section (A) and (B) cited earlier, but
controlling for confounding becomes less important since evaluation
is less concerned with proving intervention effectiveness and is
more concerned with monitoring as one proceeds through the evaluations described in Sections (D) and (E). The reason for describing the control of confounding factors in this section, however,
is not to prescribe experimental designs for intervention evaluation, but is rather to aid in judging whether a putative indicator
of nutritional status has been demonstrated to be sensitive to
changes in nutrition in individuals and populations where only a
small minority suffer the florid clinical forms of kwashiorkor or
marasmus.

We have discussed how the sensitivity of response is diminished by random errors of measurement and random variations in the indicators. These errors of measurement and other variations in the indicators are all due to factors other than those to which the intervention is addressed. They are, in that context, variations that are not specific to the purposes of the intervention. So long as these non-specific variations are random and their effects add up to zero, they only decrease the sensitivity of response. When, however, a non-specific influence changes the indicator among many individuals in the same direction, there is a danger that the resulting shift in the mean will be incorrectly attributed to the intervention.

There are basically three strategies to control for confounding factors: Controlled experimental designs; use of complementary indicators; and statistical analyses. The *classical procedure* is by experimental design where one compares the group benefiting from the intervention with a group similar in all relevant characteristics but which does not benefit from intervention (28). For instance, volunteering to participate in an intervention immediately introduces a bias if this group is to be compared to a control group which did not choose to take advantage of the intervention, because the factors which promote cooperation with the intervention program may also effect changes in the outcome indicators.

Good experimental design is the single most important factor necessary for successful evaluation. This depends upon careful formulation of the questions which the evaluation is supposed to answer. Defining the appropriate questions is facilitated if the practical consequences of alternative answers are specified. For instance, the question, "What are the correlates and consequences of participation by potential beneficiaries of a program?", is much less useful than asking, "Who needs the program? If these needy participate, is their performance, health or survival improved?" If not, "why not? What proportion of the needy participate? Why not?" Alternative answers to each of the questions in the latter series has immediate implications for program implementation. Experimental design is always slighted *in compendia*, such as this volume, because adequate treatment of the issue cannot proceed without addressing specific substantive questions. Generalizations on this issue have not been useful because apparently minor constraints on the use of "classical" experimental designs vitiate their usefulness and such constraints are the rule in field evaluation.

One particular constraint which results in falsely optimistic evaluations about a program's effectiveness, is the use of the same indicator to select those who are in need of the intervention,

and to judge the response of the intervention in those selected.
The use of such an indicator must correct for the indicator's
inevitable regression towards the mean between the time of selection and the time of evaluation (29).

Evaluations which sample different individuals in a population
instead of following individuals longitudinally must be particularly
careful to ascertain whether population movements in and out of
the intervention areas are not due to the immigrant's desire to
cooperate with the intervention compared with the emigrants' indifference. In such a case, the immigrants may immigrate into the
intervention area with better indicators of performance, health
and survival than those of the emigrants, because those better
indicators are associated with factors which promote cooperation
with the intervention program, but are not due to the intervention
program *per se*.

One of the great disappointments in evaluating intervention
programs has been the discovery that comparisons between villages
or regions often result in spurious differences due to non-specific
influences which affect whole villages and regions. Often these
effects cannot be explained, much less prevented (6). In this
context, Gordon *et al*. stated that in the nutrition intervention
studies they reported it was impossible to determine how much of
the difference in effects observed between villages was due to the
different interventions, to general secular trends which were different between the three villages, to sudden unexpected occurrences
such as epidemics which infested villages differently, and to other
unknown factors which might have affected the villages differently
(19:VIII).

For instance, it is usual practice to ascertain through baseline surveys the comparability of villages with respect to the
evaluation indicators. Figure 3, shows actual data on infant mortality rates for two villages chosen to be comparable in 1968 for a
nutrition intervention that began in 1969. Comparing the rates in
1968 suggests that the two villages were quite similar with respect
to this indicator. However, looking at the trends between 1960
and 1968 in these villages, sorely tries one's confidence in the
comparability of future infant mortality data across the villages.
Such confidence is, of course, a prerequesite for believing that
the reduced mortality after the intervention seen in village A
relative to village B is due to an intervention applied to village
A and not to village B.

Therefore, any experimental design which does not randomly
distribute the intervention and its control within a village or a

region must have sufficient villages or regions covered by each
treatment (replicates) so that one can estimate the probable contribution of non-specific influences at the village or regional
level. Adjacent villages and regions must have different treatments, and the villages and regions should be so stratified that
any other random non-specific influences are controlled for. Designs which show differences between regions or villages but do
not have these required replicates must remain suspect.

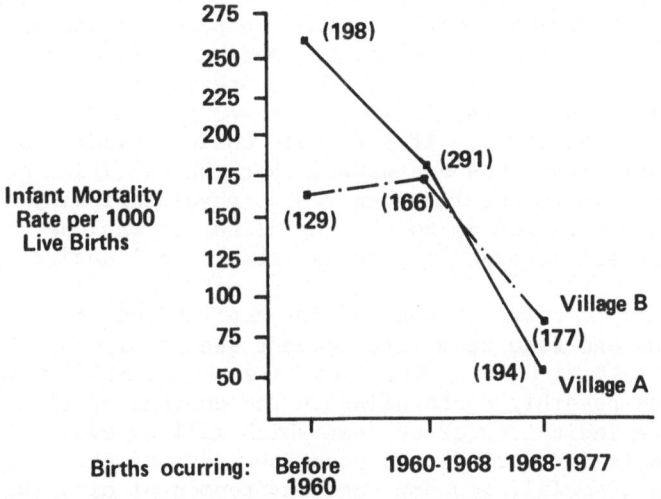

FIG. 3. *Infant mortality rate trends in two villages chosen for
a nutrition intervention.* Source: Female Retrospective Life
History Questionnaire from *INCAP-RAND Survey in Guatemala.*

Notes: Numbers of live births in each period are in parentheses.
All rates are calculated from retrospective data for comparability. We can identify no reporting bias that would have differentially affected the two villages; nevertheless, this possibility
exists.

The *second and complementary strategy* to avoid misinterpreting
a change in levels of an indicator consequent to intervention is
to measure various complementary indicators (30). Each indicator
should measure some different step between the intervention and its
outcome. For instance, if increased caloric intake of the pregnant
mother is supposed to be responsible for a subsequent improved survival of the infant, then one should find that improved caloric intake leads to greater maternal skinfolds, to a greater maternal
weight gain during pregnancy, to a greater birthweight of the infant
and to a greater infant skinfold, as well as to improved infant survival. Furthermore, all these variables should show a statistical
association with each other. The choice of these complementary indicators and their expected statistical associations requires a
clear conceptualization based on previous demonstration of the expected effect of the intervention on performance, health and survival. If influences not related to the intervention's objective
affect one of the indicators, it is unlikely that they will affect
the whole chain of indicators. Thus, for instance, if improved caloric intake by pregnant mothers was accompanied coincidentally by
improved medical care, and it was the medical care which improved
infant survival, one would not find the statistical links between
the intermediary variables linking improved maternal nutrition to
improved infant survival. If the whole chain of indicators are
congruously affected, one can assert that the nutrition or health
has been improved by the intervention or physiologically similar
influences. A decision as to whether or not it was due to the intervention itself depends on adequate statistical design.

The *third strategy* to control for confounding factors is to
measure these and take them into account when analyzing the data
(c.f. Habicht *et al.*, 31). This requires the identification of
the variables possibly confounding in the context of the intervention, and the indicators of outcome which will be evaluated. The
first consideration must depend upon knowledge of the population's
psychological, social, economic and environmental circumstances as
they relate to the intervention and to this population's participation with the intervention. Estimates must then be made of the expected effects of these behavioral and environmental biases on the
indicators. The appropriate measures of the confounding factors or
their proxies can then be chosen.

It is not possible to provide a list of confounding variables
that are relevant in every health or nutrition intervention. At
the bottom of Table II, we list the possible confounding factors
which, in our opinion, could have been measured and evaluated in
the studies reviewed there. Butz and Habicht (37) give a more complete list and discuss methodological considerations that arise in
evaluating their effects.

Table II. SUMMARY OF DESIGN AND INDICATOR CHARACTERISTICS FROM INTERVENTION PROGRAMS IN TABLE I.

References: Year of Publication	(17) (1963)	(18) (1965)	(19) (1967)	(20) (1970)	(11) (1970)	(21) (1970)	(22) (1973)	(23) (1973)	(2) (1977)
I. Choice of Intervention									
a. Unit of Intervention	Vil-lage	Child	Vil-lage	Vil-lage	Vil-lage	Child	?	Child	Child
b. Was choice of type and quality of intervention based on more evidence than dietary survey information?	No	No	Yes	Yes	?	?	Yes	Yes	Yes
II. Control of Intervention									
a. Did intervention reach central distribution center in adequate quantity? (weighed)	Yes	Yes	Yes	Yes	Yes	Yes	Yes	Yes	Yes
quality? (by assay)	Yes	?	Yes	?	?	?	Yes	?	Yes
b. Did intervention reach home by documented record of distribution?	–	Yes	Yes	Yes	–	–	–	Yes	–
c. Did intervention reach target persons in adequate quantity by documented quantitative measurement by: occasional dietary survey?	–	?	Yes	Yes	–	Yes	–	Yes	Yes
frequent record of ingestion of intervention?	Yes	?	No	No	No	Yes	Yes	No	Yes
d. Was replacement effect sought measured adequately and taken into account?	No	No*	Yes	No*	No	Yes	Yes	No	Yes
III. Choice and Measurement of Indicators									
a. Was initial level low for: Diet? Anthropometry? Morbidity? Mortality? Other?		See Table I							
b. Was analysis made of variability due to measurement and short-term intrinsic variability?									
Diet?	No	No	No	No	No	No	No	No	Yes
Anthropometry?	No	No	No	No	No	No	No	No	Yes
Morbidity?	–	No	No	–	–	–	–	–	–
Mortality?	–	–	No	No	–	–	–	–	–
Other?	No	–	–	–	–	–	–	No	–
IV. Control of Confounding Factors									
a. Adequate controls	Yes	Yes	Yes	Yes	No*	No*	?	Yes	No
b. Replication	Some	Yes	No*	Some	No	–	?	Yes	Yes
c. Analysis for Congruity									
Dietary Ingestion?	Yes	No	No	No	No	Yes	No	No	No
Anthropometry?	Yes	Yes	Yes	Yes	Yes	Yes	Yes	Yes	Yes
Morbidity?	–	No	Yes	–	–	–	–	–	–
Mortality?	–	–	No	No	–	–	–	–	–
Other?	Yes	–	–	–	–	–	–	No	–
d. Analysis Stratified by:									
Age	Yes	Yes	Yes	No*	No	No	Yes	No	Yes
Sex	Yes	No	Yes	Yes	No	No	Yes	No	Yes
Dose of Intervention	–	No	No	No	No	No	No	No	Yes
Indicators of Self-selection	No	No	No	No	No*	No*	No	–	Yes
Lactation	–	No	No	No	No	No	No	No	–
Food Supply or Home Diet	No	No	No	No	No	No	No	No	No
Income or Health	No	No	No	No	No	No	No	No	No
Education of mother or other family member	No	No	No	No	No	No	No	No	No
Medical care, disease risk or disease experience	Yes	No	No*	No*	No	No	No	No	No
Secular trend	No	No	Yes*	Yes	No	–	No	–	–

Legend: - = not relevant; ? = not clear in report; * = cause for doubting authors' inferences. Where * is associated with "No", it indicates that we consider this a serious defect which calls into question some or all of the authors' inferences. Where * is associated with "Yes", it indicates that the authors tried to take this into account but we judge either that their methodology was inadequate or that we come to a different inference from the results than they did.

It is important to emphasize that none of these strategies correct experimental design, measurement and analysis for congruence, and measurement and analysis for confounding factors can substitute for each other. They have been presented in their order of importance. There can be no possible useful conclusion without adequate experimental design. Interpretation of positive effects in an outcome indicator must be reinforced by analysis of other indicators for congruity to be persuasive. Analysis of possible confounding factors reinforces the assertion that a change in an indicator of nutritional status was, indeed, due to the intervention and not to some confounding factors (see Table II).

Presentation of Specific Intervention Studies which Tested the Sensitivity of Indicators of Nutritional Status

Tables I. a-e present results from nutrition intervention studies at the individual or population levels directed against protein-calorie malnutrition in preschool children who live at home. These Tables present those variables which have been studied often enough to be tabulated. This is a rather small subset of the many variables proposed for evaluation studies (33-35). Other variables have not been reported frequently enough in intervention literature to be able to ascertain whether they will or will not respond to nutrition intervention programs directed against protein-calorie malnutrition under field conditions.

Where possible, we have tried in Table I. to set limits or maximal ranges within which the indicator is expected to vary. The level seen or recommended in developed countries we call the "best" level. The "worst" level is that which we believe is compatible with survival of the population in its present numbers. 2/

2/ In Table I, the Worst and the Best situations for height, weight and mortality were estimated in the following fashion:
Weight and height: attained and increment: The "best" levels were data taken from a well fed population (15). The "worst" are taken from a compilation (35). In preschool children, measuring the increment from these data produces the same result as measuring the mean increment in children followed longitudinally [see comparative data in Hansman (37)], which is not the case in adolescence.

Mortality: The best levels were those reported to the United Nations Organization (38). The worst levels were taken from our guess based on our experience in underdeveloped countries, where deaths are underreported.

We convert the levels of the indicator before and after intervention to a percent of the physiological range, R, by subtracting
the value of the indicator from the "worst" level and dividing
this difference by the range R to deliver a percentage. Thus, in
Table I.c the first study measured one year increments in weight
(17).

In developed countries this one year increment is 2 kg over the
age period under consideration. Under the "worst" conditions in the
literature the one year increment in boys is 1.6 kg. The range, R,
is 0.4 kg. The control group of boys who received no supplement
gained 1.6 kg per year, no better than the "worst" expected growth.
Their percent of R was therefore (1.6-1.6)/0.4= 0%. The boys who
received the supplement gained 2.1 kg per year. Their percentage
of R was therefore (2.1-1.6)/0.4 = 125%. Thus if the indicator is
already at levels similar to those of developed countries, the percentage of range will approach 100%. If the indicator reflects conditions similar to those worst conditions reported in the literature
the percent of the range will approach 0%. A comparison between the
percentage of the adequacy before the intervention and that after
intervention gives an idea of change during the intervention.

The last column of Table I indicates whether the authors reported a statistically significant change in the indicator subsequent to intervention as compared to a control group. The next step
is to decide whether a negative finding in this column reflects insensitivity of the indicator or ineffectiveness of the nutritional
intervention.

Evidence that the Nutrition Intervention Actually Improved the Diet

Unless a dietary intervention of adequate quality can be shown
to have reached target individuals in sufficient quantity, the failure to find an effect on outcome indicators could be due to an inadequate intervention. Demonstration of adequate quantity of intervention requires that one show that individuals consume an adequate
amount of supplement (Table II. Section II.c), and that this increase
was not lost through a comparable reduction in the usual home diet
consumption. The latter is referred to as dietary substitution
(Table II. Section II.d). Only careful, well-designed surveys en-
tailing large sample sizes of about 600 person-measurements in each
comparison group can discard the possibility of physiologically important substitution of 5% or more of home diet. These calculations
are based on the fact that the day to day variability in the intake
of individuals in malnourished populations has a coefficient of variation of about 35% for protein and calories. Therefore, where the
claim for no substitution effect was made on the basis of small dietary surveys this is considered an inadequate response to the question,

"Was replacement effect sought, measured adequately, and taken into account?" In such cases the estimated "change in intake" is followed by a question mark in Table I.a. This Table presents the dietary intervention data on the nine studies reviewed. Because none of the studies presented age distribution data, we could not estimate minimum protein-energy requirements for survival ("worst" case) or for maximum growth ("best" case) so as to judge how much the intervention would be expected to improve the diet. However, one study reported such a high protein-energy intake before intervention that one wonders whether one could expect any improvement from the intervention (17). For five of the studies the data presented does not permit an estimate of improved dietary intake (see last column). The four studies which adequately measured substitution effects represent interventions which should have resulted in some beneficial outcomes for the participating preschool children inasmuch as the baseline protein and especially the energy intakes were low in all, and the improvement of the protein-energy intake was substantial: from 45% to over 140% of the energy contained in the initial diet. The latter increase seems hardly believable (21). Either the initial diet was not compatible with life or the increase was not compatible with physiological ingestive capacity.

Sensitivity of Height and Weight to Improved Nutrition

Tables I.b and I.c report the outcome indicators of growth in height and weight. Of the five studies in which one could not judge the quantity of the intervention, only one showed any consistent improvement in growth (23). Two others showed inconsistent results. On the other hand all of the four studies which presented adequate evidence of an appropriate nutrition intervention also reported statistically significant increments in growth for preschool children after infancy (2, 19, 21, 22). Of these studies, only one measured infants and this study revealed no improved growth during infancy due to supplementation of the infants or of their lactating mothers. Thus, one may conclude that the outcome indicators of height and weight are sensitive in preschool children to factors associated with the intervention. Martorell, *et al.*, reached the same conclusion in their review of post-infancy growth and protein-calorie supplementation (39).

Whether or not the effect on growth was due solely or even principally to the nutritional component of the intervention must be addressed by examining the adequacy of the control groups, the outcome of analyses for congruity, and inspection of concurrent changes in confounding variables (Table II. Sections IV. a-d). In this context one of the five positive studies selected the intervention group from volunteers and compared that group to non-volunteers (21). The results of the statistical analyses cannot, therefore, be ascribed to the nutrition intervention. Another of these studies reporting positive results is not specific enough concerning its comparison groups for one to be sure they were appropriate, although careful reading of the report inclines one to believe they were (22). A third study has inappropriate comparison groups but presents convincing data to show that the improvement in growth is not due to factors affecting consumption of the supplement (2).

Appropriate comparisons imply adequate estimates of random variability to decide if a difference is significant. One study (19) did not have enough replicate groups to do so; another (22) may have had such replicates, but did not present the necessary analyses for the reader to judge.

Congruity analysis of the five positive studies separately (Table II) results in discarding one (21) as presenting very unlikely results, and the discarding of the infant data in another (19) because the values of growth in height and weight are incompatible with infant physiology. The preschool data in the third (23) presents non-intervention data for weight increments which are so low as to appear incompatible with the survival of a stable population. The response to intervention overshoots normal growth enormously during a period of six months. This data is not, however, so incongruous with present knowledge that we reject it.

From a practical point of view, we conclude that at least certain studies demonstrate that height and weight are sensitive to nutrition intervention programs, especially if measured longitudinally in the same children. In such cases, height is considerably more sensitive to intervention in the sense of producing greater statistical significance than is weight — a fact which we have commented upon elsewhere (49).

Sensitivity of Morbidity and Mortality to Improved Nutrition

Table I.d presents the reported effects on morbidity of nutrition intervention in these studies. The only study (11) which presents evidence of any positive effect of nutrition on illness had comparison groups which were self-selected and could be expected to show this pattern without nutrition intervention. The study most cited (19) as showing a beneficial nutritional effect on mortality does not show it at all in the data as presented in Table I.d, and the argument in the report based upon a change in secular trends is not convincing, especially in view of the lack of replicability in the experimental design. This lack of a beneficial effect on the morbidity of free-living malnourished but ambulatory children corresponds to our findings of a marked effect of disease on child growth but no effect of growth stunting on the incidence of disease (7).

Table I.e presents the reported effect on mortality of nutrition interventions in two studies (19,20). The first of these is the study most cited as showing a beneficial effect on mortality from improved nutrition, but in fact it shows no greater improvement due to nutrition than is evident in one of the comparison groups. Again, the argument made in the report that the nutrition-supplemented group was in some way better is based on secular trends which are not replicated in the experimental design, a defect recognized and mentioned by the authors of these reports and brought to the attention of the reader in one (19:VIII).

Gordon *et al.*, pointed out in reporting on his field study that in developed countries only about 30% of all infant deaths occur after the first months of life (postneonatal), whereas about 60% of all infant deaths are postneonatal in developing countries. However, this ratio of postneonatal to infant mortality is influenced by so many factors that it is probably not useful for evaluation of this type of intervention. For instance, in the village receiving medical care, the ratio worsened from 54% to 69% of postneonatal deaths over all infant deaths at the same time as the total infant death fell from 136 to 88 per 1000 live births.

In the other study (20), data are presented suggesting that infant mortality is improved by nutrition intervention, but the authors could show no effect whatsoever on growth. This lack of congruity makes us believe that the beneficial effect reported was due to other causes, such as differing medical care. In practical terms we must conclude that morbidity and mortality are not sensitive enough indicators to serve as evaluation indicators for the effect of nutrition intervention in preschool children.

Sensitivity of Birthweight and Infant Mortality to Improved Nutrition of the Mother

We have reviewed elsewhere our reasons for believing that birthweight can be a useful indicator to evaluate nutritional intervention in malnourished mothers (26,27). Although many reports in the literature would contradict this belief, we found that these reports either did not substantiate improved dietary intakes or that the studies were done in well-nourished populations (25). Our conversion to thinking that birthweight could reflect individual and aggregate maternal malnutrition in malnourished populations was based on a study which controlled for many confounding factors by experimental design. The distribution curve of birthweight was more affected by maternal supplementation among the lower than among the higher birthweights, which is congruent with a physiological effect associated with supplementation rather than with biases in measurement (8). This study also examined the relative additive and synergistic effects of important influences, including nutrition, on birthweight (41), and explored which confounding factors might explain the association between intervention and outcome (31). This study found congruent dose-responses of the home diet and of the nutritional intervention (27). The dose-response was independent of when and of how long the supplement was consumed during pregnancy (42). This is congruent with efficient maternal storage of energy during pregnancy for use when the energy requirements of the fetus are greatest towards the end of the third trimester. The birthweight was more significantly affected by maternal nutrition than was the length of the newborn, in contradiction to the pattern after birth, but congruent with a transfer of more energy from the better nourished mother to her child towards the end of pregnancy. There is to date only this one study which shows such clear-cut results that birthweight will increase if nutrition is improved in malnourished pregnant women. Belief based on the results of one study border on faith, and corroborative evidence is sorely needed from an independent research team.

This evidence for an effect of maternal malnutrition on infant mortality was vigorously and eruditely denied until the nutrition community came to believe that maternal nutrition affected birthweight on the evidence of the single study reported above. Early data from that study gave some basis for hope that the clear association between low birthweight and infant mortality was mediated by malnutrition, rather than by gestational prematurity, intra-uterine infection or other similar non-nutritional courses (41). Until more definitive data is available, projected estimates of infant lives to be saved by national nutrition programs are premature. In particular it is probable that nutrition intervention which is not coupled with primary medical care (24) will not be cost-effective, nor perhaps even beneficial in terms of improved infant health and well-being (8).

In conclusion to this section, we were amazed at how little competent work has been done in the evaluation of nutrition interventions directed towards remedying protein-energy malnutrition in populations. Before much more can be said about choosing sensitive indicators for such evaluations, more candidate indicators must be tested in careful field intervention studies as described earlier in (A) and (B). This research cannot be accomplished by evaluations of pilot or large-scale interventions because such interventions cannot assure the specificity of response necessary to identify sensitive indicators of nutritional status.

CAN INTEGRATED INTERVENTION PROGRAMS BE EVALUATED?

Our discussion so far has treated issues of measurement and
evaluation of simple interventions: those in which the treatment
consists of only one or a few changes introduced as part of a single intervention. As Table II indicates, successful application of
optimal design and evaluation principles has been rare in areas of
nutrition and health, even when interventions were of this simple
type. These studies could have taken advantage of experimental design techniques for which the standard principles and techniques
were developed.

More often than not, nutrition and health interventions are
not of this simple type. Therefore, we turn now to discuss the
special measurement and evaluation complications that arise in complex integrated interventions in which intentional changes are introduced in medical, nutritional, social, political and economic
factors. Evaluation is complicated immensely in these situations.
The greater the number of factors purposely changed, the more difficult it will be to estimate the separate effect of changes in each
factor on chosen indicator variables. More importantly, replication
of the intervention also will be more complicated.

Setting for Large Scale Integrated Interventions

Before outlining the nature of these measurement and evaluation
difficulties, it is useful to ask why integrated interventions are
becoming popular. Frustration of researchers as well as policy-
makers with the meager results from simpler specific interventions
is probably an important factor. Their frustration is partly due
to several of the problems discussed above leading to failure of
many simple interventions to produce measurable and important changes
in indicators of health and nutrition in individuals and more frequent failure to produce significant results at the population level.

Health and nutrition professionals are also increasingly concerned that very specific interventions may be ineffective within
the same institutional, technological and socio-economic environment that originally led to poor nutrition and health. The concern is well founded in light of the rich interactions that char-
acterize biological, social, economic and agricultural systems in
poor populations. It is clear that nutrition and health outcomes
emerge from these interactions. However, a change introduced as
an intervention may not affect these outcomes if other factors in
the environment are in fact limiting improvements in health and
nutritional status. In addition, individuals can frequently take

advantage of these interactions to turn the effect of an outside
intervention away from that intended to a direction they prefer.

Let us illustrate the biological, socio-economic and agricultural interactions that commonly exist in economically poor environments. Consider that the nutrition and health of a family's members (and, therefore, of a population) in a poor area are influenced by the amounts and types of food produced or transported into
the region, the types and distribution of food storage facilities,
the prices of nutritious and non-nutritious foods, the prices and
availability of medical care, and people's knowledge and beliefs
concerning food and medical care. The family's income and wealth
also directly influence the family members' consumption of food
and their use of traditional and/or modern medical care. In addition, the complex of economic and other factors that influence
how people spend their time can have significant indirect effects
on nutrition and health. As an example, in communities where wom-
en have incentives to work away from home, breast-feeding is less
common and those women with the higher work incentives tend to
lactate the shortest period. These women may also spend less time
in food preparation and home health care. As another example,
changes in the amount of time children spend working and in school
may affect both their own nutritional requirements and the effectiveness of their mothers in meeting these requirements. In poor
populations family members' nutritional status also depends on patterns of food distribution within the family and on determinants
of these patterns. We discuss elsewhere the role of many of these
factors in influencing women's breastfeeding behavior (32).

It is thus clear that nutrition and health are among the many
outcomes of the biological, social, economic and agricultural systems that interact within families and communities. If these systems are equilibrating systems -- that is, if the pattern of observed outcomes reflects an optimal allocation of the family's or
community's resources given the biological, technological and economic conditions that exist -- then particular changes in the environment may, indeed, be ineffective. For example, a particular
intervention may only relax a non-effective constraint. Increasing food grain production will not increase rural people's grain
consumption nor nutritional status if facilities for storing grain
from plentiful to sparse seasons are already inadequate or if the
high cost of transporting the grain to other communities prevents
the farmers from selling their higher production for income. Reducing the price of existing means of storage and transport or introducing new technologies in these areas would enable the community to benefit from increased food production.

Similarly, families may find it in their interest to reduce
their own health- or nutrition-producing activities in response to

an intervention that independently contributes to health or nutrition. A school supplementation program cannot be expected to increase children's food ingestion by the amount of supplementation. Poor parents respond to the school feeding program as though it were a decrease in the effective price of food and therefore encourage their children to consume somewhat more food at school. They then divert resources from children's food to food for other family members and to expenditures on non-food commodities such as shelter or clothing . As long as these substitution possibilities exist, persons can be expected to make use of them in order to increase their perceived benefit from an intervention. The result is a smaller change in the indicator variables than might be expected. The less the people in a community value better health and nutritional status relative to other things, the more they will rearrange the allocation of their resources to transform a nutrition and health intervention into benefits that they value more highly.

For both these reasons there is considerable appeal to shifting from simple interventions of the classic experimental design toward integrated interventions that change a number of conditions thought to be limiting to better nutrition and health. Furthermore, an integrated intervention study may well be the most cost-effective way to elucidate critical facts necessary for effective public health policy for certain important questions.

Approach to Evaluating Integrated Interventions

When intentional changes are introduced in medical, nutritional, social, political and economic factors, evaluation is complicated immensely in these complex interventions. The greater the number of factors purposefully changed, the more difficult it is, in general, to estimate the separate effect of changes in each factor on chosen indicator variables. More importantly, replication of the intervention is also more complex. Finally, if the intervention is unsuccessful, it is more difficult to find out why -- which factors were responsible.

Unfortunately, inadequate formulation, operation, measurement or evaluation results in programs of doubtful benefit and even more doubtful replicability. It is here that a clear perception is necessary as to the nature of the program. Is it an intervention study designed to prove biological relationships between an intervention and outcome in a free-living population whose characteristics are well defined? Alternately, is the program a pilot study which is based upon the proven results of a field intervention study and which tries to accomplish an outcome which is known to be sensitive to the intervention under the expected constraints of a large-scale

public health program?   Or perhaps it may be the large-scale public health program itself.

Formulating a comprehensive intervention requires considerably
more knowledge about the structure of the complex system from which
people's nutritional status and health emerge than does formulating
a simple experimental design. In addition to following the important considerations discussed in previous sections, designers of
integrated interventions must also use procedures that maximize the
probability that the set of chosen interventions has a significant
effect on the indicators while simultaneously minimizing the losses from undesirable side effects -- and do this all on a budget.

The first goal is not so difficult. The list of things caus-
ally associated with good health and nutrition is long, and we know
how to change many of these things, from food production and distribution to water, sewage, and hygiene. By intervening in enough ways,
a significant result is nearly guaranteed. The evidence is all
around, however, that significant undesirable side effects are nearly impossible to avoid in large interventions, and often very difficult to measure. Our limited scientific understanding of the
linkages within and among biological, behavioral and agricultural
systems does not facilitate identification of the many outcomes
that may be affected by a single change in the environment, much
less by multiple changes. These issues as well as the identification of promising integrated interventions, can only be determined
by rigorous intervention studies. Only these will reveal integrated
interventions that are likely to succeed within the resources available to public health programs. Intervention studies and pilot programs will reveal the initial outcome variables and side effects
which must be measured in the evaluation of large-scale integrated
public health programs.

After an integrated intervention has been formulated and tested
in field studies, additional problems will arise during its operation
as a pilot study. Chief among these is the temptation, sometimes
explicitly encouraged, to alter the set of interventions in mid-
course as experience accumulates. The decision is admittedly a difficult one. If it is clear that an additional change should have
been added to the intervention set based on the emerging data concerning limiting conditions or the efficacy of the existing intervention, one would like to make the indicated change for the duration of the intervention. Similarly, the initial intervention set
may have been well formulated, but conditions have changed, due
either to natural responses to the intervention or to independent
changes in the environment. Making the indicated change in mid-
course increases the expected change in the indicator variables.
The result of such an operational change is to hamper the measuring of the experimental treatment and of evaluating the intervention.

The cost of the pilot study which revealed these deficiencies will, however, have been small in comparison to making these mistakes in the course of a large-scale public health program. And another pilot public health program can substantiate that the new integrated intervention is replicable and cost-effective.

    Another pitfall in the operation of integrated interventions arises when part of the intervention consists of political, social or educational activities intended to organize people or redirect their attention toward goals of the intervention. The exact nature of such interventions invariably shifts and adjusts as the intervention proceeds, making it very difficult to measure and keep track of just what the intervention was at particular times. Even if accurate records are kept, evaluation of these parts of the intervention and possibly of the entire effort is in jeopardy because the form of the intervention has become endogenous and dependent on the population's responses. How then can one examine these or related responses to evaluate the effectiveness of the intervention? In addition, political and social interventions are very difficult to replicate since, among other reasons, their outcomes generally depend on personalities and activities of the persons who are intervening. Hence, replicating the treatment across villages in the experimental design, as recommended above, is difficult. Replicating it later in other sites is even *more* difficult. However, adequate knowledge about the crucial linkages acquired through intervention studies and substantiation of the replication in pilot studies will increase the likelihood that the large-scale intervention will be successful and be adequately evaluated and monitored for maximum cost-effectiveness.

    Proper experimental design is critically important in the case of complex integrated interventions. For simple experiments there is the possibility of making inferences about cause and effect through multivariate statistical analyses if the design is flawed, as long as most conditions in the population have stayed static. When many factors are intentionally changed, on the other hand, inadequate replication and controls leave one unable to untangle the mass of changes and make statements about nutrition and health effects due to the intervention. This problem is exacerbated if the effects of the components of the intervention are not additive. Indeed, one generally acts as if they are not, since one generally tries to combine complementary interventions in the hopes that their result will be greater than the simple addition of their effects (synergistic action).

    In our opinion, the evidence that many kinds of behavioral and biological processes are interrelated does not imply the conclusion that interventions must be broad and complex to produce lasting changes in health and nutrition indicators. The implication

instead, is that the specific interventions chosen must be those
that change the conditions -- institutional, economic, biological --
that are limiting in a particular setting. By changing specific
conditions in different experimental settings, by formulating the
experiments wisely, and by measuring the treatments, major confounding factors, and indicator variables intelligently, we can accumulate understanding of the relevant mechanisms and the particular
interventions that are effective in specific settings.

One should design the integrated intervention studies so that
this synergistic effect is sufficiently understood so that it can
be applied cost-effectively. For instance, perhaps one wishes to
know which combination of medical care, environmental sanitation,
nutrition education, and food subsidies will result in cost-effective
results in health. Single-purpose intervention studies such as
those reviewed earlier, will have delivered the best indicators for
improvements in health and nutrition. By using these indicators to
evaluate different combinations of interventions one can evaluate
new additions to previous combinations, beginning with the least
expensive and most feasible first, and progressing to more expensive additions later, until the benefits no longer justify further
increments in cost. This procedure will not permit a teasing out
of the synergistic from the additive effects of the intervention,
but will reveal a good candidate for pilot testing and ultimately
for large-scale intervention. The alternative is complex large-
scale interventions that are costly to operate, costlier to replicate on a national scale, and from which little can be learned if
the intervention fails and nothing can be safely changed in the
future if it succeeds.

CONCLUSION

We conclude that an indicator must be sensitive to the intervention and be specific for that intervention. Knowledge about
sensitivity must come from single purpose intervention studies.
In these studies specificity of the indicator's response to nutrition is assured by controlling non-nutritional influences through
intervention, experimental design and statistical analyses. The
procedures, therefore, are clear for amassing the knowledge necessary
to implement and evaluate the nutritional and health impact of large-
scale integrated public health programs. It is distressing that we
have followed this procedure so little that most of the crucial indicators necessary for evaluation of interventions have not even
been properly tested. In particular, only height and weight have
been reliably shown to be sensitive to improved protein-calorie
nutrition in preschool children, and height is more sensitive than
weight. Birthweight as an indicator of maternal nutrition has so
far only been shown to be sensitive to improved nutrition in one

study -- this finding must be replicated before it can be generalized. Morbidity and mortality appear to be poor and insensitive
indicators of nutritional status in the preschool years, although
infant mortality may utlimately prove to be a useful indicator
where medical care is otherwise adequate.

The little experience to date in testing these very few of
the many indicators suggested for evaluation should be a warning
that pronouncements, even by renowned authorities, cannot replace
validation by single purpose intervention studies. Relaxing "scientific" constraints to recommend the continued use of "commonly
used" but unvalidated indicators will only result in falsely negative evaluations of valuable and useful programs. It would be better to recognize our limited knowledge about useful indicators and
to use them gingerly when we must do so now. We should proceed as
quickly as possible to focus single purpose intervention studies
to validate "commonly used" indicators and to develop other better
indicators.

ACKNOWLEDGEMENT

This is a report of research of the Cornell University Agricultural Experimental Station, Division of Nutritional Sciences.

REFERENCES

1. Habicht, J-P., and M. C. Latham. Ethics of population research
   in population. (Submitted for publication).
2. Yarbrough, C., J-P. Habicht, R. E. Klein, *et al*. Response of
   indicators of nutritional status to nutritional interventions in populations and individuals. In: S. J. Bosch
   and J. Arias (eds.). *Evaluation of Child Health Services: The Interface Between Research and Medical Practice*.
   DHEW Publication No. (NIH) 78-1066. Washington, D. C.:
   U. S. Government Printing Office, 1977. pp. 195-206.
3. Scrimshaw, N. S., and M. Béhar. Malnutrition in underdeveloped
   countries. *New Engl. J. Med.*, Part I. 272: 137-144, 1965;
   Part II, *ibid.* 272: 193-198, 1965.
4. McClure, F. J. *Fluoride in Drinking Water*. U. S. Public
   Health Service Publication No. 825. Washington, D. C.:
   U. S. Government Printing Office, 1962.
5. Habicht, J-P., J. M. Lane, and A. J. McDowell. National nutrition surveillance. *Fed. Proc.*, (in press).
6. El Lozy, M., and G. R. Kerr. Results of lysine fortification
   of wheat products in southern Tunisia. pp. 113-133. In:
   H. L. Wilcke, (ed.). *Improving the Nutrient Quality of
   Cereals*. Washington, D. C.: U. S. Agency for International Development, 1977.

7. Martorell, R. *Illness and Incremental Growth in Young Guatemalan Children.* Ph.D dissertation. Seattle: University of Washington, 1973.

8. Habicht, J-P., A. Lechtig, C. Yarbrough, and R. E. Klein. Maternal nutrition, birth weight and infant mortality. pp. 353-378. In: K. Elliott, and J. Knight, (eds.). *Size at Birth.* CIBA Foundation Symposium 27, London: Elsevier, 1974.

9. Habicht, J-P., and C. Yarbrough. Growth monitoring and nutritional assessment: antrhopometric field methods; criteria for selection. In: R. Alfin-Slater, and D. Kritchvsky, (eds.). *Nutrition: A Comprehensive Treatise.* New York: Plenum Press, (in press).

10. Habicht, J-P. Estandarización de métodos epidemiológicos cuantitativos sobre el terreno. *Bol. Of. San. Pan.,* 76: 375-384, 1974.

11. Swaminathan, M. C., D. H. Rao, R. V. Rao, *et al.* An evaluation of the supplementary feeding programmes for preschool children in the rural areas around Hyderabad City. *Indian J. Nutr. Dietet.,* 7: 342-350, 1970.

12. World Health Organization. *Methodology of Nutrition Surveillance. Report of a Joint FAO/UNICEF/WHO Expert Committee* WHO Technical Report Series No. 593. Geneva: World Health Organization, 1976.

13. Galen, R. S., and S. R. Gambino. *Beyond Normality: The Predictive Value and Efficiency of Medical Diagnoses.* New York: Wiley & Sons, 1975.

14. Yarbrough, C., J-P. Habicht, R. Malina, *et al.* Length and weight in rural Guatemalan ladino children: birth to seven years of age. *Am. J. Phys. Anthropol.,* 42: 439-447, 1975.

15. National Center for Health Statistics. 1976 NCHS Growth Charts. *Monthly Vital Statistics Report,* 25(3) Supplement, 1977.

16. Myers, L., J-P. Habicht, and C. Johnson. Components of the difference between black and white women in the USA of hemoglobin concentration in blood. *Am. J. Epidemiol.,* 1979.

17. King, K. W., W. H. Sebrell Jr., E. L. Severinghous, *et al.* Lysine fortification for wheat bread fed to Haitian school children. *Am. J. Clin. Nutr.,* 12: 36-48, 1963.

18. Bancroft, T., and K. V. Bailey. Supplementary feeding trial in New Guinea highland infants. *J. Trop. Pediat.,* 11: 28-34, 1965.

19. Series of articles written with various coauthors by Gordon, J. E., N. S. Scrimshaw, M. A. Guzmán, M. Béhar, and W. Ascoli with alternating first authorship: Nutrition and infection field study in Guatemalan villages. Guatemala: Institute of Nutrition of Central America and Panama, (INCAP), 1959-1964.
    I. Study plan and experimental design. *Arch. Environ. Health,* 14: 657-662, 1967; II. Field reconaissance,

administrative and technical; study area; population
characteristics; and organization for field activities.
Arch. Environ. Health., 14: 787-801, 1967; III. Field
procedure, collection of data and methods of measurement.
Arch. Environ. Health., 15: 6-15, 1967; IV. Deaths of
infants and preschool children. *Arch. Environ. Health*,
15: 439-449, 1967; V. Disease incidence in preschool
children under natural village conditions, with improved
diet, and with medical and public health services. *Arch.
Environ. Health*, 16: 223-234, 1968; VI. Acute diarrheal
disease and nutritional disorders in general disease incidence. *Arch. Environ. Health*, 16: 424-437, 1968; VII.
Physical growth and development of preschool children.
Arch. Environ. Health, 17: 107-118, 1968; VIII. An epidemiological appraisal of its wisdom and its errors.
Arch. Environ. Health, 17: 814-827, 1968; IX. An evaluation of medical, social, and public health benefits,
with suggestions for future field study. *Arch. Environ.
Health*, 18: 51-52, 1969.

20. Baertl, J. M., E. Morales, G. Verastegui, and G. G. Graham.
    Diet supplementation for entire communities. Growth and
    mortality of infants and children. *Am. J. Clin. Nutr.*,
    23: 707-715, 1970.

21. Kamalanathan, G., G. Nalinakshi, and R. P. Devadas. Effect of
    a blend of protein foods on the nutritional status of
    preschool children in a rural balwadi. *Indian J. Nutr.
    Dietet.*, 7: 288-292, 1970.

22. Gopalan, C., M. C. Swaminathan, V. K. Srishna Kumari, *et al.*
    Effect of calorie supplementation on growth of undernour-
    ished children. *Am. J. Clin. Nutr.*, 26: 563-566, 1973.

23. Rajalakshmi, R., S. S. Sail, D. G. Shar, and S. K. Ambody.
    The effects of supplements varying in carotene and calcium
    content on the physical, biochemical and skeletal status
    of preschool children. *Brit. J. Nutr.*, 30: 77-86, 1973.

24. Habicht, J-P., and Working Group on Rural Medical Care. Deli-
    very or primary care by medical auxiliaries: Techniques
    of use and analysis of benefits achieved in some rural
    villages in Guatemala. pp. 24-37. In: *Medical Auxil-
    iaries*. PAHO Scientific Publication No. 278. Washington,
    D.C.: Pan American Health Organization, 1973.

25. Lechtig, A., G. Arroyave, J-P. Habicht, and M. Béhar. Nutri-
    ción materna y crecimiento fetal. *Arch. Latinoamer. Nutr.*,
    21: 505-530, 1971.

26. Lechtig, A., J-P. Habicht, C. Yarbrough, *et al.* Influence of
    food supplementation during pregnancy on birth weight in
    rural populations of Guatemala. pp. 44-52. In: A. Chá-
    vez, H. Bourges, and S. Basta, (eds.). *Nutrition. Vol.
    2.* Basel: S. Karger, 1975.

27. Lechtig, A., J-P. Habicht, H. Delgado, *et al.* Effect of food
    supplementation during pregnancy on birthweight. *Pedia-*

trics, <u>56</u>: 508-520, 1975.

28. Federer, W. T. *Experimental Design*. New York: MacMillan, 1963.
29. Davis, C. E. The effect of regression to the mean in epidemiologic and clinical studies. *Am. J. Epidemiol.*, <u>104</u>: 493-498, 1976.
30. Habicht, J-P., C. Yarbrough, and R. E. Klein. Assessing nutritional status in a field study of malnutrition and mental development: specificity, sesitivity, and congruity of indices of nutritional status. pp. 35-42. In: J. Cravioto, L. Hambraeus, and B. Vahlqvist, (eds.). *Early Malnutrition and Mental Development*. Symposia of the Swedish Foundation, Vol. XII. Uppsala: Almqvist and Wiksells, 1974.
31. Habicht, J-P., C. Yarbrough, A. Lechtig, and R. E. Klein. Relation of maternal supplementary feeding during pregnancy to birth weight and other sociobiological factors. pp. 127-145. In: M. Winick, (ed.). *Nutrition and Fetal Development*. New York: Wiley Interscience, 1974.
32. Butz, W. P., and J-P. Habicht. The effects of nutrition and health on fertility: hypotheses, evidence and interventions. pp. 210-238. In: R. G. Ridker, (ed.). *Population and Development*. Baltimore: Johns Hopkins University Press, 1976.
33. Jelliffe, D. B. *The Assessment of the Nutritional Status of the Community (With Special Reference to Field Surveys in Developing Regions of the World)*. pp. 3-27. WHO Monograph Series No. 53. Geneva: World Health Organization, 1966.
34. Gordon, J. E., and N. S. Scrimshaw. Field evaluation of nutrition intervention programs. *World Rev. Nutr. Diet.*, <u>17</u>: 1-38, 1973.
35. Beaton, G. H., and J. M. Bengoa. *Nutrition in Preventive Medicine*. WHO Monograph Series No. 62. Geneva: World Health Organization, 1976.
36. Habicht, J-P., R. Martorell, C. Yarbrough, *et al*. Height and weight standards for preschool children. *Lancet*, <u>1</u>: 611-615, 1974.
37. Hansman, C. Anthropometry and related data. pp. 101-154. In: R. W. McCammon, and V. E. Beales, (eds.). *Human Growth and Development*. Springfield: Charles C. Thomas, 1970.
38. United Nations. *Demographic Yearbook 1974*. New York: United Nations, 1975.
39. Martorell, R., A. Lechtig, C. Yarbrough, *et al*. Protein-calorie supplementation and postnatal physical growth: a review of findings from developing countries. *Arch. Latinoamer. Nutr.*, <u>26</u>: 115-128, 1976.
40. Yarbrough, C., J-P. Habicht, R. Martorell, *et al*. Anthropometry as an index of nutritional status. *Adv. Exp. Med. Biol.*, <u>49</u>: 15-26, 1974.
41. Habicht, J-P., C. Yarbrough, A. Lechtig, and R. E. Klein. Relationships of birthweight, maternal nutrition and infant mortality. *Nutr. Rep. Int.*, <u>7</u>: 533-546, 1973.

42.   Habicht, J-P., A. Lechtig, C. Yarbrough, and R. E. Klein. The
      effect on birth weight of timing of supplementation during
      pregnancy. p. 71. In: P. Arroyo *et al.*, (eds.). *Suma-
      ria - IX International Congress of Nutrition*. Mexico,
      1972.

COMMENTS

A. Pradilla, *Fundación para la Educación Superior*
*Cali, Colombia**

L. F. Fajardo, and G. Acciarri, *Universidad del Valle*
Cali, Colombia

INTRODUCTION

It is apparent that many health and nutrition interventions
are made without recognition or clear definition of the ways they
should produce an impact. Often they are based on general impres-
sions such as "to give food is good", "to have a Health Center is
good", "to have one doctor per 1000 inhabitants is good", with the
expectation that these activities will have beneficial impacts. In
a sense, the reaction is "to do things" instead of determining what
the problem is and what is necessary to solve it. For instance,
national goals for decreasing malnutrition often are based on recu-
peration centers which cover at best 10% of all malnourished people.
Similarly, goals for decreasing the prevalence of diarrhea are
implemented by increasing the number of health centers and hospitals
in systems where not more than 25% of the population has any access
to them. It becomes difficult to evaluate programs such as these
without a clear understanding of the problems they were designed to
solve.

As an alternative to the "shotgun" or "do good" approach to
large-scale interventions, many people emphasize the value of pilot research programs to precede national or regional programs.
Most well-designed pilot interventions have a positive effect or
produce instructive data. However, success in a pilot research
area is very often impossible to replicate in large-scale service
programs. Usually the pilot project controls several variables
that are not easily controlled in the real world. Workers in a
research project are selected primarily for their demonstrated capabilities; this may not be possible in real life where political
and social characteristics may influence their selection. Important decisions are made unilaterally in the pilot project, whereas
in a public health program, decisions cannot be taken without previous consultation with the many others who may be involved. Thus,

*Mailing adress: c/o World Health Organization, G.P.O. Box 250
Dacca, Bangladesh

it is highly desirable to learn as much as possible from real life
experiments (national interventions) by means of careful evaluation
of the process by which a program fails or succeeds.

Another problem causing difficulties, not only in the implementation of health and nutrition programs but also in their evaluation, arises from the necessarily vague definitions of the abstract terms health, well-being, and nutrition. These terms must
be considered dynamic closely associated to prior history and current environment, and thus very difficult to quantify for purposes
of evaluating the effects of interventions. However, if health,
nutrition or well-being are taken as the sum of more concrete components, it becomes possible to describe the flow of activities,
tasks, functions, and their check-points with appropriate indicators which will quantify and measure impact and explain the reasons
for success or failure. For the purpose of evaluation, then, health
in developing countries could be defined as the lack of intestinal
infection and preventable diseases which in turn are often important components of nutritional status. Thus, nutritional status
is a function of several variables which must be defined specifically for different circumstances and is not synonymous with feeding or food consumption alone.

Many of the critical issues of indicators and experimental design for pilot projects are fully described in several of the other
presentations in this volume. Habicht and Butz in particular have
provided a detailed and thoroughful analysis of potential indicators of nutritional status. In our discussion, we will emphasize
only the points referring to the evaluation of large-scale governmental interventions, as emphasized in experiences we have had in
Colombia.

ESTABLISHING A CAUSE-EFFECT RELATIONSHIP BETWEEN AN INTERVENTION
              AND THE CHANGES IN THE MEASURED VARIABLES

The central role of evaluation is to assess the results from
a given set of interventions. If only the design and organization
of a program can be studied, evaluation becomes meaningless. Planning and evaluating an intervention requires understanding of the
pre-existing situation and the associated factors (causal diagnosis),
the needs to be met by the intervention, a detailed account of the
components of the program, a theoretical analysis of what results
can and cannot be expected of a given intervention, an indentifi-
cation of the intermediate outputs necessary to reach the stated
goal, and the selection of appropriate indicators of success or
failure. The following scheme (Figure 1), summarizes the process
of evaluation which is being followed by the Nutrition Group, at
the Fundación para la Educación Superior (FES).

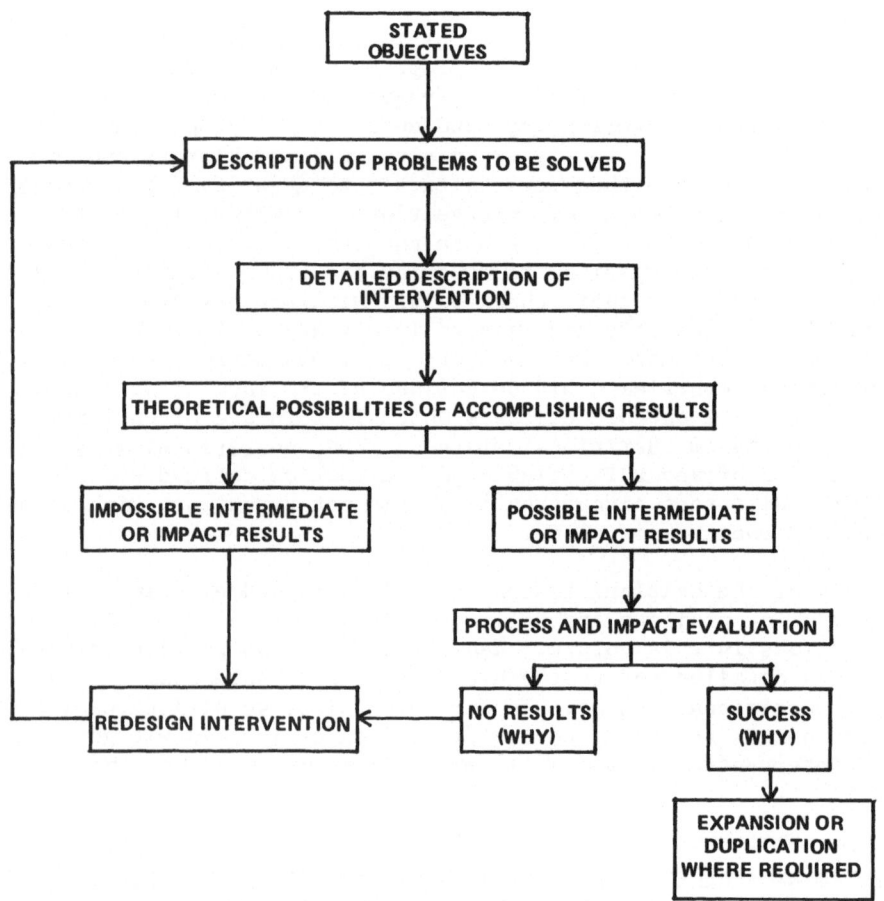

FIG. 1. Evaluation scheme

Ideally, the choice of interventions should follow the same method.
The utilization of conceptual or epidemiological models based on
known or derived associations will facilitate planning and evaluating for both simple and integrated interventions, as the latter
represents the sum of simpler ones.

The epidemiology of most common diseases is well understood today although the exact weight for some modifier variables requires more investigation.

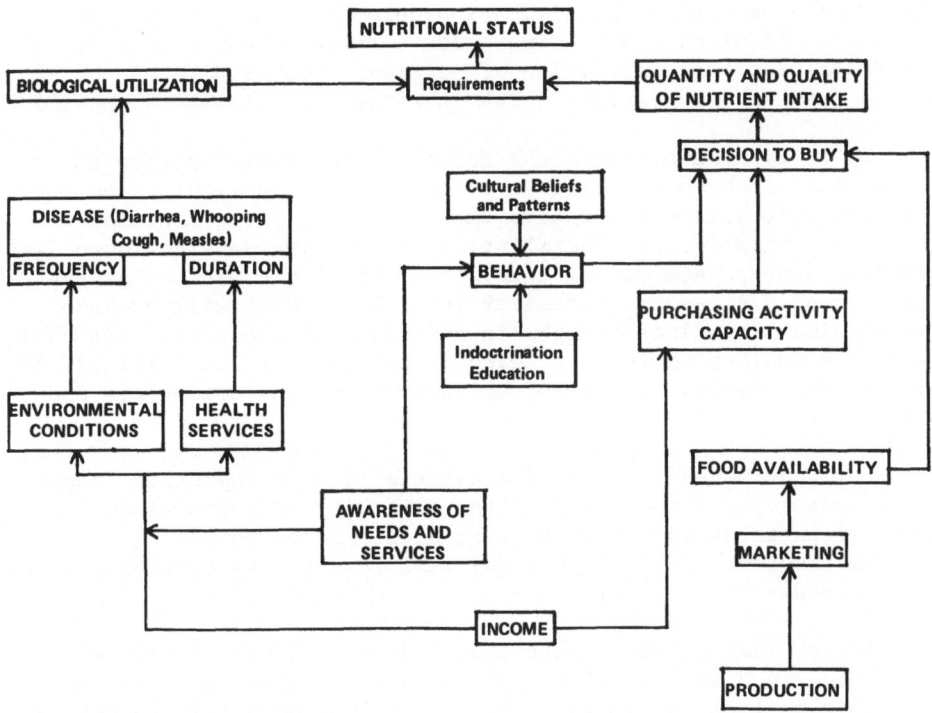

FIG. 2 *Conceptual model for nutritional status*

A comparable conceptual model for nutrition is presented in Figure 2 as it has been used for nutrition assessment in some countries (1), and for a proposed continuous evaluation of an integrated nutrition plan in Colombia (2). The model has served as a diagnostic tool which, when contrasted with proposed interventions, allows a prediction of possible and impossible outcomes. Also, by the definition of the restrictions for the accomplishment of a given result, it aids in selecting indicators for measuring the intermediate outputs and outcomes.

In this simplified model nutrition is presented as a function
of food intake and biological utilization of food. The former is
a function of purchasing capacity, food availability and culture.
For example, food programs exert their effects primarily through
food availability and augmentation of income. Only when appropriate changes in consumption behavior are made by the individual or
groups may the effects be attributed directly to food intake. On
the other hand, if the nutritional problem is caused by a high
prevalence of disease which increases nutrient requirements or decreases biological utilization of nutrients, no results can be expected from an intervention which increases food intake alone (3).

By fully understanding the nature of activities during an intervention, it becomes possible to define the intermediate outputs,
identify appropriate indicators and the timing for collection of
them. For example, the installation of curative services associated
with the appropriate use of them by a community could change the
duration of disease and mortality (4), although it will produce
only minimal immediate changes in nutritional status (5). In this
case, the indicators must be selected to quantify accessibility of
the health service, the use of the service by the community, and
mortality.

Low and inadequate use of available service indicates inappropriate service for the needs of the community or cultural and behavioral patterns that must be evaluated and reconciled in redesign-
ing the program. Only in this way will long-term nutritional gains
be achieved.

Direct indicators of nutritional status which are available
and needed in research pilot projects become laborious and costly
to obtain in large programs. It is sometimes necessary to rely on
indirect indicators of probability or risk. A large amount of data
is usually collected in most countries which permits development of
indicators and indices measuring probabilities of communities for
specific risks. Abnormal response to a given intervention calls
for specific surveys to explain it. It is perhaps in this area of
indicator responses and the relationships between concrete variables
where more research is needed.

CONVERTING THEORY INTO PRACTICE

In the past several years, the Nutrition Project at The Universidad del Valle and F.E.S. has been concerned with the development of a model for evaluating the impact of nutrition and related
health programs. A more complete report of it is available elsewhere, however, it may be helpful to discuss it briefly in this
presentation.

This organizational system, called the Nutrient Flow Model, may be described in sections, the first of which consists of three variables: nutritional status, health status, and the nutrition gap. These three variables are interrelated as shown in Figure 3.

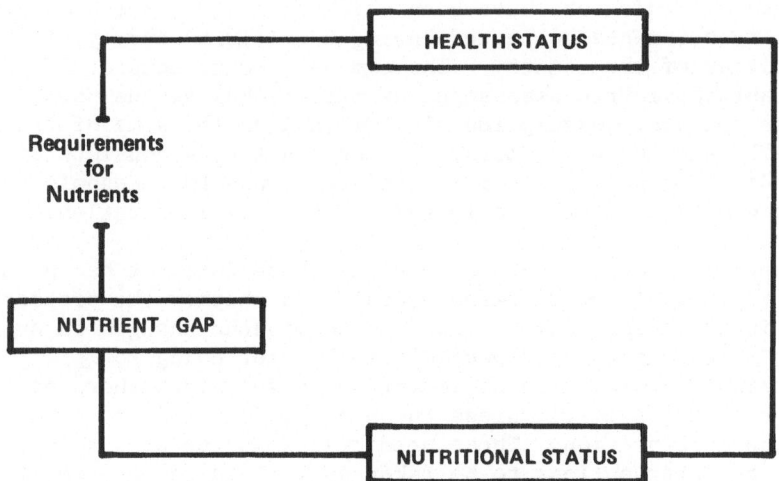

FIG. 3 *Nutrient flow model*

This model simply states that nutritional status is a function of the nutrient gap (the difference between requirements for nutrients and consumption of nutrients) and of health status. In theory, a reduction in the nutrient gap will improve health status, and improved health status will reduce overall nutrient requirements. The reduction in nutrient requirements for one cycle leads to a further reduction in nutrient gap, etc. for another cycle.

The utilization of this framework is currently being explored in the development of a national food and nutrition surveillance system for Colombia. Key to the Colombian system is the use of existing data resources to minimize cost, combining these data into appropriate indices or indicators that will serve both diagnostic and evaluative purposes. Analyses of these data will provide a basis for close monitoring of any changes over time as social programs are implemented as part of the National Nutrition Plan.

The Colombian National Nutrition Plan consists of four separate activities: a) food supplements to pregnant women and infants; b) distribution of food coupons; c) extension of simple

preventive health care; and d) integrated rural development projects designed to increase family income. These are to be implemented singly or in combinations in different areas of the country.

In the preliminary stages of planning the surveillance system,
two sources of indicators have been utilized. The first consists
of direct measurements collected during nutritional surveys in 54
municipalities of the country. These measurements consist of clinical and anthropometric assessment of nutritional status, health
conditions and food consumption along with data for some of the related family and social factors. The second source consists of indirect indicators derived from agricultural, health, economic and
demographic data regularly collected by official institutions.

By applying the conceptual model to these data, it has been
possible to predict for different localities whether the proposed
official interventions may be expected to produce changes in nutritional status, and the expected time lag for doing so; i.e.,
food distribution will have no impact in those places where poor
health conditions prevail unless these conditions are improved as
part of the intervention. These predictions may be used to guide
the types of interventions to be taken as well as the nature of
the evaluation performed. These in turn will verify the correctness
of the underlying assumptions. In the long run, such conceptual
approaches to planning and evaluation will contribute to improved
services to families and to populations.

An example will be presented here to illustrate how these predictions may be made. The relationship between nutritional status
of a population segment, average dietary intake in the population,
and infection rate in that population or community conforms to the
following equation (derived from data from longitudinal studies in
Colombia):

$$N = B_o + B_i \times \frac{1}{R(p)}$$

N = nutritional status

B_o= constant proportional to the minimum requirements to maintain life in the population in
question.

B_i= estimate of biological utilization under the
cultural and environmental conditions of the
community.

$R(p)$= nutrient requirements (R) as a function of the probability of being infected (p).

I = intake

Simple examination of the equation indicates that when (p) is very high it will not be possible to change N by increasing intake (I) alone. This can be graphically presented in Figure 4.

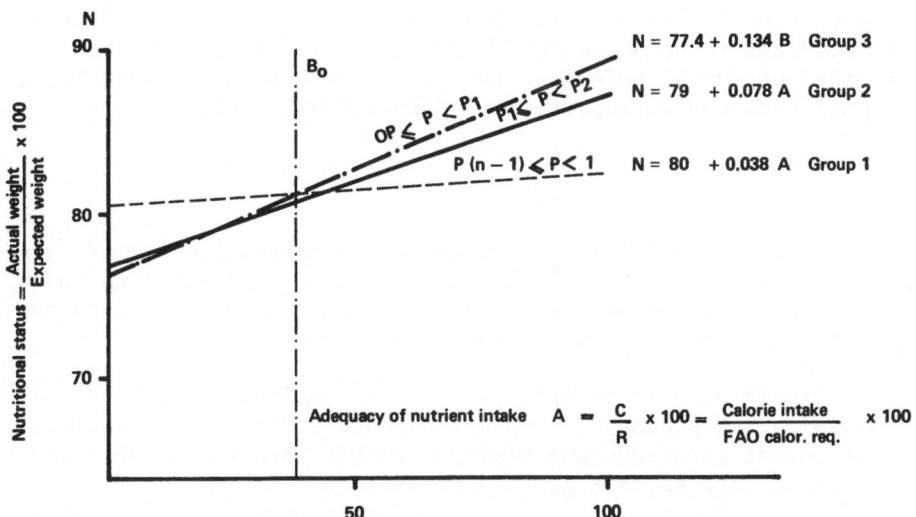

FIG.4 *Relationships between nutritional status and adequacy of nutrient intake as a function of Infection.* (See text for explanation of symbols and groups).

For this presentation data from twelve municipalities were used. The municipalities were divided into three groups based upon morbidity data and the quality of sanitation. Group 1 had the worst conditions (higher p), and Group 3 had the best conditions (lower p).

Graphically, it can be seen in Figure 4 that for Group 1 it is impossible to improve nutritional status by increasing nutrient intake alone (slope 0), thus the food distribution intervention will not show any nutritional impact. Failure in this case would not be due to a "bad program" but to the fact that this program was not directed to the real problem. In Group 3, nutritional change would be expected with the same program (e.g.nutritional supplements). Changes in nutritional status in Group 2 could result either from food supplementation or improved health care. Thus, no change would be interpreted as a result of failure in design or execution of the program. These alternate explanations would be sought by exploring other indirect indicators available in the surveillance system.

In undertaking evaluation, the indicators must be selected depending on the specific process being analyzed. In certain cases, the information is required for the community as a whole, in others it is necessary to select specific families or individuals. Here again, the conceptual model can facilitate selection of indicators, their analysis, and interpretation of resultant changes.

CONCLUSIONS

1. It often is helpful to define the terms health,nutritional status and well-being as the sum of many factors and conditions which are more concrete and measurable. Evaluation will need to be designed using these quantitative measures.

2. For simple as well as integrated interventions the use of epidemiological schemes or conceptual models serves to illuminate the causal processes underlying a problem and to indicate the expected effects of a given intervention.

3. Direct or indirect indicators can be selected for the evaluation based on the conceptual model and the anticipated operational and impact outputs.

4. Evaluation must adapt itself to reality. Impact and process evaluation is meaningless if it cannot explain the reasons for failures and success.

5. Pilot projects have an important role in the development of indicators and in increasing our understanding of the relationships among a variety of program factors. On the other hand, government programs present opportunities for process and impact evaluations and thus represent a very important tool for testing the applicability and shortcomings of existing knowledge.

REFERENCES

1. Pradilla, A., M. T. Menchú, J. del Canto, and V. W. Bent. Planificación de las actividades de nutrición a nivel de los servicios descentralizados de salud. pp. 33-45. In: J. Aranda-Pastor, and B. Breuer, (eds.). *Programas de Nutrición en los Servicios Descentralizados de Salud en América Central.* (Seminario Sub-Regional, 1975). Guatemala: Talleres Gráficos del INCAP, 1978.

2. Pradilla, A., I. Beghin, J. del Canto, *et al.* Modelos interpretativos para la selección de prioridades en nutrición. Nivel nacional. *Arch. Latinoamer. Nutr.,* 27 (Suplemento 1): 89-107, 1977.

3. Acciarri, G., D. Wilson, J. Eckroad, *et al.* Requerimientos nutricionales y saneamiento ambiental. Presented at: *IV Congreso Latinoamericano de Nutrición, Caracas, Noviembre, 1976.*

4. Habicht, J-P., and Working Group on Rural Medical Care. Delivery of primary care by medical auxiliaries: techniques of use and analysis of benefits achieved in some rural villages in Guatemala. pp. 24-37. In: *Medical Auxiliaries.* Scientific Publication No. 278. Washington, D.C.: Pan American Health Organization, 1973.

5. Mata, L. J. *The Children of Santa María Cauqué: A Prospective Field Study of Health and Growth.* Cambridge, Mass.: The M.I.T. Press, 1978.

GENERAL DISCUSSION

The discussion opened with a recapitulation that there are a number of widely accepted indicators of protein-energy malnutrition in preschool children: height, weight, arm and head circumferences, skinfold, weight/height ratio, morbidity, mortality, and rates of clinical malnutrition (e.g., Gómez classification). Four of these (height, weight, mortality and morbidity) have been explored as to whether they respond directly to changes in nutritional status under field conditions; only height and weight have been proven to have a direct relationship. It is possible that the other two may relate also but long periods of time (5-10 years) will be necessary to demonstrate this relationship. In any given situation, however, any indicator may be appropriately used if it satisfies the following criteria: 1) it responds to the type of intervention under study; 2) it is sensitive to nutritional change over the range expected in the field setting; and, 3) it is responsive primarily to nutritional factors, or the confounding contributors are understood.

Dr. Habicht noted that his presentation dealt primarily with indicators of nutritional status in preschool children. He was in agreement with other participants in the conference that birthweight is a good indicator of maternal nutritional status, at least in populations with a high prevalence of low birthweight. Even here, however, it is necessary to know some background characteristics of the mother, the sex of the infant, etc., to use these data correctly. More research is clearly needed. It is highly probable that infant mortality may also serve as a useful indicator of maternal and infant malnutrition but the evidence is not yet complete. In fact, a major problem facing evaluators today is that much of the basic research relating early variations in indicators of nutritional status with later outcomes has not been done. There is an urgent need to do such research with the best available current techniques.

In using anthropometric measures, much concern centers around which standards to use. The FAO/WHO height and weight standards are widely employed. Depending upon which height or weight standards are selected, politicians may claim more or less of a problem or need for interventions. In this context it must be emphasized that improved nutrition is more than merely increased height or weight; it has much wider functional or social significance for the well-being of people. Finally, it is important to recognize the educational value of height and weight data in working with mothers of young children, as a demonstration of progress or change.

In some countries and populations, indicators of iron nutrition, for example, are needed as there are major nutritional problems independent of height and weight. Thus, different indicators may well be needed for different communities or individuals.

It is readily recognized that health interventions rarely are univariate, and yet they may well impact directly or indirectly on nutritional status so that the latter may serve as a useful though crude measure of impact. To illustrate this, a conceptual model (Table I), was presented to illustrate the evaluation of the expected nutritional impact following the introduction of potable water. A comparable conceptualization could be utilized with immunization, preventive medical care, or other programs.

This model shows that one should not only evaluate the intervention and the final outcome but also many of the intermediate steps between the intervention and the outcome. Some of these steps are clearly related to administrative activities but others could be considered, in other circumstances, ultimate outputs in their own right.

At the beginning of the project it is necessary to identify the appropriate indicators of nutritional status which should be

Table I. *VARIABLES TO BE MEASURED IN ASSESSING THE IMPACT OF*
          INTRODUCTION OF POTABLE WATER

Steps in Evaluation Process	Items to be Evaluated
Assessment = Diagnosis	Indicators of nutritional status Existing water resources Environmental factors
Evaluation of resources and structure	New resources and administrative structures needed to attain goals
Projection of activities to meet goals	Training, funding, building and services required
Planned results:	
Units produced	Personnel, pipes laid, water purification centers built
Coverage + quality	% population covered, volume and quality of water available
Usage	% population using only this water
Planned impact:	
Health effect	Diarrhea: incidence, duration, severity
Nutrition effect	Indicators of improved protein-calorie nutrition
Unplanned results:	Immigration to region drawn by water availability
	Decrease in % coverage
	Increase in diarrhea
	Decline in nutritional status

measured. Due to the complexity of nutrition problems, it is impossible to use a single nutritional indicator which alone would permit enough information about nutrition to be useful. An extensive list of indicators of nutrition has been presented in a WHO/FAO/UNICEF Expert Committee report (1).

Considerable attention was focused also on methods for testing the effectiveness of alternate delivery systems. It was agreed that comparisons of delivery systems could be accomplished only if:

a. An adequate, uniform measurement system were available. The extent of the intervention, intermediate variables, confounding variables and outcome variables would all have to be measured in the same way for each delivery system.

b. Sufficient community replications were possible. To obtain sufficiently accurate and precise estimates of outcome variation peculiar to the test communities, it would be necessary to achieve extensive community replications for each delivery system.

c. Delivery systems and control status were randomly assigned.

d. Control communities were assigned. Without applying the measurement system to communities receiving usual public health measures, it would not be possible to determine whether any delivery system yields a result better than no delivery system at all.

REFERENCE

1.   Report of Joint FAO/UNICEF/WHO Expert Committee. *Methodology of Nutritional Surveillance*. Technical Report Series 593. Geneva: World Health Organization, 1976.

FAMILY COMPOSITION AND STRUCTURE IN RELATION TO NUTRITION AND HEALTH PROGRAMS

Susan C. M. Scrimshaw
　　University of California at Los Angeles
　　Los Angeles, California

and

Gretel H. Pelto
　　University of Connecticut
　　Storrs, Connecticut

INTRODUCTION

Purpose

The purpose of this paper is to aid in conceptualizing and predicting outcome variables for studies of the impact of nutrition and nutrition-related health programs on family composition and structure. An attempt is made to emphasize outcome measures of potential utility to action programs. After a discussion of the relevance of the problem, this paper presents a model of the impact of health and nutrition programs on family size and structure. This model focuses on the most pertinent variables and relationships in the experience of the authors. Section three delineates some basic methodological issues, while section four presents some concrete suggestions for data collection and analysis. A true methodological manual would run to book length. We have merely highlighted several important aspects of data collection and refer the reader to other sources on methodology that we feel are particularly useful.

Relevance

During the course of the conference many questions were raised about the validity and utility of evaluation efforts. Many of these

comments were directed at the difficulty of "proving" that a given
program had a specific impact. For example, how can one know whether
an observed drop in morbidity in infants was due to a supplemental
feeding program when other factors such as lowered exposure to patho-
gens due to behavioral changes, vaccinations, etc. may have been
operating? There is no question that the objectives of many health
and nutrition programs may be realized through a multiplicity of
factors which are difficult or impossible to distinguish. A "perfect" evaluation, which explains everything, may be impossible or
possible only at great cost. Such comprehensive evaluation may not
be a reasonable goal, but the other extreme of rejecting evaluation
leaves a program with no parameters to guide it. But it may be possible to understand a great deal about a given program with 20% of
the effort of the most comprehensive evaluation. An empirical asses-
ment of the impact of a program, based on as much evidence as possible, will be better than assuming you are on the right track without ever looking for evidence to support or disprove your assumption.

There appear to be several types of evaluation possible where
the impact of health programs is concerned. One type measures the
extent to which program goals are achieved, and the extent to which
those achievements can be attributed to the program (program impact).
A second type measures the effectiveness of the delivery of the
services offered. This is actually a measurement of program process, but that process in turn affects the degree to which the program is used, and thus affects its impact. A third, less usual
type of evaluation attempts to measure the unintended consequences
of a program, its impact in areas other than the distinct program
goals.

An example of the type of goal measured in the first type of
evaluation would be "to lower the infant mortality to level 'x' or
below". In this case, questions are asked about the best way to do
this (vaccinations, food supplementation, treatment of infection,
improved economic status of the family, health education for the
mother, etc.). However, the type of experiments (such as treatment
for one group and not another) which planners would like often are
difficult to carry out for ethical and practical reasons. Often,
scarce resources dictate "natural" experiments where a type of program may be tried first in one region. Many other times, the outcome of components of the program can be predicted, thus aiding in
the assessment of the impact. For example, if you know a measles
vaccine is highly effective and it is administered to roughly 80
percent of the children in a given population, a drop in the incidence of measles very likely may be due to the program efforts.
Mortality as well as morbidity may be affected, since it is also
known that the death rate for measles is higher in a poorly nourished
population. Thus, you might also be able to hypothesize that an

observed drop in the infant mortality is due, at least in part, to the vaccination program.

The second type of evaluation mentioned above is not of *what* you decide to do, but how well you do it. This is the evaluation of the *efficiency* of a program in delivering services. In many ways, this type of evaluation is easier than the first. It is possible to find out who is using the services, how they feel about them, and how to improve the services so that more people will use them and find them easy to use. The value of this type of evaluation should be clear. Obviously, you want to make the most efficient use of your resources. (Unless your goals also include factors such as employing as many people as possible even though that is a less efficient way to deliver services.) Obviously, if your program is poorly delivered, that will affect its impact. Not incidentally, that would also make it more difficult to assess the value of a given course of action. A good example of this type of complication is when you assume that people did not use a contraceptive services program because they did not want to space or limit their family size, when in fact, the women in that society happened to be extremely reluctant to be examined by male physicians, and the program staff included no female physicians.

As discussed previously, impact evaluation has another dimension as well as the two just described. Whatever your goals, your course of action, and your health care delivery system, any or all of these can have unintended consequences. The example of the measles vaccination program described above may be taken a step further. If the infant mortality rate has dropped (supposedly due in part to lower rates of infection), then more children will survive than did previously. If this is not perceived by parents immediately, or if it is perceived but fertility is not reduced accordingly, then the completed family size will be larger. Depending on economic and other circumstances, this may be either an advantage or a disadvantage to the family. In any case, the growth rate for the population will be higher and this in turn will have a set of impacts such as increased need for jobs, education, food, health services and other resources. This is an example of the impact of health programs on family size and structure which went largely unpredicted during the early decades in this century when great emphasis was placed on reducing morbidity and mortality. This prediction could have helped societies plan for these changes in population size and structure. While causality can never be proved, such analysis and predictions of likely outcomes are essential for planning, and for feedback to programs. For example, an attempt to improve the nutritional status of families may be thwarted by the increase in family size as more children survive so that family resources must be shared among more people, thus lowering the amount of food available per capita, and lowering the

nutritional status of the family once more. Clearly, unintended
consequences can be either negative or positive, and they may be
either related or unrelated to program goals.

These unintended consequences of programs call for a broader
type of evaluation than has been previously the rule. Family composition and structure are among the variables influencing and
being influenced by health and nutrition programs and have received relatively little attention. Because they both affect
health behavior and are affected by health programs, it becomes
doubly important to measure them and their relationship to such
programs.

There is abundant comparative evidence from the wide range of
different human societies that familial social groups play an
exceedingly important role in human life ways. From the very
earliest period of human history, the primary domestic or household unit has been a major component of human adaptation. In
many societies it is the primary unit for procuring, preparing,
and distributing food. The maintenance and socialization of
children, as well as the provision of affective bonds among adults,
appear to require stable, long-lasting family clusters, and every
human society for which we have adequate data is founded on strong
family units.

Without downplaying the importance of larger social groups --
the band, village or more complex city, state and national communities, it is clear that the household is a very basic element
in the successful maintenance of human life systems. It is to be
expected that the nature of this unit, in terms of its organization, composition, and structure, will vary in relation to particular ecological-economic requirements. That is, different types of
environments require different kinds of family organization for
their successful exploitation. For example, the division of labor
between adult male and female within the household will take quite
different forms in an Eskimo band, as compared with a Mexican
farming community or an Amazonian horticultural village. Moreover, intra-cultural differences in family or household structure
reflect this same principle. For example, rural households often
have different composition than their urban counterparts, even
when cultural origins are the same for both groups.

Many human groups have families that are quite different from
the monogamous, nuclear family structure that Euroamericans tend
to regard as "normal". Widespread in human societies one finds
varying types of extended family households that contain more than
one marital bond among adult members, often with generational continuity as well. For example, an extended family structure may
consist of an older-generation husband-wife pair, plus one, two,

or more married sons and/or daughters (and their spouses), with
their children, all living in the same residential unit and sharing
economic resources. Other variations include polygamy (marriage
with more than one individual at a time), matrifocal or female-
headed households, and the inclusion of non-kin or fictive kin
(such as *compadres*) in the household.

These variations in social group membership suggest that we
should distinguish between the concepts of "family" and "household".
Typically, social scientists define the household as "a group
of people living together in a single domicile, sharing food and
other resources, whether or not consanguineously related". Families,
on the other hand, do not necessarily all live together. Furthermore, different cultures and subcultures may have very different
conceptualizations of what a "family" is and who is included within
it. Even within a society the definition may vary with context.
In North American usage, for example, the phrase "just the family",
(used in connection with a ceremonial event) may mean husband, wife,
and unmarried children or a wide network of kinspeople, including
aunts, uncles, cousins and so on. For many theoretical and practical purposes (including evaluating the impact of health and nutrition programs) the household, rather than the family, is the relevant unit of attention.

In order to focus on the impact of health and nutrition programs on households, the important underlying concept of human
adaptation must be taken into account. The basis of this concept
is that much of human behavior is not random, but represents an
adaptation to a particular environment (socio-economic as well as
physical). Anthropological ecologists theorize that beliefs and
behaviors that affect fertility, death, and disease rates are major
factors in the adaptations of human societies. Over time, every
society develops behavioral strategies which maximize gains and
minimize losses in its population size relative to particular environments (1). "Good" mini-max strategies improve these relations
in terms of the numbers of individuals that particular environments
can support and are, therefore, adaptive in strictly biological
terms. There is good evidence that human societies have always had
some control over fertility and mortality. Polgar (2), Dumond (3),
and Hassan (4), present important evidence that both were lower
during prehistoric (neolithic) times than previously thought.

Looking at modern peasant populations, we find very few examples of reproduction at the biologically possible maximum (one
child every two years throughout the woman's reproductive span).
For example, an anthropologist working in Haiti found that peasants
in the cul-de-sac region needed at least two sons and two daughters
to survive economically. Given the high infant mortality rate,
the mean number of pregnancies (around nine) per woman over 40 years

old was about right to achieve this. Obviously, the women were
not having the biologically possible maximum number of pregnancies
(5). On the other hand, the mean number of pregnancies for women
over 40 in highland Ecuador was seven, resulting in the "right"
number of living children for that economic system given the prevailing infant mortality rate, which is lower than in Haiti. Under
a different, more generous subsistence system in lowland Ecuador,
the mean number of pregnancies was nine (6). For a more detailed
discussion of adaptation in relation to morbidity and mortality
see reference 7.

Given the importance of human adaptation as an influence on
individual, familial, household, and societal behavior, health
and nutrition programs which alter fertility and mortality patterns
may strongly affect these social groupings. These effects are all
the more important to note because many adaptations and the behaviors which sustain them are often not overtly recognized by the
individuals and groups which practice them. That is to say, the
behaviors seldom result from a societal meeting where somebody
says: "Our death rate just went down because we improved our agricultural production, so its time to lower the birth rate". Most
behaviors evolve over a long period of time, and persist because
they are part of a successful adaptation to a given environment.
Our assessment of such behaviors is complicated by the fact that
environmental conditions may change, but the development of appropriate new behaviors takes time. For example, malaria may be
eradicated but certain areas may still be designated "unhealthy"
and people will not hunt or fish there, thus neglecting a new resource area. Still, it is essential to *observe behavior* and not
merely ask questions because many behaviors do not result from
decisions at the conscious level and, therefore, may not be reported accurately.

On the other hand, even though many behaviors may not be
overtly recognized as influencing mortality and fertility, program
planners must be aware that programs are not being introduced into
a vacuum, but that considerable behavioral change may be necessary.
These changes may have unforeseen consequences which are not always
favorable in economic or health terms. For example, introducing
supplementary feeding to a breast-fed infant might reduce its
demand on maternal milk to the extent that the mother might begin
to ovulate sooner than otherwise, resulting in the closer spacing
of the next pregnancy with possible detrimental effects on the
mother and both children (8). Obviously, a program would not with-
hold the supplement in this case, but would inform the mother of
the potential early resumption of fertility and offer her the means
of avoiding an unwanted pregnancy.

In this paper we focus on the household as the primary unit of
analysis in evaluation. However, it should be clear from other

papers in this volume that this is but one of several units that must be examined in evaluating programs. Furthermore, the household unit should be regarded as neither the major etiologic agent in nutrition and health problems, nor as the major obstacle to successful change. However, in some situations it may be necessary to change health threatening aspects of household organization. For example, if high quality protein foods are very unevenly distributed *within* the household unit, improving the nutritional status of all members may require a shift in food distribution patterns. Similarly, in many instances family planning and natality reduction may be an essential aspect of a health action program in order to improve the health status of children and women of childbearing age.

Our main theoretical assumption is that the household, through its collective resources, is a key mechanism within which individuals organize their efforts to meet basic needs. Even in nutrition and health programs that do not directly set out to change some aspect of family structure and organization, the changes that are instituted will often bring about structural reorganization of the household unit. Thus it follows that careful monitoring and analysis of changes in this unit, in relation to intervention programs, should be an essential aspect of evaluation.

A MODEL FOR CONCEPTUALIZING THE IMPACT OF HEALTH AND NUTRITION PROGRAMS ON FAMILY COMPOSITION AND STRUCTURE

Evaluating the impact of health programs necessitates consideration of many variables and their complex interrelationships. Even when the discussion of impact is limited to family composition and structure, multiple relationships are involved. The following model (Figure 1) is an attempt to conceptualize some of these relationships in order to define and clarify measurements. We have not included all possible variables, but have selected those that appear to be most significant for the purposes of this conference. The model is constructed around independent variables that describe program inputs, and dependent variables that may reflect the impact of those programs. The intervening variables represent the conditions through which the program may act, and the context variables reflect the effects of larger social forces that also influence changes in the dependent variables over time. It should be noted that the division of components into "dependent", "intervening", "independent" and "context" variables is for heuristic purposes only. In other situations (e.g., epidemiological research) the status of these components may change with respect to their categorization as "independent", "dependent" and so on. In reality these components are related in a *systematic* fashion, with multiple and complex interactions.

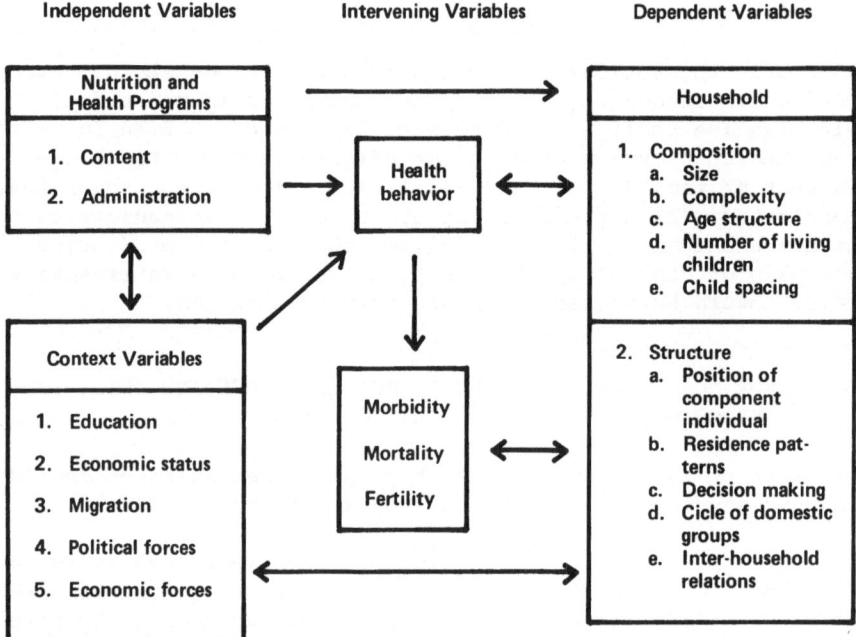

FIG. 1. A model for conceptualizing the impact of health and nutrition programs on family composition and structure.

Independent Variables in the Model

Programs. In the usual case, programs of planned change in the health field involve some intervention (e.g., in the form of education, medical technology, health aides or a service facility) that introduces aspects of modern, biomedically-based health care into areas of high infant mortality, chronic malnutrition, specific serious diseases, or combinations of these. The interventions, or inputs, are often introduced into a defined geographic area, especially when they involve day-to-day activities of health professionals and paraprofessionals. Thus, the independent variables are, in principle, observable in the form of specific administrative procedures such as food supplements, numbers of immunizations, measures to eradicate mosquitoes and introduction of specific family planning education by identifiable personnel.

Despite the apparent clarity of such inputs, it is important to realize that programs with presumably similar inputs may have differential impact depending on the local acceptability of the program content and the ways in which the program is presented or administered. "Medicine and Politics in a Mexican Village" by Oscar Lewis and several other articles in the same anthology (9), provide excellent examples of this point. Because of such differential program impacts, input variables must always be carefully observed *at the point of impact* in terms of both content and administration (mode of delivery). Scrimshaw presents a detailed discussion on the assessment of these two factors as they affect program acceptability (11).

Context Variables. There are many variables that may affect (and be affected by) nutrition and health programs, which for the purposes of this paper can be called context variables, as they are part of the wider community picture. The most relevant of these for nutrition and health programs include: education, economic status, migration, political and economic forces. A clean separation of variables is often not possible. Under the circumstances within which families and groups live, behavioral outcomes are often the results of complex interactions of economic, psychological, cultural, biomedical, and other factors. Even the best research designs cannot cope with all the "extraneous" variables that can affect outcomes.

In one example, Marchione developed a rigorous before-and-after design to test the effects of a health aides program in a Caribbean country (12). During the period of the study (1973 to 1976) the people affected by the health aides program showed improvement in nutritional status (as measured in the heights and weights of small children). After careful statistical assessment of the results, Marchione concluded that the improvements were

indeed real, but they were apparently brought about by factors
beyond the program, notably changes in cropping patterns in response to world-wide price fluctuations, as well as national land
use policies. Economic forces, especially as they impact on food
production, are often the most significant contextual variables.

     Within the household, both economic status and educational
status are important variables which often influence factors such
as the use of health programs and the effectiveness of intervention at the household level. Other important variables that affect
household composition and related characteristics are migration,
and patterns by which additional persons (kin and non-kin) are
incorporated into household units.

     There are very few places in the world that remain unaffected
by urban migration. In many areas of Latin America, as elsewhere,
practically every family is affected directly, usually through
emigration of younger members (13, 14). Research on the impact
of health programs on family composition and structure must, therefore, somehow take into account the effects of this migration.

     At the receiving end of the migration patterns (in towns and
cities) there is often the development of households with
multiple additions, as relatives from the rural homelands arrive to
seek their fortunes. Ugalde and associates documented the striking
importance of kinship in the entire pattern of cityward migration
noting that "among migrants (to Mexico City)....53 percent received
help in finding housing, and 48 percent received temporary food
and shelter from their Mexico City relatives"(15). The large
household sizes they documented in Ciudad Juarez, Mexico City, Cali
and Barranquilla reflect the influx of kinfolk rather than high
birth rates in the city. In Mexico City (six neighborhoods) 38
percent of households had nine or more people; in Barranquilla
the figure was 15 percent; while 27 percent of households in a
"suburb" of Ciudad Juarez had nine or more persons.

     In another study, focused on Ecuador, urban households were
larger than either coastal or mountain rural areas. Also, more
than half the urban households consisted of extended families, as
compared to 40 percent of the rural coastal households and 24 percent of the mountain households. The same study revealed a great
deal of communication and visiting between family members in rural
and urban areas. Clearly, these interchanges can be hypothesized
to influence the acceptability of programs focused on changing
health behavior, through people's increasing exposure to new
ideas (6).

Intervening Variables

Health behavior. Program use, as reflected in actual health behavior, is classified as an intervening variable for the purposes of this analysis. The content and administration of programs and the context variables are all seen as affecting program use. Health behavior, in turn, affects rates of morbidity, mortality, and fertility as well as household composition and structure. However, it may be affected by them as well.

Morbidity, mortality and fertility. The inputs from health and nutrition programs are generally expected to have a direct impact on rates of morbidity, mortality and fertility. In almost all cases *reduction* in these rates is the hoped-for outcome. The reductions in illness, untimely deaths, and unwanted pregnancies in their turn have effects on a variety of social, cultural and economic features. Therefore, as indicated in Figure 1, we consider the changes in morbidity, mortality and natality to be *intervening variables*, although they may also be considered dependent variables since they are affected by health behavior and by household size and composition.

Household size and composition. For the purposes of this analysis, household size and composition are mainly considered dependent variables. However, it must be emphasized that these variables may affect and be affected by the context variables, health behavior, and by morbidity, mortality and fertility. Thus, in some cases they act as intervening variables.

Dependent Variables

As noted above, we have selected a set of concepts from the general domain of household (family) composition and structure for discussion here. This list is not a comprehensive set of all potentially relevant variables that could be categorized under the general rubric of "composition and structure" Rather, it represents a number of main elements that appear to us to be of some significance.

However defined in particular societies, household or family composition includes the following variables:

1. Size
2. Complexity
3. Age structure
4. Number of living children
5. Child spacing

These variables are frequently measured in research projects and in action programs concerned with health and nutritional status. However useful such data are, additional meaning can be acquired through the examination of other variables. The broader understanding of the basic household composition variables is particularly important to the question at hand, which seeks to understand the impact of programs on households. These additional variables deal with household structure.

Household structure is a more abstract conceptualization that can refer to a variety of features of households. We have chosen to focus on the following:

6. Relative position of household members
7. Patterns of residence
8. Dominance or decision-making patterns
9. The cycle of domestic groups
10. Interhousehold relations

Household composition. A household can range from one individual to many, representing several generations. Frequently the smallest unit consists of a woman and her dependent children. Complexity, on the other hand, refers to the types of people or relationships that are represented in the household. A household may include people who are related by marriage, by consanguineous (blood) ties of varying degrees of closeness, and by people who have no biological or sanctioned sexual relationships with other household members. Households will also vary in terms of their age structure. They may include a wide distribution of individuals across the age range from infancy to extreme old age, or a much narrower range, as would be the case when the household included only one or two generations.

While the variables of household size, age range and complexity may be difficult to separate, it is sometimes necessary to do so in order to assess the impact of health and nutrition programs. For example, it can be assumed that household size is not totally random, but has some relationship to efficiency in the feeding and maintenance of the group. Health programs may create changes in efficient household size. For example, some dietary patterns are facilitated by the presence of several meal-makers, thus encouraging extended family organization. If new, more individualized food preparation is introduced, households may tend toward smaller size.

Family composition may be affected if a program undermines the authority of an individual, which then leads to conflict in the family. For example, if a grandmother's advice on child care and feeding is considered wrong by the program, the result may be that the mother gives in to the grandmother (the health program loses) or the grandmother is defied (grandmother loses). A classic example of a program affecting family composition is the welfare system in the United States, where less aid (or no aid) is given to households that include a healthy adult male. Families may split up to get aid, or the adult male may attempt to live with his family secretly.

Since health and nutrition programs often focus on only some members of a household (e.g., children under five, pregnant women), it is important to assess the impact of this feature. Does this focus alienate other members and discourage program use by favoring only some individuals? Does it improve health for some members leaving the others free to spend scarce resources on their own health and feeding? Is the program concentrating on the right individual to achieve its goals?

An example of the latter question is provided by some recent research on the energy expenditures and nutritional needs of adult males in a Latin American country based on the assumption that improving their nutritional status would permit them to work harder and earn more money, which would then be used to improve the nutritional status of the entire family. In our opinion, it is impossible to make this type of assumption without further investigation. How does the program director know that additional energy will go into economically productive labor? If it does, how does one know that any extra money earned will be spent on food, or even on the rest of the family? It may go towards other items, such as a radio, lottery tickets, or beer.

Concerned about this issue, one investigator in Guatemala did a comparative study of male and female activities (16). She found that although men did considerable economically productive work, they had much more free time than the women. The women in the same community started their day much earlier than the men, getting up to make tortillas and prepare other food for the family. They also invested some time in animal care (mostly pigs and chickens) and small garden plots. Then, they did agricultural work on a plantation (often walking long distances to work). At some times of the year this agricultural work was identical to the work the men did (e.g., picking coffee). All this was done in addition to child care, washing and other household work, and frequently, pregnancy or lactation. Obviously, this situation calls for a careful assessment of who will benefit the family most through inclusion in a nutrition program.

Two components that health and nutrition programs can be expected to affect are the number of living children and child spacing. To accurately assess program impact these variables should

be derived from carefully collected fertility histories. These
histories should include all pregnancies and their outcomes (induced or spontaneous abortion as well as stillbirth), perinatal,
neonatal, and subsequent deaths. While the number and spacing of
living children relate to the *current* household size and composition, health and nutrition programs are likely to alter these
variables through the reduction of mortality at all stages from
conception on. A further complication in assessing program impact
is derived from evidence that differences in spacing between
births can affect child survival. In Ecuador this has been observed for both the first and the second child in a birth interval
pair, although the second child was more strongly affected than
the first. For example, the second child of a closely-spaced pair
had a slightly higher probability of not surviving *if* its older
sibling was alive when the second child was conceived (8). Thus,
it is possible that a program could increase the chances for survival for some children while decreasing them for others, especially
if one of the program impacts was closer spacing. Clearly, the
biomedical and behavioral factors behind such mortality differentials need to be more thoroughly explored.

Another important aspect of both the number of living children
and birth intervals is that cultural norms about them are not
always overtly recognized by individuals or groups (7). The categories of behaviors which affect family size and spacing have
been described as "intervening fertility variables" by Davis and
Blake. Their article on the subject is an essential guide to any
researcher attempting to measure behavior related to fertility and
family size (17).

The significance for health and nutrition programs of the
intervening fertility variables and both overt and covert norms
about family size and spacing is that these norms and behaviors
may be affected by and affect program use. For example, if cultural norms and behaviors lead to an average completed family size
of five children (with about eight pregnancies in order to end up
with the five), and the program succeeds in reducing mortality so
that more of the eight survive, families may find themselves emo-
tionally and financially overwhelmed. If cultural norms are recognized, the program may be able to substitute the option of child
spacing or limiting to maintain the previous economically feasible
size of five.

Conversely, mortality rates may have been so high prior to
the program that the community needs and welcomes the additional
children who are surviving. What is their impact on family and
household structure, and on the economic situation of the family?
In some instances, their labor may improve the household's economic
situation (18). In a Javanese case, Benjamin White has argued that

wetland rice cultivation provided good opportunities for intensi-
fying agricultural production whenever additional labor, even child
labor, became available (19). In such a situation the psychological
and economic costs of child and maternal morbidity and mortality
were apparently balanced off against the need for greater economic
productivity and the advantages of a large family labor force.
Similarly, in Latin America the steady migration of young people
to the cities may provide strong motivation to maintain large families in order to increase the likelihood of economic largesse
from urbanized offspring, as well as to improve the possibility of
keeping one or two at home to insure one's old age.

At this point not enough is known about family and community
responses to rapid drops in infant mortality and changes in pregnancy spacing. The collection of data to help understand these
factors should be an important part of the assessment of program
impact on family size and structure.

Household structure. In a cross-cultural perspective, the
matter of where a newly married couple resides is of some significance for understanding a number of aspects of familial and
societal functioning. In the contemporary urban world, the preference is overwhelmingly for *neolocal* residence; that is, the new
couple establishes an independent household, apart from relatives.
More common historically, was the pattern in which the new couple
resided either with the young husband's people (patrilocal residence) or the bride's people (matrilocal residence). In some
societies the couple spends a period with each "side" of the family. Other variations (more frequently encountered in Africa and
Oceania) include residence with the groom's maternal uncle or the
bride's mother's brother.

Whether a couple sets up an independent household or is incorporated into an on-going household as part of a matrilocal or
patrilocal extended family may have important effects on natality
patterns, as well as other aspects of health (17, 20, 21). While
the debate about the relationship of extended family structure to
high fertility is as yet unresolved, there can be little doubt that
health, nutrition, and other development programs should be examined for possible influences on residence patterns.

The concept of family power structure or patterns of dominance
in decision-making has been of interest to sociologists, anthropologists and other students of family organization. It is also
often directly relevant to the interests of health care workers and
administrators, for in many situations the nature of family decision-making can significantly inhibit (or facilitate) the utilization of services. For example, in families in which adult women
do not have the authority to make decisions about health matters,

failure to have children vaccinated or to seek prenatal services
may reflect the viewpoint of the male household head, rather than
the female. In such circumstances, securing the confidence and
the cooperation of the male decision-maker is a prerequisite to
expanding the utilization of the program.

There is a general tendency to assume that the nature of family decision-making is culturally determined and homogenous within
a community. Thus, the concept of *machismo* is widely regarded as
the "cause" of male dominance in Latin American family power structure. Without denying the contribution of cultural ideas such as
machismo, it is also important to explore the extent to which the
composition of the family influences family decision-making. For
example, there is considerable ethnographic evidence from many
parts of the world to suggest that the status of a woman, within
a family, is drastically altered by age, motherhood, and becoming
a "mother-in-law". In many communities, the low status mother immediately becomes a high status person with considerable decision-
making authority and control over resources when her son marries
and brings his bride to her household. Recent analyses of women
as decision-makers in Latin America demonstrate this same increase
in power with age and status changes, as well as a certain amount
of covert decision-making (for example in the allocation of family
resources for children) which is concealed from men (22, 23, 24).
Thus, we may hypothesize that the composition of the family may
have considerable effect on family power structure and, hence,
health and nutrition programs that alter family composition can
also have an impact on decision-making.

Furthermore, it is important to note that health and nutrition programs can directly affect family authority under particular
kinds of administrative circumstances. As mentioned previously,
in the United States the federal program of Aid to Dependent Children, which is available only to children in fatherless homes,
apparently leads to a situation in which a woman must assume authority with respect to the government agencies, although her husband
or male partner may actually be present in the household. Alternatively, when mothers of young children are designated as the
recipients of extra food in a supplementation program, a mother's
status as "procurer of food!' for the family may change her role
in decision-making in other aspects of household and family life.

Another family component whose position may be influenced by
health programs is the elderly. Not only may their authority be
althered by programs, but changes in family size or structure may
affect other factors such as migration, leaving an older and
economically marginal segment in traditional villages.

Unfortunately, even in areas with available modern health services, the chronic diseases of the elderly often receive relatively less attention. In part the investment in medical attention for the elderly is not made because it has little economic payoff; on the other hand, the infirmities of old age are often beyond the reach of even advanced medical science.

More detailed study of the effects of health programs on the roles of elderly people in families is much needed. Such studies should include attention to the changing roles of the elderly within household structures, and the effects of differential health strategies in which certain types of health care become widely available (e.g., immunizations) while specialized long-term care and treatment of chronic disease is neglected.

The concept of the cycle of domestic groups is widely used in anthropology to denote changes through time in the structure and composition of households (25). Parallel to the idea of the life cycle of the individual -- from childhood to maturity to senescence -- households can also be said to have a cycle. In many contemporary situations the cycle begins with marriage and ends with the death of the spouses, but in systems with extended family organization the cycle is one of expansion and contraction, without a clear "beginning" or "ending".

From the foregoing description it should be clear that health and nutrition programs that alter longevity, fertility, or age of menarche will have, over time, an impact on household domestic cycles. In the event that improved health and nutrition standards, along with other changes in living standards, increase *both* the number of offspring *and* the life expectancies of people, then some aspects of this cycle may be extended, with a longer post-child-bearing period for the senior generation and a longer overall adult career during which families and individuals may expand and "improve" their lands, domiciles, and other economic holdings. Such a lengthening of the family career may, however, produce serious new problems if it is accompanied by increased dependency. One of the solutions to the prospect of longer careers *and* heavier economic burdens (or lack of locally available resources) is out-migration to urban centers, which creates yet another set of problems in both rural and urban areas.

Linkages Between the Independent, Intervening and Depending Variables

Although the public health and social sciences literature is full of hypotheses and conjectures about the effects of health and nutrition programs, very little research has been directed to the documentation and analysis of their impact on families and house-

holds. Therefore, many of the suggestions in the preceding discussion and in the examples below are hypotheses and hunches to
be explored, although isolated and inconclusive evidence supports
some of these effects.

Increase in family size. There is one clear and relatively
unambiguous effect of health and nutrition programs that has been
documented widely. Throughout most of Latin America, as in most
of the world, dramatic decreases in infant mortality have been
recorded, followed by rapid population increases. The following
example, from Ecuador, can be duplicated for many other countries.

Ecuador's 1975 birth rate was 41.8, while the death rate was
9.5, resulting in a growth rate of 3.2 (28). At that rate, Ecuador's population can be expected to double every twenty-two years.
It should be noted that the birth rate actually declined slightly
over the period covered, but the growth rate increased dramatically
as a result of falling infant mortality rates. Retrospective
fertility histories collected in 1971 revealed another interesting
occurrence. As infant mortality rates fell during the 1960's, so
did the percentage of live births. The difference was reflected
in increased rates of induced abortion. This is a clear indicator
of attempts to regulate family size. In this case, spacing was
also a factor as abortion began to be induced for the second pregnancy and was most frequent for the second through sixth pregnancies. This is clearly not a population of desperate grand multi-
paras, but of younger women of lower parity making decisions about
their fertility before it becomes a serious problem (8).

Increased ratio of dependents to adults. As infant mortality
rates decline rapidly, there is a net increase in the percentage
of children per family unit or per adult "breadwinner". For example,
in Ecuador in 1975, 46 percent of the population was under fifteen.
The demographic assumption that individuals under fifteen are all
"dependent" is, of course, an unrealistic view of the world in
terms of the ages when children in many societies become economi-

Table I. FERTILITY AND MORTALITY IN ECUADOR (26, 27)

Year	Birth Rate (per 1000)	Death Rate (per 1000)	Growth Rate
1920	47.9	30.9	1.7%
1940	47.1	25.9	2.2%
1960	47.3	14.9	3.3%
1965	44.0	11.7	3.2%

cally productive. In most cases, children contribute to the household long before age fifteen (18).

Increased morbidity burden in families with hereditary illness. Modern health programs include some instances in which improved medical systems add to family burdens of caring for the
sick. One example of this is the problem of thalassemia (Cooley's
Anemia), which is especially prevalent in the Eastern Mediterranean and certain other parts of the Old World. In earlier times
children with thalassemia usually lived for only a few months or
at most three or four years. Now, with extensive programs of blood
transfusions and drugs, individuals can often be maintained into
adolescence and beyond. Families with two or even three living
thalassemic children are, therefore, now possible with the new
medical procedures. Families with such children often carry heavy
burdens of psychological tensions (guilt, anxiety, etc.), as well
as the financial and logistic costs of caring for the children who
usually become progressively more deformed and sickly in their
terminal years (29). There are other diseases comparable to that
of thalassemia.

Outmigration and loss of household members. Earlier we treated
outmigration as a context variable, but in many areas population
pressures brought about by sharply decreased infant mortality may
directly force outmigration as families and individuals seek solutions to their economic circumstances. Outmigration, for economic
reasons, has most probably followed as a direct consequence of
health programs in many parts of the world. In some areas the
first to migrate are the young men and women, a practice that not
only affects family structure but community life as well (6).

Migration due to population pressure is not generally separable
from the movements of people responding to other factors, so it is
perhaps nearly impossible to analyze the direct contribution of
health/nutrition programs to changes in family composition. In
Marchione's study of a Health Aide Program in Jamaica, he
suggests an interesting effect of household structure based on
a factor analysis of household and socio-economic variables (12).
His factor of "family cohesion" was correlated with nutrition levels
of the young children in the sample. While the relationship may
be one in which greater family cohesion affects chidren's health
and nutritional status, he also poses the hypothesis that, at least
in part, the health and nutritional status in households may be
contributing to improved cohesiveness among the parents. In this
case the factor of "family cohesiveness" included items such as
"presence of father in the home", "contribution of father to support of child", and "presence of mother in home".

Clear demonstration of the effects of health and nutritional status on household cohesiveness, including reduced divorce and separation rates, will require a very tight research design, probably incorporating before-and-after measurements in order to properly assess the chronological sequences of changes.

Summary. The actual effects of a health and nutrition program will, of course, be determined by a variety of factors that will vary from one cultural-ecological situation to another, and from one type of program to another. Since the primary purposes of this paper are to develop a framework for assessing impact and methodological guidelines for carrying out such assessments, we are less concerned with predicting outcomes before programs are instituted. That is, the extraordinarily difficult problem of accurate prediction of the impact of a health program is not a central focus of discussion here. This more appropriately would follow from basic research that monitors existing programs and programs that are about to be initiated. In the following section we will take up the methodological issues of impact studies.

BASIC METHODOLOGICAL ISSUES

Most current health and nutrition programs have developed out of western medical and public health traditions. As discussed by Rosenfield, there is no single system which can be described as "western" medicine (30). Nonetheless, what today is known as "western" medicine is largely derived from European and American practices. In addition, it is only relatively recently (the past fifty years) that this medicine has had a "scientific" basis, has been able to systematically understand many diseases, and has produced what Dubos calls "the magic bullets of medicine" (30, 31). In a relatively short time, western medicine has come to dominate many of the responses to health and illness throughout the world (31, 32). However, there remain many health problems that do not yield to western biomedicine for a variety of reasons.

Many dedicated practitioners of western medicine find themselves uncomfortable with the levels of disease that continue to coexist with western medicine. For example, John Bryant states that "large numbers of the world's people, perhaps more than half, have no access to health care at all, and for many of the rest the care they receive does not answer the problems they have" (33). One reason for the latter problem is that programs based on western medical premises may run into problems when applied without consideration of the relevant cross-cultural variations. Paul provides an excellent set of case studies on this problem (10). For example, an early INCAP program had difficulty due to several factions in the village of which the health workers were unaware and

to which they did not relate equally, thus alienating part of the
community. In the same program, beliefs about the intention of
the project (e.g., they are fattening our children so they can send
them to the United States to be eaten) and about the nonreplicabi-
lity of blood drawn for analysis also created problems.

Although many elements of Latin American culture are closely
related to elements of European culture, many are also based on
pre-Hispanic cultures. There has been a blending and an evolution
of cultural traits which results in much variation between and
within countries. In addition, there is much variation between
socio-economic groups in Latin America, as elsewhere. PAHO has
long been aware of this as an important factor in health care for
this hemisphere. In fact, this conference reflected the need felt
by PAHO representatives and health professionals in general to go
beyond the evaluation techniques which currently predominate and
to produce sensitive cross-cultural measures of program impact.
This task is made all the more difficult by the fact that there is
an inherent contradiction between the concept of "sensitive cross-
cultural measures" and the use of a single, absolutely identical
research technique in all cases. Because the cultures vary, one
technique will not measure the same thing across all cultures no
matter how badly uniformity may be desired. The same approach does
not have the same meaning or yield comparable results in every
situation. The question, then, is how to come as close as possible
to the goal of measurements that are both meaningful and accurate,
and applicable cross-culturally, so that comparisons can be made
between programs and their impacts.

A Qualitative-Quantitative Approach to Data Gathering

One answer to the problem of achieving measurements that are
both meaningful and accurate is to attempt to take advantage of
the more qualitative methods that have been developed by ethno-
graphers and to wed these with the quantitative techniques that
have proved to be indispensable to the development of verifiable,
scientific knowledge. A period of intensive participant-observation and informal interviewing in the community or communities in
which the evaluation is being carried out serves several important
functions:

a.   It provides information from which to generate hypotheses
about program impact at the local level that may not be apparent
from the outside.

b.   It provides information on culture patterns and family
lifestyles on which specific questions in formal quantified surveys
can be based.

   c.   It yields insights about local language usage and helps
the evaluator to design questions that will be understood and will
not offend or confuse respondents. For example, one of the authors
(Scrimshaw) found that among Puerto Rican women in New York City,
the question: "Sabe como evitar los hijos?" elicited the information about whether or not the respondent had knowledge of contraceptive techniques. In Ecuador the same question brought a response from women that was a vigorous denial that they practiced
abortion: "No me sacaría un hijo". In order to find out about a
woman's knowledge of contraceptives, the question had to be re-
phrased as: "Sabe como evitar quedar encinta?" Also, in nearly
every culture there are some subjects which are not openly discussed. Chen and Murray present an excellent discussion of this
based on research in Haiti which should be consulted by anyone
planning survey research in Latin America (34).

   d.   It produces data on local conceptions of health and illness that may influence people's responses to formal questions.
For example, a mother may say that her baby is currently "well",
but the local definition of a well child includes a child with
parasites ("all children have worms"), edema ("a plump baby is
healthy"), and so on.

   e.   It provides the evaluator with general information about
life in the community that is extremely helpful in interpreting
the statistical results of the quantitative data.

As suggested by the last item, qualitative, descriptive information is important not only in the early phases of evaluation
research but in later phases as well. Usually the results of the
quantitative data analysis will be presented in the form of correlation coefficients, tests of independence, tests of significance
and sometimes in the form of multivariate analyses, with complex
causal modeling, path analysis or other similar techniques. If
the research has been carefully done and the data base itself is
valid, then the patterns that emerge from the statistical analysis
should be referable back to the reality of life in the community.
That is, it should be possible to identify cases (households and
individuals) that exemplify the patterns revealed in the statistical analyses. Thus, the use of "case studies" or "case histories"
(a type of qualitative data) not only provides a check on the statistical manipulations, it also gives a sense of reality to the
evaluation report and helps planners and administrators to interpret and judge the intervention program. In projects which have
used and compared a combination of quantitative and qualitative
methods, both the reliability and validity of the results have been
judged higher (6, 34, 35).

Initial Considerations

When the central aim of the research is the examination of changes in household composition and structure, there is no practical methodological substitute for direct and intensive interviewing in samples of households. Furthermore, from the discussion of the variables in the preceding part of the paper, it would appear that a considerable amount of data on age, economic status, migration history, social activities, as well as fertility and morbidity history must be collected from each household if one is to sort out the effects of the program from the welter of competing and confounding variables. Effective household interviewing under such circumstances may call for a complex interview schedule that may require several hours or several visits to administer.

Given the need for intensive interviewing in households, it is often necessary to settle for fairly small samples. This is not the only research strategy available, but except for unusual circumstances of abundant research resources, it appears to have the most likelihood of success, given the complexities involved. That is, when the choice must be made between a large sample and less intensive coverage vs. a smaller sample with more intensive interviewing, the latter is preferable in the matter of evaluating impact on the dependent variables discussed above.

Basic Methods of Data Collection

As mentioned above, a paper of this length cannot be a manual for field research. However, we feel that it may be useful to offer some suggestions regarding specific methods that are important in the evaluation of the impact of health and nutrition programs.

Interview schedule design. Interview schedule design is a fine art, a fact which is frequently ignored in the haste to conduct surveys. High quality in interview schedule design is essential. Data based on poor and poorly organized questions is misleading and inaccurate no matter how large or random the sample, or how sophisticated the analysis. In-depth knowledge of the culture to be studied is very important, and pretesting of interview schedules is essential. Much thought must be given to the wording of questions, the order of questions, and their appropriateness. In general, the least sensitive information is collected first, the more sensitive questions are asked after some rapport has been established. Care must also be taken to ask only questions which are really necessary for evaluation, in order to keep the interview from becoming too long.

Another important aspect of survey research is great care in interviewer selection, training, and supervision. The interviewer

must be acceptable to the community in terms of age, sex, status
and mode of interaction. He or she must be thoroughly familiar
with the interview schedule and the concepts behind it. The training should emphasize accuracy in data collection and respect for
the interviewee. We have found that optimum motivation and accuracy are not found by paying the interviewers by the interview,
nor at a fixed rate (daily, weekly or monthly) alone. Instead,
half-salary (the going rate for social workers is one possible
guideline for establishing salary) should be paid during training,
with the understanding that the best of the trainees will be hired
and the others will be standbys. Then, the basic salary should be
paid with a bonus (the amount depends on the duration of the survey) to be paid upon *successful* completion of the survey. The
interviewers are clearly informed that their performance is evaluated on the basis of accuracy (first priority) and quantity (a
reasonable amount of work per day). Individuals who perform poorly, particularly on the first count, should be dismissed, thereby
losing the bonus. Interviewer team spirit is also important. This
can be encouraged by involving them in the content of the project
and holding periodic feedback sessions on the progress of the data
collection. Supervisors are also needed for leadership, checks
on accuracy of interview, and trouble-shooting. Using these approaches, one of us was able to run a survey with thirty interviewers and six supervisors, which involved two months of data
collection under difficult conditions (urban high crime areas,
swamps, extremely hot weather, etc.). Only one person was dismissed (a supervisor who was unwilling to proceed accurately with
the sampling). All others completed the work, saying that it had
been difficult, but that their involvement in the project and the
final bonus had been important incentives (35, 36, 37, 38 and 39).

   Open-ended questions. Many of the interview techniques essential to research on household composition require quite structured, even pre-coded questions. In complex interviews it is preferable, where possible, that questions be pre-coded for computer-
ized processing (after careful pretesting). On the other hand,
significant areas of household structure, concerning topics such
as male-and-female roles, the place of elderly people in household interaction, and other topics, may need to be explored by
means of other techniques.

   Open-ended questions may produce a wide array of responses
with content much different from that obtained with pre-coded response categories. In those many communities where people are
fairly open about discussing such topics it may be quite productive to frame open questions such as:

   "What are the daily activities of the grandfather in your
   household?"

"Could you tell me about how your life and activities are different now from ten years ago?" (Direct question to elderly person).

"What are the differences between males and females in deciding things and organizing the work of the family?" (Direct question to adult women of household).

If open-ended questions of this sort produce lengthy replies, the data can be extremely useful if structured content analysis of the replies is carried out. Often researchers can establish lists of "themes" or "positive and negative attributes", with clear rules for coding, in order to convert the qualitative statements into quantifiable enumerations of such contents as:

a. "Frequency of joint male-female tasks"
b. "Positive emotions toward others"
c. "Number of mentions of death"
d. "Ratio of instrumental vs. non-instrumental tasks" and others.

Pictures and other controlled stimuli. Many researchers have found it useful to employ indirect methods in seeking information, especially about more sensitive subjects. One standard technique is to show each respondent some pictures, asking them to construct fictional narratives such as: "Tell me what is happening in this scene, and tell what will happen afterwards....". This picture technique is sometimes used for eliciting psychological data, but it serves equally well to provide direct expressions about family roles, interfamily interactions, and other topics. The general assumption is made that people will usually project quite realistic and true-to-life content into their fictional narratives. It is best operationalized with pictures (even photographs) tailored to details of local conditions and cultural patterns. The Spindlers used used this technique to gather information about "instrumental activities" among the Blood Indians in Alberta (40). Their pictures show individuals engaged in various instrumental tasks such as farming, office work, roping cattle, as well as more traditional roles including healing and ceremonial activity.

Participant observation. Participant observation is discussed in detail elsewhere (35, 41). For the collection of the type of data discussed in this paper, participant observation is useful during the pre-survey design stage, for observing use of health programs and health behavior (11), and in observing interactions among household members related to aspects of family structure and dynamics. In sum, participant observation is important for the understanding of human behavior, and for comparison with data

collected by other methods. It is particularly important for researchers and administrators in terms of helping them develop a
clear and understanding perspective on the users of health programs.

Direct observation. In general it is advisable that research
data for testing complex questions about effects on family composition and structure be drawn from *several different sources*, in
order to provide cross-checking of significant relationships and
descriptive (contextual) data. Some important data are available
through direct observation, including location of household, number
of rooms, "type of neighborhood", "socio-economic level" (as estimated from house construction, furnishings, etc.). Often it is
possible to construct "material style of life" ratings for households and families from direct observation, in the course of interviewing on other significant variables.

Archival data and other public records. Archives, particularly church records, hospital records, and civil registers, can
be major sources of data about births, deaths, marriages, and other
family data. In most cases, however, such archival records of
family data *are inadequate by themselves* for testing significant
applied questions, even though they can be extremely important as
supporting contextual information. In some cases archival data
may be useful for comparing and contrasting different communities
that are targets in health and nutrition programs. Records of
people using health centers, lists of participants in nutrition
programs, and a large variety of other secondary data sources
can be useful in comprehensive study of impacts on families and
households.

Given the ever-expanding scope of long-term and short-term
migration, plus the complex problems of legal and illegal domiciles in *barrios, favelas*, and other kinds of new settlements, it
is obvious that in most areas the official census records, church
records, and other recorded data are seriously incomplete resources
for assessing and evaluating the impact of health and nutrition
programs.

Rating and ranking tasks of households and communities. In
many instances it is very important to ascertain *locally* appropriate
ranking (e.g., in prestige or political power) of families ,
social groups, occupations, or other categories. Highly useful
and consistent results have been demonstrated by a number of researchers using quite direct and simple ranking techniques. Simon
(1972) asked three of her most reliable local informants to independently rank order a large series of households in a community
in terms of prestige or "categoria" (42). Their rankings were
similar enough to demonstrate that some sort of unspoken community-

wide assessment of familial prestige was operating. This same
method of ranking of families or households has been widely used --
in Italy, India, and other places -- to establish the locally relevant dimensions of social stratification and differential prestige
(43, 44).

In many cases it is important to compare different communities
in a health program in terms of their institutional complexity,
"modernization", or other qualities. One way to establish a rank
ordering among communities is through key informant interviewing
in the range of selected communities. That is two or three key
informants in each community (or neighborhood of a city) can be
asked questions about significant local facilities, ceremonial
events, elected officials, and physical structures. Communities
can then be rank-ordered in terms of the presence or absence of
key characteristics. Poggie and Miller used this method to rank-
order a series of towns and hamlets in rural Mexico in relation to
a study of modernization (45).

Use of existing knowledge and resources. In most situations
involving health care delivery, resources exist that can be helpful in the assessment of the program. These resources can provide
important data complementary to information collected through
quantitative and qualitative community studies. However, resources
are not always available for a systematic analysis of program impact through community, household and family studies. Under such
circumstances, using information available through other means is
a good deal better than no assessment at all.

Other research projects can be an important source of information even when their primary focus is not on the most central
variables most relevant of the health project. Fields which are
likely to provide helpful information include epidemiology, anthropology, economics, psychology, and sociology. For example, in
many cultures midwives not only attend deliveries but provide prenatal care, postpartum care, and pediatric care as well. An anthropological study of midwives may include data about the impact of a
health and nutrition program on the community, since some of the
same variables are involved.

It hardly needs to be said that programs need to work with
community groups on all aspects of program impact. Most programs
need to be planned and implemented with the knowledge and participation of relevant community groups (as discussed in other papers
in this volume). To do otherwise can lead to disastrous opposition (9). While the data obtained from these groups are important,
the researcher or administrator must keep in mind the goals and
concerns of each group in the sense that they will affect the groups'
perceptions of the program's impact. Thus, a predominantly male

group of community leaders that considers itself politically radical will differ in its assessments from a "*club de madres*".

.Whether an evaluation is conducted by individuals responsible
for the program or by outsiders, it is extremely important that
the input of program staff at all levels be obtained wherever possible. In addition, program staff often have an excellent sense
of many things involved in evaluations, particularly in the evaluation of program process. Discussion should not be confined to
program staff at the top of the hierarchy, but should also include
people in daily contact with program users. For example, community
workers (e.g., *promotoras*) may be particularly useful. It is
their job to know what is going on at the family and other levels
within the community, and if they are doing their job well their
insights can save a great deal of trouble. One obstacle to obtaining these insights may be the hierarchies which exist in any program. The community workers are often low in the hierarchy, and
may be hesitant to communicate with their superiors. Another difficulty is in assessing the accuracy of their information (e.g., are
they covering up their own shortcomings?). Despite these problems these individuals are an important resource for evaluation.
With sensitivity and common sense, discussions with them can be
helpful in planning intensive and extensive research, as well as
in getting a sense of the program's impact. In more than one
instance, a team of foreign evaluators has been called in to "solve"
a problem which could have been equally or more clearly understood
by talking with the program staff.

Data analysis: focusing on intragroup diversity. In the
matter of data analysis we would like to stress the importance
of paying close attention to *within*-group differences for understanding the impact of a program. In experimental research, comparisons are usually made between "control" and "experimental"
groups, and in epidemiological studies, data is typically presented in terms of the mean or normative standards from which segments of the population are said to deviate. It is, of course,
very valuable to be able to categorize populations with respect
to particular parameters and to be able to specify whether an intervention had a "statistically significant effect". At the same
time, however, analysis of the range of variation *within* the experimental and control groups can yield important insights about
the processes through which the program is having an impact.

The work of Muñoz de Chavez, et al (46) exemplifies the advantages of an intragroup focus in etiological studies. Their
comparison of families with well nourished children and families
with malnourished children in a small farming community led to the
identification of a series of variables that appear to be implicated
in the etiology of malnutrition in that area. A similar approach

can be applied to studying the impact of a nutrition program. For
example, in the matter of household composition and structure, it
is very likely that some housholds will be strongly affected,
others only moderately and still others will apparently be unaffected.   In such a situation, it is useful to attempt to identify
patterns of association that help to explain the differential impact.   Is the degree of change related to differential program
use; to characteristics of households prior to intervention; to
geographical or ethnic factors; etc.?

.   This type of analysis is especially useful when the evaluation procedure is in the form of on-going "process evaluation".
In such a situation it can provide important feedback to the program, which can, in turn, guide future activities. However, it
is also valuable in *post hoc* evaluation for it can help to identify those segments of the population that are most likely to benefit
from a particular type of intervention, as well as those who are
most difficult to reach.

SUGGESTIONS FOR OPERATIONALIZING THE MODEL

Many suggestions on data collection and references to good
sources on research design have been made throughout this paper.
A detailed variable by variable, question by question guideline
would prove far too lengthy in this context. As has been discussed
in the previous section, we feel that most research will benefit
from the multi-method approach. For example, the relative status
of individuals in the household should be determined by asking one
or more (preferably more than one, independently) household members,
and by observing how individuals in the household actually behave
towards one another, and how decisions appear to be made. Brief
suggestions will be made below on data collection of the various
categories of variables, and guides to research design.

Independent Variables

Scrimshaw provides a more complete discussion of cultural
factors in the delivery of services than can be presented here (11).
Therefore, the reader is referred to that paper. Similarly, educational, economic and political factors are covered in other papers
in this volume. For the type of investigations proposed here, the
data on migration should focus on what is happening (e.g. who mi-
grates, do they send money back, do they return, is there visiting
between country and city, how do urban migrants fare, etc.) rather
than on the dynamics of migration and the reasons for it *except*
where changes in household compositon and structure as hypothesized

outcome of nutrition and health programs are suspected to influence migration. This means that data collection on migration should probably be confined to relatively few interview questions. The assessment of political and economic forces, on the other hand, should probably be done mostly through informal means such as conversations with individuals and groups, observation, and study of national and local political and economic situations.

Intervening Variables

Health behavior is best assessed through a combination of program records, observations of program use, observations of use of other health resources besides the program (e.g., other western-oriented programs or practitioners and indigenous practitioners such as lay midwives), interviews and conversations on health behavior ("When is a baby sick?", "What do you do when....?"), and observations of behavior (e.g., seeing a mother dilute milk to feed a baby). Clearly, the focus should be on behavior which is hypothesized to affect family composition and structure. Of course, this could mean all behavior affecting fertility, mortality and morbidity, which leaves the area for investigation fairly broad. This is where the qualitative data collection becomes useful, as the information gathered can provide a basis for focusing the study design.

Although this paper concentrates on program effects on household composition and structure, the effects of household composition and structure on health behavior should not be neglected by evaluators. In a common example, if one partner (for instance, the man) makes most of the health related decisions in the household and a program is aimed at women (as maternal and child health programs often are), the program may be underutilized. In another example, mothers who have relatives in the household (extended family) or nearby, may be more likely to use health services because they have someone to leave children with when they take one child for health care or go for care themselves. More than one health program has improved attendance by providing child care services at the health center in places where extended families are not common. In much of the discussion on household and family throughout this paper, it should be easy to hypothesize the effects of various types of households and families on health behavior and program use.

Data on mortality and fertility can be collected through vital registrations (usually of limited accuracy) and as part of a survey. Data on morbidity may be available through the program, but should also be part of a survey. Where possible, repeat

morbidity surveys (several visits to a household over a period of
time) or morbidity surveys of the entire community or a very large
portion of it are useful.

Dependent Variables

Household composition. Data on household composition can be
used to determine household and family size and structure. One
of the most efficient ways to collect such data is to elicit information for a diagram of the household. In such a diagram, males
are represented by a triangle, females by a circle. Generations
are separated vertically. Each individual in the diagram is assigned a number and relevant information is recorded next to that
number on a list below the diagram. We have found that the diagram
often involves the person interviewed in a positive way, and is
well accepted.

Data on fertility and mortality are most easily collected with
some adaptation of the fertility history form proposed by Donald
Bogue (47). Other manuals in the same series provide techniques
for the analysis of the fertility history data and other related
data. The series is available in Spanish as well as in English.

Sexual union (marriage, common-law marriage, visiting relationship) histories can be collected using a grid form similar to
Bogue's fertility history form. In the past, it has been most
common to only collect such histories for women. We suggest that
careful thought be given to collecting them for men as well. For
example, in cultures where men have more than one family either
serially or simultaneously, a man may be supporting more than one
household. Estimates of family income by the nutrition or health
program (for purposes of fee setting, helping people plan how to
spend income on food, etc.) will need to take into account how
many families or at least children are being supported.

Obviously, the data collected using grids for fertility histories or union histories must be supplemented by questions and
observations which collect data on attitudes, and reasons for attitudes and behaviors.

Household structure. The most frequent method for operationalizing the concept of family power structure is to ask a series
of questions about hypothetical or actual behavior with respect to
a series of typically-encountered family decisions. Questions
can range from the domain of mundane, day-to-day activities to
significant life-altering decisions. Researchers often try to get
responses, separately, from male and female household heads, and
sometimes from children as well, in order to assess the extent of

agreement in individuals' perceptions of the decision-making process. Responses to the questions can be scored by combining them
into a simple, arithmetic index, or particular items of greater
significance from the perspective of the researcher may be weighted
more heavily. Alternatively, two indices can be constructed, one
which measures decision-making in day-to-day affairs and another
that deals with more significant life events.

Some researchers have attempted to measure family power by
means other than question-response in an interview. There is
little doubt that behavioral observation is often highly productive
of insights or more accurate information since it is less subject
to the problems of distortion and misinformation that typically
accompany an interviewer-respondent form of data gathering. In
order to gather data on family decision-making behaviorally, it is
usually necessary to set up some type of standardized situation
in which decision-making can be observed. By creating a standardized situation the problems of comparability of observation and
scoring procedures are minimized and efficiency with respect to
the amount of time required to obtain the data can be maximized.
On the other hand, not all communities are readily amenable to
this type of data gathering, which requires a particular kind of
cooperation on the part of respondents. However, a "game" designed by Murray Strauss and associates to measure family power
structure was apparently successfully administered in several
different cultural contexts such as India and Sri Lanka, as well
as the United States (35). Measures similar to those discussed
for power structure can be applied to the other variables related
to household structure.

                              CONCLUSIONS

While it is difficult to be certain of precise causality in
the assessment of program impact, the evaluation of nutrition and
health programs is extremely important in order to assess and
improve the running of the program (process), and to get a sense
of both specific and broad program effects. Without this, a program runs the risk of completely missing the means of achieving
its goals. In the case of broader impact, the achievement of short
and long run assessment, the basic groupings of families in households, and the dynamics of these groups, are a necessary consideration.

This paper has attempted to provide a basis for understanding
and studying the impact of nutrition and nutrition-related health
programs on family and household size and structure. The relevance
of such an approach was discussed, and a model of the important

variables related to health programs and social structures and their possible interactions was presented. Throughout the paper, examples of important linkages were provided as were suggestions for data collection. The latter touched on important methodological issues and considerations, and presented some suggestions for the collection of information related to specific variables. Because of the complex nature of research design, the methodological sections provide only a beginning of research tools, along with leads to appropriate sources containing more detail.

This paper, then, should be seen as a springboard for the conceptualization and design of projects to assess the impact of nutrition and health programs on family size and structure which will provide helpful information as to the role of such projects in positive changes in individuals, households, and communities.

ACKNOWLEDGEMENTS

The authors wish to acknowledge the important input of Pertti J. Pelto and Danile M. S. March in both the conceptualization and critical review of this paper.

REFERENCES

1.   Alland, A. *Adaptation in Human Evolution: An Approach to Medical Anthropology*. New York: Columbia University Press, 1970.

2.   Polgar, S. Population history and population policies from an anthropological perspective. *Curr. Anthropol.* 13(2): 203-211, 1972.

3.   Dumond, D. E. The limitation of human population: A natural history. *Science* 187:713-721, 1975.

4.   Hassan, F. A. On mechanisms of population growth during the neolithic period. *Curr. Anthropol.* 14(5):535-542, 1973.

5.   Murray, G. Personal communication. 1972.

6.   Scrimshaw, S. *Culture, Environment, and Family Size: A Study of Urban In-migrants in Guayaquil, Ecuador*. Ph.D. Dissertation. New York: Columbia University, 1974.

7.   Scrimshaw, S. *Cultural Values and Behaviors Related to Population Change*. New York: Institute of Society, Ethics and the Life Sciences, Hastings on Hudson, 1977.

8.   Wolfers, D., and S. Scrimshaw. Child survival and intervals between pregnancies in Guayaquil, Ecuador. *Population St.* 29(3):479-495, 1975.

9.   Lewis, O. Medicine and politics in a Mexican village. In: B. Paul (ed.). *Health, Culture and Community*. New York: Russell Sage Foundation, Inc., 1955.

10. Paul, B. D. (ed.) *Health, Culture and Community*. New York:
     Russell Sage Foundation, 1955.
11. Scrimshaw, S. *Cultural and Other Practical Considerations
     in the Evaluation of Maternal and Child Health Programs*.
     n.d. Revision of *Anthropology and Population Research:
     Application in Family Planning Programs*. New York:
     Center for Population and Family Health, Columbia Uni-
     versity, 1972.
12. Marchione, T. J. Food and nutrition in self-reliant national
     development: The impact on child nutrition of Jamaican
     government policy. *Med. Anthro.* 1(1), 57-80, 1977.
13. Balan, J. Migrant-native socioeconomic differences in Latin
     American cities: A structural analysis. *Lat. Amer.
     Res. Rev.* 4:3-29, 1969.
14. Davis, K. and A. Casis. Urbanization in Latin America.
     Millbank Memorial Fund Quart 24(3):186-207, 1946.
15. Ugalde, A. *et al.* *The Urbanization Process of a Poor Mexican
     Neighborhood*. Austin: Institute of Latin American
     Studies, University of Texas Press, 1974.
16. Scrimshaw, M. W. Personal communication. 1976.
17. Davis, K. and J. Blake. Social structure and fertility: An
     analytic framework. *Economic Development and Cultural
     Change* 4 (April):211-235, 1956.
18. Nag, M. The economic value of children in agricultural so-
     cieties. In: J. Marshall and S. Polgar (eds.). *Culture,
     Natality and Family Planning*. Monograph 21. Chapel Hill:
     University of North Carolina Population Center, 1976.
19. White, B. Demand for labor and population growth in colonial
     Java. *Human Ecology* 1(3):217-236, 1973.
20. Lorimer, F. *Culture and Human Fertility: A Study of the
     Relation of Cultural Conditions to Fertility in Non-
     industrial and Transition Societies*. Paris, UNESCO,
     1954.
21. Nag, M. Family type and fertility. In: *United Nations World
     Population Conference, 1965*. Vol. 2. New York: United
     Nations, 1967.
22. Scrimshaw, S. Stages in women's lives and reproductive deci-
     sion making in Latin America. *Med. Anthro.* Vol. 2,
     In Press.
23. Jaquette, J. Literary Archtypes and female role alternatives:
     The women and the novel in Latin America. In: A.
     Pascatello (ed.). *Female and Male in Latin America*.
     Pittsburg: University of Pittsburg Press, 1973.
24. Maynard, E. Guatemalan women: Life under two types of patri-
     archy. In: C. J. Mathiasson (ed.). *Many Sisters*. New
     York: The Free Press, 1974.
25. Goody, J. (ed.). *The Developmental Cycle in Domestic Groups*.
     Cambridge: Cambridge University Press, 1971.
26. Enderica Velez, R. Dinamica y estructura de la población.
     Rev. Ecuatoriana de Higiene y Medicina Tropical 25(1):
     61-74, 1968.

27. Merlo, P. *Estructura y Crecimiento de la Población*. Quito,
        Ecuador: Junta Nacional de Planificación y Coordinación,
        1967.
28. Myers, P. *World Population Data Sheet*. Washington, D. C.;
        Population Reference Bureau, 1975.
29. Book, P. A. Thalassemia in Cyprus: Coping with chronic
        disease. Paper presented at the *Northeastern Anthro-
        pological Association Annual Meeting, Providence, 1977*.
30. Rosenfield, A. Modern medicine and the delivery of health
        services. *Man and Medicine*. In press.
31. Dubos, R. *Mirage of Health: Utopia's Progress and Biological
        Change*. New York: Harper and Row, 1959.
32. Illich, I. *Medical Nemesis*. New York: Pantheon Books, 1976.
33. Bryant, J. *Health in the Developing World*. Ithaca: Cornell
        University Press, 1969.
34. Chen, K. H. and G. Murray. Truths and untruths in a Haitian
        village: An experiment in Third World survey research.
        In: J. Marshall and S. Polgar (eds.). *Culture, Natal-
        ity and Family Planning*. Monograph 21. Chapel Hill:
        University of North Carolina Population Center, 1976.
35. Pelto, P. J. and G. H. Pelto. *Anthropological Research: The
        Structure of Inquiry*. New York: Cambridge University
        Press, 1977.
36. Scrimshaw, S. *Migration, Urban Living and the Family: A
        Study Among Residents in the Suburbios and Tugurios of
        Guayaquil, Ecuador*. Report prepared for the International
        Institute for the Study of Human Reproduction, Columbia
        University, New York, 1973.
37. Babbie, E. R. *Survey Research Methods*. Belmont, California:
        Wadsworth Publishing Company, 1973.
38. Backstrom, C. H. and G. D. Hursh. *Survey Research*. Evanston:
        Northwestern University Press, 1963.
39. Lazarfeld, P. F. *Qualitative Analysis: Historical and Crit-
        ical Essays*. Boston: Allyn and Bacon, Inc., 1972.
40. Spindler, G. and L. Spindler. The instrumental activities
        inventory: A technique for the study of the psychology
        of acculturation. *Southwestern J. Anthropol*. 21:1-28,
        1965.
41. Crane, J. G. and M. Angrosino. *Field Projects in Anthropology:
        A Student Handbook*. Morristown, New Jersey: General
        Learning Press, 1974.
42. Simon, B. *Power, Privilege and Prestige in a Mexican Town*.
        Ph.D. Dissertation, University of Minnesota, 1972.
43. Silverman, S. F. An ethnographic approach to social strati-
        fication: Prestige in a central Italian community.
        Am. Anthropol. 68(4):899-921, 1966.
44. Freed, S. A. An objective method for determining the collec-
        tive caste hierarchy of an Indian village. *Am. Anthropol*.
        65(4):879-891, 1963.

45. Poggie, J. and F. C. Miller. *Social and Cultural Aspects of Modernization in Mexico*. Minneapolis: University of Minnesota, 1968.
46. Muñoz de Chavez, M. *et al*. The epidemiology of good nutrition in a population with a high prevalence of malnutrition. *Ecol. Food Nutr*. 3:223-230, 1974.
47. Bogue, D. J. *A Model Interview for Fertility Research and Family Planning Evaluation*. Family Planning Evaluation Manual No. 3, Rapid Feedback for Family Planning Improvement. Chicago: Community and Family Study Center, University of Chicago, 1971.

COMMENTS

Nelson Amaro, *Banco de Vivienda Popular*
Guatemala City, Guatemala

This paper presents a model of the factors to be considered when measuring the impact of nutrition and health programs on family structure and size. It also describes a variety of ways to measure this impact. This commentary includes various suggestions concerning the substantive content, and offers suggestions to broaden the ideas offered in the paper by Scrimshaw and Pelto.

TYPES OF EVALUATION

When one is trying to introduce evaluation techniques in developing countries it is necessary to consider the values being promoted by the specific programs and projects. The question of values is often omitted both in text books, and in the paper by Scrimshaw and Pelto because it is considered irrelevant to the specific research project or program. This exercise might be called "evaluating the evaluation".

In societies which are in the process of change, the values which maintain the given structures are being questioned; nevertheless, they frequently prevail. This means that, from the evaluation point of view, the only alternatives available for the beneficiaries are those which the existing system provides. Undoubtedly, health and nutrition programs for the household are inserted in this system with all the value implications that orient any social action. Figure 1 in the paper by Scrimshaw and Pelto provides the classic example of this concept: a state, an agency, or an administration which offers services, and a population which receives them. This is a hierarchical relationship which does not consider possible alternatives which may be offered by service

recipients and which may solve their own problems with a minimal
and temporary intervention from state or private agencies.

   Naturally, there might be many programs for which their Figure 1 is appropriate because it assumes that the state provides
services as an obligation. However, there are projects where the
community and the family play a more active role, (e.g., the "bare-
foot doctors" in China, self-therapy psychology in the United States
mental health field, or the communal gardens in Panama (1)). These
are some alternatives to traditional approaches that have only recently been considered and which may offer new and imaginative
solutions to escape from static and rigid situations. We would
like to see models which address unexplored dimensions in this
field while still taking advantage of previous experience. The
model presented by the authors does not touch these points.

   In the area of health, as well as in other sectors, there are
key values related to the wider social structure which result in
institutional arrangements that implicitly or explicitly guide different projects, programs and activities. An example would be the
extent to which a health system places more emphasis on curative
rather than preventive care. In developing countries this policy
would be associated with more specialized education at the university level, a greater degree of differentiation in medical personnel, a greater concentration of medical services in the urban areas
where they are demanded, etc. From the perspective of program planning and evaluation such specialization may be effective and efficient. However, we would all agree that the values which underline
such an organization may not be consistent with social development.
Quite often, the values and their corresponding social consequences
are not readily seen. They can be made obvious through a qualitative
rather than quantitative analysis. In developing countries this type
of analysis is necessary to relate the process of evaluation to those
alternatives which offer solutions to pressing problems. This type
of analysis was elaborated for the education field by Rama (2).

   The attainment of what Campbell has called an "experimental
society" is perhaps more applicable to societies with greater potential for change (3). Not included here are the less developed countries which within months could alter their power structure and
could undertake major social changes, (i.e., the situation in many
Third World countries). There is little doubt that a scientific
evaluation of the problems that give rise to such social changes
could have two important consequences: first, it could modify the
status quo in favor of new solutions; and second, it could avoid the
development utopias proposed by social activists which, although
well-intentioned, imply a high cost for the society involved. These
are the kinds of problems that must be dealt with if what is presently called "evaluation", as it has been developed specifically in
the United States, is to be applicable on a world-wide basis.

THE PROBLEM OF THE THEORETICAL FOCUS

In spite of efforts by many writers to convince us that the Third World's problems are human adaptations to environmental modifications, we remain unconvinced that this is true at the family level. The facts presented are always *post facto* and, to a large extent, the theories assume the model of the "rational man" which is likely to be found only in urban areas of the developing world where behaviors with respect to population size are based on decisions made at the family level. It can be seen that these are made in terms of ends and means. In this case, for example, the couple decides on the desired number of children and then use known methods to achieve the desired number. This is typical behavior of middle and upper classes of much of the developing world. Some point to this strategy as the cause for the decline in fertility in industrial countries (4, 5).

However, even in urban areas of developing countries, the lower classes only begin to plan their families when they already have the desired number of children, when the mother is older, and when the number of children is beyond the limits which they can afford (6). Practically speaking, this is survival family planning, and not particularly rational. In the rural peasant cultures we fail to see the "rational man" anywhere. The limited research in this area documents the following contradictions:

a.   Desired number of children and the real number are rarely in agreement.   1/

b.   The great majority of women have not even talked with their husband about the number of children they want to have.   2/

1/   In his study of human fertility in Latin America, Stycos concludes: "The Projective Technique revealed that family size is a matter of very low salience for most of the Haitian men and women interviewed, that norms concerning the appropriate family size seem nonexistent and inappropriate for most subjects, and that an attitude of religious fatalism about number of children is characteristic". (7)

2/   In a study which my colleagues and I conducted in Guatemala, women were interviewed to determine what percentage of them had never spoken to their husband about the number of children desired (8). The results obtained in four different areas were as follows: Urban planned area with level land and traced streets -- 35%; urban unplanned areas on broken terrain -- 45%; fully "ladino" western-oriented municipality -- 60%; and fully Indian municipality -- 77%.

c.   The explanations given about "machismo", the "economic
         help" which children provide, and the "insurance" for
         old age provided by the children fail to specify, from
         the couple's point of view, the number of children con-
         sidered necessary for fulfilling each factor.

What is seen here is not rational behavior. These data contrast with the authors' conclusions like "through time, each society develops strategies which maximize the benefits and minimize
losses in the population size according to the environment in
which it happens". Compare this statement with George C. Homans:
"What has been called the "rational-choice model of human behavior"
coincides in part with the body of propositions of behavioral
psychology. The coincidence has not always been recognized, because the rational theory has usually been put forward not by psychologists but by other scholars such as economists and mathemati-
cians interested in explaining the process of decision-making.
The main proposition of the national theory in one of its forms
may be stated as follows: "in choosing between alternative courses
of action, a person will choose the one for which, as perceived by
him, the mathematical value of p x v is the greater where p is the
probability that the action will be successful in getting a given
reward and v is the value to the person of that reward" (9). This
criticism is valid even when the subjects are not aware of the
bases for their decisions, such as the market mechanism which reg-
ulates supply and demand. Individual buyers and sellers are not
searching for specific market goals, yet one expects to find mechanisms for rational behavior (e.g., in the market economy the "in-
visible hand" and in the authors' theory the "biological factors")
which do not alter the nature of the theory.

Our criticism of completely rational models has already been
expressed. The authors fail to recognize that contemporary development is not a problem of autonomous changes but a series of ex-
changes and confrontations in an integrated world system (10).
Lastly, one could argue that what the authors say takes place over
a long period of time to which one could respond "in the long run
we will all be dead". We think that this theoretical burden is
unnecessary with respect to the concrete model which was presented.

PROBLEMS OF THE MODEL

We cannot overcome the problems of creating a model without
reference to time and space. Evaluation of programs should always
be based upon the concrete objectives defined by the responsible
agencies. Sometimes, it is the evaluator's job to make explicit
those objectives which have not been defined. For example, in the

cotton growing areas in southern Guatemala, health programs which
have been designed for areas with low population density have been
applied to the large coastal migration centers. The model does not
encompass such situations even though it could, at the risk of be
coming tremendously complicated by the number of variables to
consider.

It seems necessary also to distinguish between quasi-models
and models. In the former, the program could be massive and the
target population would not have precise limits, while in the
latter, the administration would control the intervention and the
target population would be well defined. Obviously, evaluation
is more difficult in the first case, where the number of variables
may be infinite. We would have liked a presentation about the
second type of program. Nevertheless, the model presented would
seem to better fit the characteristics of the first. This stems
from the author's need to deal with the "contextual variables"
which in the absence of detailed prior knowledge becomes pure
speculation at a very general and abstract level.

The research of Marchione in the Caribbean illustrates our
previous assertion by demonstrating that although indices of health
improved following implementation of a program of health care, they
did so because of factors beyond the program itself -- such as
changes in cropping patterns and the politics of land distribution (11). One of the aspects which will probably need more
specification in the future, from the methodological point of view,
is the impact of these historical events on program results. For
example, production and price structures fluctuate regularly in
developing countries. It is necessary to develop a methodology
which would allow us to creatively deal with this problem.

In addition, the use of a control group and pre and post
measurements makes the "contextual variables" almost useless. This
kind of design assumes that the groups having been randomly assigned
to the experimental and control status do not significantly differ
on these variables. The treatment of the "contextual variables"
only becomes relevant when it is not possible to be very rigorous
in the design or where there are factors beyond the control of the
evaluator. It is well known that the actual use of health services depends, to a large extent, on these kinds of variables.
If the program administrator cannot determine who receives the
program services, controlling for these factors becomes extremely
important. This is why it is so important to understand the difference between models and quasi-models, or between experimental
research and quasi-experimental research (3).

While considering how to control variables, the problem of
the causal ordering of the variables emerges. What affects what?

Where is there interaction or reciprocal causality? These relationships are not clearly established in the model. In this case,
it would be necessary to identify the direction and degree of the
interrelationships between the independent variables. Furthermore,
the authors fail to explicate the relationship between program
administration adn program content; between decision-making at the
program level and the "contextual variables" at the research level.
It could be that these are acting indirectly, making the relationship assymetrical rather than interdependent as Scrimshaw and
Pelto's Figure 1 indicates. Lastly, it is difficult to understand
the scheme from a causal perspective.

If we agree that the crucial point is how the program delivers
its services, then why do we talk about content and administration
when there are so many variables involved? If what is crucial in
"health behavior" is the use of the program, why is it not defined
that way?

Finally, regarding the design of studies of health program
impacts on family composition and structure, we should remember
that the possible measures are secondary to the health objectives themselves. It seems that additional designs would be necessary to identify the relations before and after the impact of the
program. To the extent that we depart from an experimental design,
the strategies and methodology are going to vary in infinite ways
which are hard to anticipate. Nevertheless, the variables listed
in this paper might be seen as a point of departure but as far as
we do depart from an experimental design, it is necessary to control for extraneous variables, thus approaching a causal model.
The techniques for regression and path analyses then should be
included as the most rigorous in the field (12). All the other
possible alternatives fall between these two poles.

CONCLUSIONS

The points covered above could be summarized as follows:

a. In the developing world it is necessary to identify the
values which underlie the programs and then seek options that favor
alternatives which go beyond the mere relationship between a
service agency and a recipient population. Program evaluation
should be carried out in this context.

b. The theory behind the models that attempt to represent
the evaluation of the impact of health programs must take short-
term factors into account. Above all, theories must remain cog-
nizant of those factors which contradict traditional theoretical
orientations and which are at odds with the data from developing
countries.

c.   The specification of variables within a model should derive from empirical data. These variables and the relationship among them must then be put to empirical test. Only in this fashion can we accumulate data in the context of a functional model.

The distinction between experiment and quasi-experiment should be made and the direction of causality should also be made clear. In this sense, the model presented by the authors is only a point of departure.

REFERENCES

1.   Ugalde, A. Los procesos de toma de decisiones en el sector sanitario y sus implicaciones políticas. *Revista de Sociología* 5:101-124, 1976.
2.   Rama, G. W. Educación, imágenes y estilos de desarrollo. *UNESCO-CEPAL-PNUD Proyecto: Desarrollo y Educación en América Latina y el Caribe.* DEALC/6, 8 September, 1977.
3.   Campbell, D. T. and J. C. Stanley. *Experimental and Quasi-Experimental Designs for Research.* Chicago: Rand McNally, 1966.
4.   Banks, J. A. *Prosperity and Parenthood.* London: Routledge, 1954.
5.   Beshers, J. M. *Population Processes in Social Systems.* pp. 44-47, New York: The Free Press, 1967.
6.   Berelson, B. National family planning programs: A guide. In: *Studies in Family Planning, No. 5 (Suppl.),* The Population Council, New York, December 1974.
7.   Stycos, J. M. *Human Fertility in Latin America,* pp. 116-132, New York: Cornell University Press, 1968.
8.   Instituto Centroamericano de Población y Familia. *Fecundidad en Guatemala.* p. 265, Guatemala City, 1972.
9.   Homans, G. C. *The Nature of Social Science.* pp. 38-39, New York: Harcourt, Brace and World, 1967.
10. Portes, A. On the sociology of national development: Theories and issues. *Am. J. Sociol.* 82(1):61-68, 1976.
11. Marchione, T. J. Food and nutrition in self-reliant national development: The impact on child nutrition of Jamaican government policy. *Med. Anthrop.* 1:Part 3, 1977.
12. Duncan, O. D. *Introduction to Structural Equation Models.* New York: Academic Press, 1975.

GENERAL DISCUSSION

The discussion of this paper repeatedly touches on the enormous complexity of family structure and composition as contextual and as outcome variables. Some general correlational data relating nutrition and health to family structure and composition were discussed.

It was pointed out that the incidence of severe malnutrition is reportedly higher in families with more children and that presumably this is due to poorer child care practices as well as to economic factors. However, correlational studies of the relationship between mild-to-moderate levels of malnutrition among preschool age children and family size frequently report contradictory findings. Undoubtedly there are a variety of additional factors which must be taken into account when discussing such relationships as these.

Several discussants remarked on the statistical difficulties in handling family structure and composition variables. Specific examples were presented in which family structure, used as a contextual variable in analyses of evaluation studies, proved to be extremely difficult to handle. Frequent changes in family structure and composition in some of these studies further complicate the picture.

Several discussants commented that they felt that too little use has been made of family contextual information in revealing important interactions in health and nutrition studies. They urged that data from existing surveys and evaluations be analyzed to quantify how different family characteristics affect health and nutritional status, or act as constraints on outcome variables of interest.

THE ECONOMIC THEORY OF THE HOUSEHOLD AND IMPACT

MEASUREMENT OF NUTRITION AND RELATED HEALTH PROGRAMS

Dov Chernichovsky*
     The World Bank
     Washington, D. C.

INTRODUCTION

As a theory of choice, household economics offers a conceptual framework in which to investigate the family's responses to changes in its environment. This framework can be useful for policy-makers and planners in formulating hypotheses about the effects of intervention programs. Econometrics, the complementary statistical extension of economic theory, furnishes a versatile statistical framework for testing these hypotheses and quantifying the effects of such programs, as well as increasing our basic knowledge about the interactions between the program and their social environments.

This paper conveys, in broad terms, an economist's approach to the evaluation of nutrition and related health programs. It emphasizes the close link between economics as a behavioral science and the measurement of the impact of intervention programs. In the first section, the basic working assumptions and framework of household economics are introduced and related to the concept of an intervention program. This relationship serves to highlight the economist's conceptual point of departure in analyzing nutrition and health-related interventions and measuring their effects. In the second section, the household's behavioral objectives that are used to specify and measure the outcomes of intervention programs are discussed. These objectives provide the conceptual framework for considering various properties of outcome variables and measurement problems in section three. Section four discusses the econometric approach to socio-economic studies in nutrition, and section five discusses the basic differences between an experi-

---

*Mailing adress: Medical, Economics, Health & Welfare Administration, Beersheva 84 120 P.O.B. 653, Israel

mental approach and an econometric approach in measuring program
impact.

INTERVENTION PROGRAMS AND HOUSEHOLD ECONOMICS

Health-related environmental programs, like malaria eradication, and largely mandatory programs, like smallpox vaccination,
apparently have been relatively successful in meeting their objectives (1), while many personal health and nutrition programs appear
to be less successful. A common feature of the environmental programs and the mandatory programs is that their implementation does
not require individuals or households to choose how to respond. The
environmental programs do not deal directly with individuals or households, and mass vaccinations may leave little or no room for individual or household choice. Programs in health and nutrition, on
the other hand, often require active decision-making and behavior
change at the family and individual level. Measurement of success
or failure of such programs becomes complicated due to several factors including lack of data, relevant statistical tools, or most
importantly, the response of the target population to the program.

Malnutrition results largely from a combination of individual
and household consumption behavior and hygienic decisions and practices. This fact limits the feasibility, economic and otherwise,
of mandatory and effectively controlled nutrition programs; that is,
these programs are most likely to leave to individuals and households the choices of whether to participate in a program and how
to use resources that become available through it. The fact that
families and individuals are required to make choices makes an e-
conomic theory of the household a useful evaluation tool.

The household, whether a nuclear or an extended family, is the
basic socio-economic unit that makes most decisions about investment in human beings and about consumption. 1/ The significance
of a household and an individual to the community is not limited to
their role as components of a sum. An individual's education, and
particularly his health, often affect the well-being of others in
the community; communicable diseases exemplify the interdependence
between an individual and his community. This interdependence and
certain cultural norms concerning the distribution of well-being
among households in the community provide much of the basic rationale for health-related intervention programs.

Economists usually view the household as a harmonious micro-
cosm that makes deliberate and rational decisions. This is a

1/ It is important to realize, however, that in some traditional
cultures, tribal or village governing entities might make important
decisions about investment in human capital.

basic working assumption employed to identify the systematic part
of human behavior by using conceptual parameters and measurable
variables. This assumption is eventually "modified" in econometric analyses by taking into account unsystematic variations of
behavior. The economic analysis of household behavior can be
summarized as follows. 2/ Households and individuals engage in
activities to produce "ends", or consumption commodities, that
have utility. 3/ These ends compete for the household's scarce
human and nonhuman resources because producing more of one commodity implies producing less of others. A change in the household situational environment can change (a) the household's income
or wealth, which determines how much a household can produce, (b)
the commodities' relative costs or prices, which determine the
relative attractiveness of different commodities, and (c) the
household's tastes and preference structure. Modifications in
household behavior are derived from changes, which an intervention program can promote, in one or more of these. An economic
conceptualization of the household's decision-making process is
sketched in a simplified manner in Figure 1.

From the viewpoint of household economics, an intervention
program has at least one inherent problem: such a program "dis-
putes" the household's ability and even willingness to realize the
social consequences of its choice and to meet some specified
social objectives. This is equivalent in many instances to ques-
tioning the rationality and social adequacy of the household's
decision-making process and objectives. There are two critical
implications of this problem. First, an effective demand for, or
utilization of, program services by the target population cannot
be guaranteed; second, even when adequate demand exists, it may
stem from private objectives that are not congruent with program
or social objectives.

Therefore, a basic requirement for evaluating program impact
is to identify the "nonprogram" parameters that determine the
household's demand for program services. This identification
should help to indicate how much a household will use the program,
when it will do so, and what use it may make of the program's
resources.

2/   The approach presented here, in broad terms, is based on traditional demand theory and some extensions of this theory by Becker
(2) and Lancaster (3). Differences in approach, which bears on
the conceptual framework, do (and should) not affect more practical
measurement issues.

3/   Those commodities can be abstract as are, for example, "good
health" and "services from children".

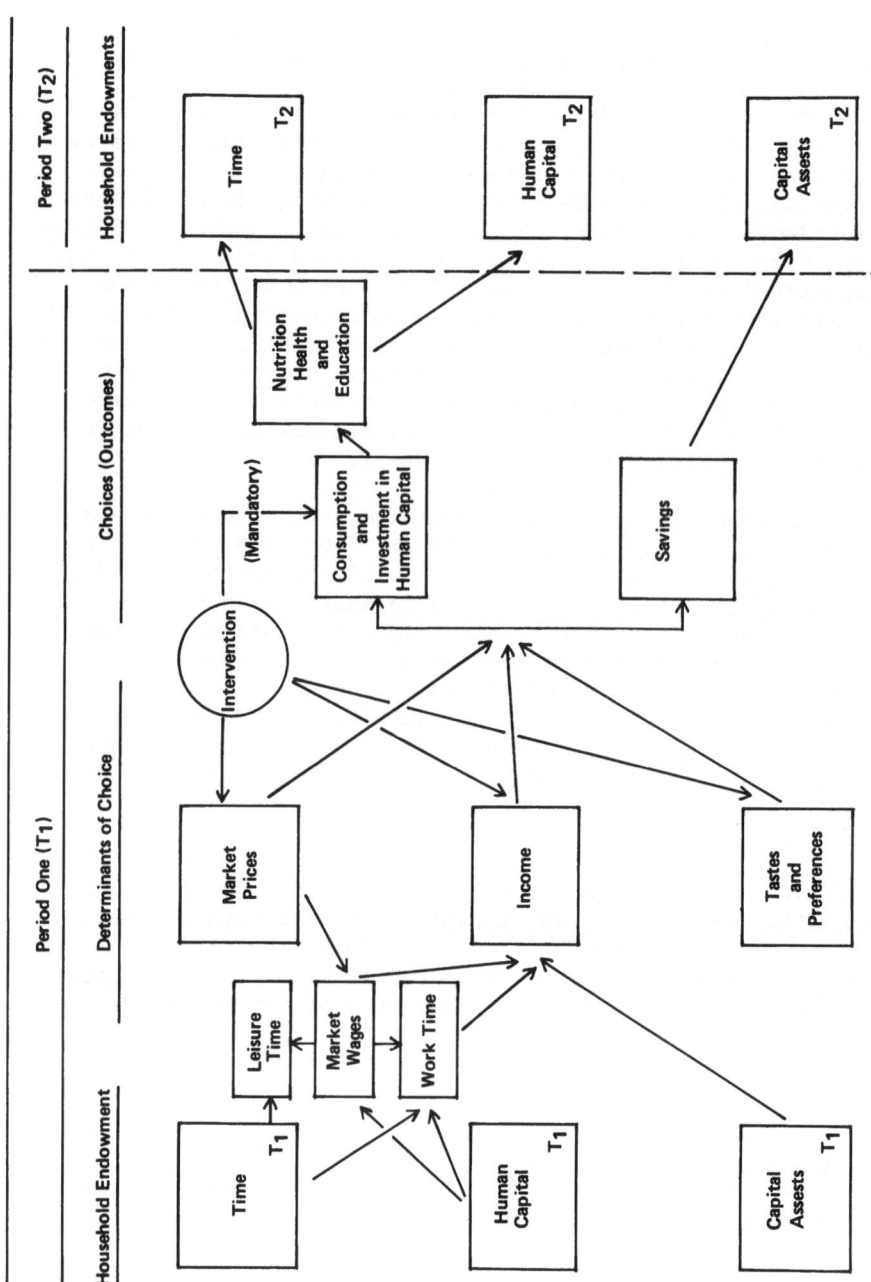

FIG. 1.   An economic conceptualization of the household's decision-making process.

Program utilization is a function of (a) the degree the program serves the household's objectives; (b) the degree it draws on household resources; and (c) the relative attractiveness of subjectively conceived substitutes for program services that meet the household's objectives. These points can be illustrated by common examples. Preventive medical care programs, particularly nutrition programs, are often hard to implement because the target populations may not recognize their usefulness. In many situations, health services may compete with traditional practices that households perceive as substitutes. Program services may not be used, even when people recognize their usefulness, because of the relatively lower costs, or higher benefits, of presumed or proven substitutes, and because of the burden the program may impose on a household's immediate welfare, as when people cannot afford the time and transportation costs to go to a "free" clinic.

Program utilization need not be dependent, however, on program objectives. A target household has the capacity to reallocate program resources to reach its own rather than the program's objectives. For example, a mother may feed a particular child less than she feeds other family members because that child participates in a school feeding program. Thus, the mother may attenuate and offset the program's specific objectives and may "spread" its impact. Further, through the effect on one aspect of household life, say child mortality, the program may have an impact on other aspects, say fertility behavior. Although these other aspects may not be among the original objectives of a particular program, nonetheless, one should consider them as possible benefits or costs of the intervention.

By relating program services to household resources and objectives, the economic analysis of the household can help to identify (a) the potential uses of program services; (b) program substitutes; (c) the relative attractiveness of the program; and (d) the extent the program draws on household resources. One can thereby hypothesize who program users will be, how they may utilize the program, and subsequently, what the program's impact may be. The formulation of testable hypotheses about program impact aids in identifying variables and relationships that may measure program impact.

AN ECONOMIC FORMULATION OF HEALTH RELATED OUTCOMES

Program "impact" or "outcome" variables must be identified and discussed in conjunction with households' objectives or ends. This section deals with the household's behavioral objectives, around which we can model family responses to health intervention programs,

and on the basis of which we can identify and discuss appropriate
outcome measures.

Economists have long sought to establish adequate measures of
welfare, which is taken as the ultimate goal of man's economic
activity. In the absence of better measures, monetary income
has been used as a measure of welfare. Income, which flows
from labor and accumulated stocks of assets or capital, serves
as a proxy for welfare because higher levels of income mean higher
levels of production and, thus, more commodities that possess
utility. Measured incomes, however, ignore many utilitarian nonmarket household activities such as leisure. Furthermore, higher
levels of income do not necessarily correlate with greater lifetime well-being when all dimensions of human welfare are considered; the health and nutrition problems of affluent societies
are evidence of this last point (4).

Health status is itself a key element as well as a good proxy
measure of other aspects of human welfare; it can be considered
both a consumption item and an investment item (5, 6). Good health
is "consumption" because it is an end in itself, accounting for a
considerable part of that human welfare not measured by income.
Health is also an "investment" because it is a key component of
human capital that determines the level and duration of one's
market and nonmarket activities. As such, it can be linked to some
measurable components of earning and nonmonetary income.

This discussion focuses on the investment aspect of health
because this sets the lower limit of potential benefits from health
programs. 4/ The discussion is structured around the concept of
expected lifetime earnings. In a simplified way, one can define
for an individual of age A the present value of his lifetime expected earnings for N years henceforth by

$$E = \sum_{1}^{N} P_i^S \cdot P_i^H \cdot W_i \quad (1 + r)^{-(i)} \quad ,$$

where $\left[P_i^S \cdot P_i^H \cdot W_i \ (1 + r)^{-(i)} \right]$ states the present value of the
earning an individual "expects" at period i. It is given by his
(conditional) probability to survive to that period, P_i^S ; by the
probability of his being physically able to work that year, P_i^H ;
and by his average anticipated productivity -- or returns, psychic

---

4/   A rate of return on a health program as an investment will
always understate the actual return by excluding the unmeasurable
(consumption) utility derived from good health.

and other, from his time -- during that year, W_i. Given a particular time discount rate r, each time-specific expected earnings
component is discounted by $(1 + r)^{-i}$, which is the present value
of a unit of earning at a particular future period. 5/ Each
term P_i^S, P_i^H, or W_i can be regarded as a health outcome; together
they encompass the "investment" dimensions in health. 6/ P_i^S is
based on age-specific mortality rates, P_i^H is based on age-specific
morbidity rates measurable by lost working days, and W_i can be
measured by one's average daily wage rate.

The productivity measure or wage rate, W_i, may warrant more
attention because, unlike the other terms, it is not usually assumed
a direct outcome of nutrition and health. In a given economic
setting, defined by the available technology, land, and capital,
an individual's wage rate can be taken as a function of his innate
physical and mental abilities, and of his physical and mental
capacities acquired through education and work experience (7).
Since educational achievement and work experience are outcomes of
a process that depends partially on health and nutrition, man's
productivity, or W_i, can be viewed as a function of his health and
nutrition, at least in situations of severe malnutrition.

Once expected earnings, as specified, are regarded as an
individual's or a family's objective, the economic analysis can
derive certain predictions about the household's behavior. The
common approach is a maximization procedure by which the household is assumed to enhance P_i^S, P_i^H, W_i, and other utilitarian
ends, subject to various constraints. This procedure sets the
trade-offs among different ends, defines behavioral optima for each,
and thereby provides the analytical framework to deal systematically
with the relevant aspects of household behavior and to generate a
set of refutable hypotheses. 7/

5/ W_i can be regarded as a term net of investment in health and
education that affects the levels of all three terms.

6/ For simplicity, we ignore the interdependence among the three
terms.

7/ Anthropological insights into, as well as prior evidence about,
the household's view of the underlying investment process are
essential for adequate modeling. That is, for example, particular
household members may get substantially better diets and "health
investment" than others because their (lifetime) earnings are
important from the household's viewpoint. Some discrimination in
feeding among household members to protect the actual or potential
breadwinner is apparent in subsistence settings.

IMPACT MEASURES: BASIC PROBLEMS AND SOLUTIONS

The specification of the ultimate outcome variable -- expected
lifetime earnings -- and its components is also important for discussing some key statistical issues that relate to impact measurement and to some basic properties of impact measures.

Time lags are critical in measuring program impact and present
a key statistical problem inherent in intervention programs. The
longer the time between the intervention and the measurement of
its outcome, the harder it is to link the program to its hypothesized impact, because one must also account for environmental,
biological, and behavioral changes that may also affect the outcome. This issue, which is discussed in more detail in the next
section, is frustrating because the impacts of health and nutrition programs take time to manifest and are often spread over
individuals' lifetimes.

This problem of time lags warrants both a conceptual and a
practical distinction between two types of programs. The first
type is a program aimed at enhancing the stock of human capital
by an intervention during some critical period of human physical
and mental development. Programs involving mothers and children
are of this type. The second type is a program aimed at increasing the efficiency of a flow of services from an existing stock
of human capital. Programs involving adult workers are of this
type (8).

The first type of program has long-run outcomes that are
often not practical to measure because of the long time lag. Consequently, one must resort to proxies for measurements. The second
type has shorter-run objectives, primarily increasing productivity
and reducing absenteeism, that are immediately observable for
adult workers. Termination of a program of the second type should
end its effect and thereby provide another means of testing impact.
Thus, selecting appropriate outcome measures is more problematic
for the first, and more common, type of program. Consequently,
this discussion focuses on outcome measures for the more general
type of program with long-run impact.

In evaluating a potential outcome variable one should consider
these questions:

a.   How does the variable relate conceptually to the ultimate
     outcome, or any component thereof, and to the program
     under study?

b.   How does it relate statistically to the ultimate outcome
     variable, or any component thereof, and to the program
     under study?

    c.   How reliably can it be measured?

    d.   What complementary data are needed?

    e.   What are the costs of obtaining and using those data?

The first question is important because it relates an observed variable to the conceptual framework and to the specific hypotheses to be tested. The other questions bear largely on the statistical aspects of potential data for testing program impact. When all these questions are considered, trade-offs among particular types, or categories, of variables may appear.

We can classify outcome variables by three categories: inputs, intermediate outcomes, and ultimate outcomes. The use of program inputs as proxy measures of program impact is common. For example, the impact of a school feeding program is estimated by the amount of calories and protein the program delivers to the target population. This approach has the merit of being directly related to the program, and also is probably least costly since it is integrated with the program. However, it also tends to be the most presumptive since it may depend on hypotheses yet to be tested about relationships between inputs and eventual impact, and it may ignore program-induced behavioral changes beyond program control. This last issue depends critically on the delivery method; an income transfer to the household is easier for the household to divert from program objectives than, say, a directly administered vaccine.

Intermediate outcomes can be measured by a variety of variables: child morbidity, intellectual development, school achievement, and anthropometric measures including birthweight. These measures apply largely to children because theory and evidence suggest that they predict, and thus approximate, eventual health outcomes (9). Although they are not ultimate outcomes, such intermediate variables are "outputs" and in most cases they approximate ultimate outcomes better than program inputs do. Birthweight, for example, predicts relatively well a child's physical growth, at least during the first years and can be used as an outcome measure for maternal care programs (10). A child's physical growth and morbidity at an early age may indicate his future morbidity, survival probability, and productivity. A child's intellectual development, which to a degree may be nutritionally determined, is believed to be manifest eventually in his productivity and wages, primarily through mental development and school achievement (11-13).

These intermediate outcome variables raise the problem of lagged program impact since basically they are manifest over time.

Hence, linking the intermediate outcomes to the program inputs
is even more complicated than using inputs as proxies for outcomes. Complementary data on non-program variables that affect
the outcome may become critical for identifying the impact of the
program. Consequently, collecting data that relate to the intermediate outcome variables requires more elaborate data collection
instruments and statistical tools than when program inputs serve
to measure outcomes.

Ultimate outcome variables involve issues similar to those
of the intermediate outcomes, but they are more difficult since
they pertain to full lifetimes. Outcomes and related variables
can be measured on the basis of individuals, households, and communities. The choice of the measurement unit depends on the
specific measurement objectives. Policy-makers and program administrators are eventually interested in variables that summarize
their efforts on a community level. Students of household behavior are also interested in understanding and explaining the
distribution of outcomes in the household or the community. Or,
they may seek to understand why identical program inputs have a
varying impact across individuals and households of different
characteristics.

While critical for identifying the circumstances under which
programs are beneficial, differences in impact may be concealed
when we aggregate or, at times, disaggregate data. This possibility must be recognized when we define the unit of measurement.
One cannot always distinguish household variables from variables
pertaining to individuals. At times a variable can be based on a
particular household member; at other times, it can be based on a
few members. The definition of a household variable based on more
than one household member may be complicated because of the low
incidence of health-related events at the household level. Identification of the target population is a key criterion for the
selection and definition of a household variable. If the target
group consists of, say, mothers or potential mothers and we are
interested in their nutritional status, then the observation is
the mother -- an individual, as well as the household because in
most societies we observe one mother per household. This household then can be described by other common household variables
such as religion, income, size, or location, etc. The same reasoning applies when the target group consists of children of given
age and sex.

A problem usually arises when one must aggregate within households or other units that share the same socio-economic endowments.
This problem appears particularly acute in measuring some intermediate nutritional outcomes. For example, when the nutritional
status of all school-age children in a household is of interest,

one needs to define a summary variable summarizing the nutritional status of these children in that household. The problem is that the number of children as well as age and sex distributions vary across households. This problem can be handled in various ways; however, while aggregating within the household, one must consider the possibility that not all children are treated equally in a given household.

The same problem applies to other household variables. For example, two mothers or two family units may live in one household and share a common income. Splitting such a group's income between the two family units, and subsequently treating them as separate units for statistical purposes, may be erroneous if behavioral patterns in extended households differ from the patterns in nuclear households. In most cases, when data are treated by averages, a few critical behavioral issues are assumed: that individuals are not discriminated against, and that the behavior of aggregated social units is the sum of the behavior of some other individual units. Before aggregating or disaggregating data, even at the household level, one must see whether these assumptions lead to different predictions.

AN ECONOMETRIC APPROACH

We turn now, before discussing program measurement, to outline some basic features of econometrics that draw on mathematics, statistics, and economic theory to delineate economic relationships empirically. The development of econometrics has been largely influenced by economists' traditional use of non-experimental data to test hypotheses and to verify economic relationships. 8/

Economic theory attempts to describe the nature of particular causal relationships, or "structures", by identifying the parameters encompassed by them, and by indicating the particular functional relationships among those parameters. As indicated previously, these relationships attempt to account only for what is believed to be the systematic part of man's economic behavior. In reality this behavior also has random elements and may be determined by parameters that we fail either to identify and observe, or to measure accurately. Consequently, the econometric equivalent of

---

8/   The term "econometric approach" used here is substantially the same as the "structural equations approach" (14). That is, it is a general application of mathematical statistics not necessarily restricted to "economic" variables. The reader familiar with this approach may bypass this section.

TABLE 1. *REGRESSION COEFFICIENTS, CARBOHYDRATES, AND VITAMIN A AS DEPENDENT VARIABLES*

(t statistics in parentheses)

Independent Variables	Dependent Variables (Nutrient)	
	Vitamin A * I. U.	Carbohydrates * g.
Family Income*	0.1542 (6.9459)	0.0085 (0.6250)
Family Size*	0.5130 (4.1073)	0.9135 (11.8791)
North: Urban Elementary School (Intercept)	10.7470	7.8833
Region (South)**	−0.1310 (−4.6454)	0.0579 (3.3276)
Urbanization		
Non-Farm**	0.0229 (0.5313)	0.2657 (9.9887)
Rural-Farm**	−0.0030 (−0.0864)	0.1489 (6.9906)
Education		
High School**	0.1852 (4.4095)	0.0486 (1.5837)
College**	0.1279 (3.7289)	0.0308 (1.4597)
Adjusted R^2	0.743	0.920

*   The logarithms of the variable values were introduced in the estimated equation.

** Denotes the use of a "dummy" variable which takes the value of 1 when an event occurs and the value of 0 otherwise.

the relationships suggested by theory include a "disturbance" or error term added to the "systematic" part of a particular relationship. This term summarizes the random, omitted, and unidentified or inaccurately measured elements of man's behavior. For example, if a particular simple economic relationship is characterized by

$$Y = f(X),$$

its econometric equivalent is

$$Y_i = f(X_i) + v_i \quad (i = 1.....n \text{ observations})$$

where v_i is the disturbance or error term.

Thus, econometric relationships also are *causal* relationships and are stated with one or more equations, depending on the underlying structure, each having a single dependent, or "outcome", variable and one or more independent variables (15); also see Annex, Sections A and B. Estimating such equations involves obtaining, usually by means of "statistical control", at least unbiased estimates of the particular effect on the outcome variable of each independent variable. 9/ Such estimates are possible when there is no, or only a "small", correlation between the error term and any of the right-hand variables, and between any two of these variables.

Given a particular economic model, at least three considerations are pertinent in specifying and interpreting econometric relationships: (a) choosing explicit functional relationships; (b) controlling for variables not suggested by theory; and (c) dealing with different and, therefore, competing hypotheses consistent with a particular estimate. The specification of a particular functional relationship can be based on common sense, theoretical and empirical knowledge, and experimentation. For example, we expect caloric consumption normally to level off as income rises, because of saturation and also because of substitution away from calories and carbohydrates to more "luxurious" proteins. Hence, the specifications of a functional relationship between caloric consumption and income should allow for a nonlinear relationship.

The two estimated equations shown in Table I are a simple example of econometric equations; the effects of certain household variables on household consumption of vitamin A and carbohydrates

9/ The common estimation procedure is regression analysis, which is also a useful descriptive tool. For biological applications of regression analysis, see for example (16).

are estimated. 10/ These estimates are based on a relationship
like that shown in the Annex, Section B. This relationship allows
for the expected nonlinear effect on consumption of nutrients by
employing the logarithms of intakes of carbohydrates and vitamin
A, and the logarithm of household income. This functional relationship was also chosen because it allows for a comparison between the sensitivity of the intakes of carbohydrates to income,
and the intakes of vitamin A to income, regardless of the different units by which the two nutrients are measured, grams or
international units. Such a relationship may impose various restrictions on the estimates; for example, the relationship specified presumes no consumption when the household has no current
income. Nevertheless, such an unrealistic presumption and other
restrictions do not outweigh the advantages of using this particular relationship. Another example of choosing functional relationships involves measurement of child growth by weight and height.
Again, nonlinearity concerning age is appropriate here. The estimates shown in Tables 2 and 3 use a quadratic functional relationship that allows for this nonlinearity. These examples show how
particular functional relationships are chosen on the basis of
prior knowledge as well as practical considerations.

Controlling for variables not originally suggested by theory
may be a useful means for improving the precision of the estimates,
standardization, and adding information. 11/ An economic model of
behavior may ignore biological factors by assuming them constant.
For example, a model that deals with parents' choices of their
children's diets and, therefore, child growth (18) might assume
that the analysis is confined to a hypothetical age and sex group
and, therefore, disregard the age and sex variables in explaining
variations in child growth. However, for an econometric analysis
based on a relatively small sample of children of both sexes and
across age groups, one should control for age and sex as illustrated

---

10/ This table is drawn from (17) where an attempt is made to use
economic theory and econometrics to predict and measure the effects
of household characteristics on its diet. The coefficients on the
logarithmic variables show the percentage change in household consumption of the particular nutrient due to a given percentage
change in these variables. The coefficients on the dummy variables
show the same but compared with variables which were "left out",
or included in the intercept term. These estimates and others are
used here for illustrative purposes only.

11/ Note that inclusion of omitted variables, which are not perfectly correlated with other independent variables, will increase
the multiple correlation coefficient, or "explained variance" of
the dependent variable. This increase should not be a goal by
itself.

in Table 2, Equation 2. Otherwise, the relationship between child
weight and age will be entirely approximated by the correlation
between diet and weight across children of different age groups.
12/ This means of control is an alternative to various standardization procedures, like weight for age, used by nutritionists.
It is also informative because it depicts growth curves directly
across age and sex groups -- controlling for other effects -- and
can be based on relatively small samples.

     The problem of dealing with competing hypotheses is major.
The first and basic issue to address is whether the line of causality implied by a particular relationship is correct. For example,
in Table 2, Equations 2 and 3, the effect on children's weight
of caloric intakes is estimated. However, the case can be made
that the causality also operates the other way: heavier children
consume more calories *ceteris paribus*. In a case like this it is
reasonable to assume a structure where child weight and caloric
consumption are codetermined. Therefore, one must use appropriate
estimation techniques to allow for this codetermination or simultaneity. The estimates reported in these equations exemplify a
case like this. The estimated effect of caloric consumption on
weight in the third equation is based on a procedure that accounts
also for the effect of weight on caloric consumption. This estimated effect differs from the estimate in the second equation where
the estimation procedure does not account for simultaneity. 13/

     The second issue is to ascertain that the variables indeed
measure (or approximate) what they are meant to measure. In the
context of nutrition interventions, a good example is the behavioral
change in food consumption of families under observation due to
presence of an interviewer. Thus, the variable that was supposed
to measure the effect of program inputs measures instead another

-----

12/ This procedure can be elaborated to account for interaction
between the age or sex variables and other variables; that is,
when, for example, a given diet has a different effect on children
of different age and sex.

13/ Two or more variables are simultaneously determined when they
are outcomes or endogenous variables belonging to a structure where
one of these variables affects the other in some relationships and
viceversa in others. Failing to account for this codetermination
while estimating one particular structural relationship may result
in a "simultaneity bias" which means that the estimated effect of
one endogenous variable on the other may be under- or overstated.
On how to deal statistically with such cases, see (15); for specific
application in a nutrition study from which this table is drawn,
see (19).

TABLE 2. *REGRESSION COEFFICIENTS, CHILD'S WEIGHT IN KG AS*
A DEPENDENT VARIABLE, ORDINARY LEAST SQUARES (OLS)
AND TWO-STAGE LEAST SQUARES (TSLS) ESTIMATES

(t statistics in parentheses)

Equation No.	Type of Estimation	Intercept	"Biological" Variables				
			Age	Age^2	Sex Male*	Age Sex	$(Age\ Sex)^2$
1	(OLS)	-0.63771	0.609 (6.628)	-0.008 (-4.736)	7.533 (5.526)	-0.563 (-4.280)	0.011 (3.708)
2	(OLS)	3.173	0.245 (3.559)	-0.019 (-1.261)	0.708 (2.994)		
3	(TSLS)	1.788	0.112 (1.246)	-0.0001 (-0.077)	0.169 (0.272)		

(Equations continued from above)	Economic Variables				
	Occupation			Diet	
	Land Owner*	Agri. Labor*	Civil Servant*	Calories	R^2
1	0.860 (2.559)	0.038 (0.110)	0.745 (1.851)		0.61
2				0.001 (4.125)	0.55
3				0.004 (3.235)	

* Dummy Variables

behavioral change induced by the program, thereby founding the measurement of the program impact. Similarly, the estimated effects of the sex variable on children's nutritional status may measure parents' behavioral discrimination between sons and daughters, as well as genetic differences between sexes. In a case like this, it may be impossible to discriminate statistically between the two competing hypotheses. 14/ Such cases put an added burden on the scientist beyond getting unbiased estimates; he must be careful in interpreting his findings in light of a variety of behavioral and other relationships that can produce particular statistical results.

Some cases of competing hypotheses are more predictable and statistically manageable than others. These cases can be generally characterized as those in which one has some notion or knowledge about correlations between only two independent variables. For example, the United States food stamp program is designed for low income groups. Consequently, a variable representing household participation in the program is expected to be negatively and highly correlated with the income variable in an analysis of this program's impact across income groups. Therefore, statistical discrimination between the effect of the program as opposed to the effect of income on a particular outcome variable may present a significant problem. A correlation between the disturbance term and one or more independent variables may have similar consequences.

Econometrics is concerned with the problems briefly described here and other related ones. The solutions offered are geared, however, to existing data and, consequently, are largely based on statistical control.

IMPACT MEASUREMENT: ECONOMETRICS AND SOCIAL EXPERIMENTS

An illustration based on one of the major "experiments" in nutrition can be helpful to the more general discussion that follows about the use of econometrics in measurement of program impact and the relationship between econometrics and social experiments.

The estimated regression coefficients shown in Table III are based on the Narangwal experimental project (21). The first equation -- which is equivalent to comparing the mean outcomes of an experiment -- shows the estimated effects on child weight of various

---

14/ For a technical discussion on related issues in the context of a nutrition project, see (20).

TABLE 3.   REGRESSION COEFFICIENTS, CHILD'S WEIGHT IN KG   AS
*   A DEPENDENT VARIABLE*

   (t statistics in parentheses)

| Equation No. | Intercept | "Biological" Variables | | | | Socio-Economic Status |
		Age	$(Age)^2$	Sex Male	Higher Caste (JAT)*
1	7.96897				
2	3.18148	0.00967 (10.81462)	−0.00001 (−4.59184)	0.51932 (4.00037)	0.52166 (3.85227)

| (Equations continued from above) | Types of Intervention | | | |
	Nutrition Supplement*	Medical Care*	Nut/Supp. + Med. Care *	R^2
1	−1.12432 (−2.45703)	−0.08715 (−0.18166)	0.27777 (0.69498)	.064
2	0.77071 (2.76640)	0.22200 (0.80560)	0.76378 (3.34425)	.707

* Dummy Variables

interventions, without controlling for other variables that might
affect the outcome (see Annex, Section E). The second equation
shows the same, but with statistical control for age, sex, and
socio-economic status approximated by caste. The first equation
shows that nutritional supplementation has a negative and statistically significant effect on child weight, while medical care and
a combination of medical care and nutritional supplementation had
no effect. Once we control for the other variables, intervention
by nutritional supplementation and by nutritional supplementation
combined with medical care show a positive and statistically significant effect on child weight.

The Narangwal experiment was not a "true" experimental design,
but for that matter, it probably could never be. 15/ Moreover,
it represents well the constraints of the kind most field programs
face. Treatments were applied to entire villages because random
assignment of the treatments within villages was socially and
practically inconceivable. Randomization on the basis of a population of villages was impractical because it would inflate the program to proportions beyond its financial and logistic means. 16/
Two issues had to be considered before estimating program impact.
First, although similar, the villages may have been different also
in aspects other than the treatments. Second, there was scope for
behavioral "self selection"; different people could, by choice,
avail themselves differentially of the services, and for that matter, could benefit differentially from given services.

Indeed, the combination of these factors is evident in the
results presented here. The first equation shows merely a negative
correlation between child weight and nutritional supplementation.
This is consistent with either or a combination of the following

---

15/ "Experimental design" refers to use of a "control" group and
"treatment" group (or groups) selected entirely by a random process. In the purest and simplest type of randomization or experimental design, as opposed to an econometric approach, one is not
concerned with identifying and specifying particular causal and
structural relationships and with estimating their various parameters. Full discussion of experimental design is beyond the scope
of this paper. The discussion here is based on (22-24).

16/ Almost none of the major other field experiments, like those
undertaken by INCAP, meets the requirements of experimental design.
The same is true, for that matter, in the field of family planning
(25). It appears that researchers attempted, for practical and
ethical considerations, to approach a situation where they have
"matching groups".

hypotheses. First, the village where children received nutritional supplementation could have had children with a lower average weight, possibly because of nutritional reasons as well as the children's age and sex composition. Second, higher caste and better caring mothers, who have heavier children, could have used the nutrition program more, and more efficiently, than others. 17/ Once we control for these possibilities, by adding the other variables to the estimated relationship, we get better estimates of the interventions' impact in the short run as measured by child weight.

This example can be useful in outlining a general (and pragmatic) approach as well as specific criteria for assessing statistical requirements for evaluation research. However, we must first agree on the following points: (a) on pure statistical grounds, (randomized) experimental designs based on large samples are superior to any other approach for "netting out" impact; (b) quantitative evaluation of programs must be, however, socially efficient; and (c) to meet the efficiency requirement we must always weigh the value of the additional (marginal) gain in statistical evidence and accuracy versus the marginal costs involved. The last point is a general efficiency criterion that may dictate the use of experimental design, econometrics, and a combination of the two. The combined use of econometrics and experimentation is emerging in economic studies, for example, the New Jersey Graduated Work Incentive Experiment (26).

Returning to the Narangwal example with the above points in mind, we must first address what it represents, and then consider what the results mean in terms of the relative efficiency of social experiments. With respect to the first question, it represents what economists call a "revealed preference": the best that could, and probably can, be done, given objectives and constraints. This does not mean that we cannot have better field experiments. It merely puts a question mark on their economic and political feasibility.

On the issue of the relative efficiency of social experiments, the results obtained by means of statistical control are most likely biased, or lack "internal validity", at least because of the nonzero correlations between any two of the right-hand variables. However, these biases do not appear serious, and the results are fairly "reasonable". 18/ That is, it is highly probable that a

---

17/ Other possibilities not discussed here are also plausible.

18/ The results indicate that using the short term outcome, child weight, nutritional supplementation had a measurable effect. Due to this particular intervention child weight in the sample used

full-fledged (and costlier) experiment might not improve the results substantially. While this is a testable proposition, which
warrants an experiment, the author is willing to conclude that to
determine the impacts of the Narangwal project, the mix of "semi-
experimentation" and a subsequent econometric approach prove sufficient.

To outline an econometrician's general approach to data requirements for impact measurement, let us consider three interventions aimed at increasing caloric consumption: (a) a national
food subsidy program to reduce the prices of cereals to all consumers; (b) a national food stamp program for everyone; and (c)
a national food stamp program with randomly selected participants.
Assume that the three programs will give participants identical
price reductions. 19/ Program (c) can be evaluated simply and unambiguously just by collecting caloric consumption data after the
fact, if we are content merely to answer two questions: Did the
program increase caloric intakes? If so, what was the average
increase per family? The answers to these questions could be un-
equivocal, assuming we gather accurate data and we draw a large
enough sample. But this approach would tell us virtually nothing
about why some families respond to the program more or less than
the average or in the case of program failure, why there should
have been no significant impact. In more general terms, the experimental program (c) lacks "external validity". Moreover, apart
from cost considerations, the administration of this program poses
social and other hazards that may jeopardize the validity of the
experiment.

Programs like (a) and (b) may be more realistic and are more
common than an experimental program like (c). Taking this reality
as a constraint, we stress how one can measure impact using an
econometrician's perspective. Although programs (a) and (b) cause
identical reductions in prices, there is a fundamental difference
between them. Under the first program, households can buy the
cereals only at the subsidized price. Under the second, households
can exercise choice in buying cereals with or without food stamps,

---

here increased by .77 kg., or 9.7%, at the sample mean. The highest zero-order correlation between two of the right-hand variables
was .34. It should be noted that a more careful econometric treatment of the data presented here may improve the results.

19/ Other differences between the programs are ignored. For a
discussion of the different implications of programs, like (a) and
(b), see (27).

and they can even sell the stamps. 20/ This difference between
the programs is also of key statistical significance. For the
first programs, all we know is that it started at some particular
point in time and existed to a subsequent point. But for the
second, additional important information is potentially available:
whether or not, and possibly to what extent, a household used the
program stamps for buying cereals.

To determine impact in the first instance, panel data are
necessary. Pre-program, or "baseline" data, should include the
variables believed, on theoretical and other grounds, to affect
the outcome. These data serve to estimate the basic relationship
between, say, caloric consumption and its nonprogram determinants.
Once this relationship is estimated, we may also be able to estimate the added program effect (c.f.Annex, Section D). For example,
suppose the food subsidy is introduced in an agricultural economy
and reduces prices of cereals. However, if farmers' incomes fall
during the program period because of bad weather, for example,
the farmers may consume less cereals even at the lower prices.
Hence, such a fall in incomes may offset any positive effect of
the program. Therefore, by accounting for changes in incomes (or
even weather conditions), one can estimate program impact, provided
no event significantly affecting the program outcome occurs simultaneously with the program in a way to confound our inferences.

In the second instance, the national food stamp program (Program B) baseline data may not be needed if we can analyze statistically the variance in households' utilization of the program.
This possibility depends on the relationship between program utilization and other variables. At least from a behavioral standpoint,
it is almost inconceivable that households of different characteristics will use, and even benefit from, the program identically.
Therefore, it may be possible to study the determinants of program
utilization as well as the interaction between program inputs and
household characteristics. That is, what are the effects on utilization of various income and education levels? How do households
of different levels of income and education benefit from given
program inputs? If consistent answers should emerge, it might be
relatively straight forward to infer about the impact of the program
itself (c.f. Annex, Section C).

20/ Although the food stamps are available to all, one must consider the time and trouble of getting them. For example, a mother
with five small children, living at a distance from where food
stamps are sold, may find it less attractive to obtain those stamps
than a mother of five grown children living nearby that selling
station, *ceteris paribus*. See Annex, Section C.

A program involving a target population identified by socio-
economic characteristics, geographical location, or nutrition
status can be regarded as a special case. Such a program differs
from those already discussed in that it is for a population identified by one or more of the non-program variables affecting the outcome. Hence, there is a built-in correlation between the measure
of participation in the program and some other determinant(s) of
the outcome. Most policy programs fall into this category. Impact
measurement in such cases must be confined to the target population and involves essentially identical considerations to those
relating to the non-experimental programs discussed above. When
within the target population, there is no (or not enough) variation in the program (input or utilization) variable, panel data
will be required to measure impact. For example, impact measurement in a particular intervention village of the Narangwal project
is not possible if all that is known is that that particular village
was exposed to that intervention. However, when there is sufficient variance in the program variable within the target population, this variance can be used to measure impact. For example,
the United States food stamp program is designed for low-income
families. Within that population, however, some families do not
use the program at all and other families use the program to different degrees. This variation may permit estimating program impact.

Within the perspective taken in the preceding paragraphs, an
experimental approach is warranted when it is less costly, or when
there is reason to believe that, given the available statistical
techniques, panel data are insufficient to measure impact. Two
basic situations may undermine the use of panel data. The first
is when the underlying structural relationships are believed to
change over time. Such a change may prohibit estimating the added
effect of the program. The second situation is one where there
is reason to believe that one or more of the non-program determinants
of the outcome will change during the monitoring period in a way
that will confound any inference. Hence, experimental design may
be used as a precautionary measure against foreseen and unforeseen
circumstances. However, taking the view that social experiments
are costly, financially and otherwise, we must look for ways (a) to
reduce their costs and (b) to maximize their usefulness.

To reduce costs, we must protect the measurement procedure
against uncertainty rather than against ignorance because protection against ignorance can be unnecessarily more costly. To elaborate, uncertainty is defined here as a situation where one has
good reason to believe that some *known* non-program determinants
of the outcome may change significantly during the program and
potentially have a confounding effect. For example, when an outbreak of diarrhea may confound the measurement of the impact of a

child-feeding program, implementation of experimental child-feeding
programs in two or more areas will lessen the risk that diarrheal
disease will confound the results and obscure a possible treatment effect. Ignorance is defined here as a situation when one
does not know the determinants of the outcome variable. In this
case, one may wish to have an experiment by a random assignment
of the intervention to "protect" the evaluation from all possible
confounding effects. Unfortunately, this may be nearly impossible
and unnecessarily costly.

When considering the use of experimental design, the economic
theory of the household and econometrics may help to reduce the
"costs of ignorance" by suggesting which non-program variables might
confound the evaluation and need to be controlled for. Alternatively, prior considerations should help to stratify and reduce
the evaluation sample. 21/ The first step is to understand, possibly by some modeling, the behavioral and other determinants of
a particular outcome. This effort should be coupled with anthropological observations as well as a pilot survey. Once key non-
program determinants of the outcome have been identified, the
number of variables for which the experiment has to be controlled
may become manageable. The second step is to protect against uncertainty by limiting the control variables to those that may
change during the life of the program. This step may further reduce the cost of the evaluation. Obviously, in reality the researcher confronts both uncertainty as well as ignorance. However,
given the costs of evaluation research based on experimental design,
the benefits from careful *a priori* modeling may be substantial.

When experimental design is selected, an econometric approach
to the data can help maximize its usefulness. As already mentioned,
from a statistical viewpoint, impact measurement in a well-designed
experiment can be satisfied just by comparing the means of the outcome variables between the treatment group(s) and the control
group(s). This approach, however, reduces the acceptability and
the universality of the results and has serious shortcomings in
experimental contexts where policies are tested for future and
wider applications. To increase the generality, or "external validity", of an evaluation based on experimental design, the researcher should include other variables or controls that affect the
outcome measure and apply econometric techniques to the data (cf
Annex, Section E). In this way, one can test some basic behavioral
hypotheses and perhaps show explicitly how a program relates to its
environment.

21/ This approach comes close to a "quasi-experimental" design.

CONCLUSION

The basic postulate of this paper is that although health related interventions aim to increase household and individual welfare, they may be inconsistent with the household's and individual's own objectives and opportunities. Where households can exercise choices *vis-a-vis* the program, studying these objectives and opportunities and relating them to particular interventions must be the first steps in understanding and predicting a program's potential impact. While analyzing household behavior is no mean task, it is nevertheless essential. By relating the concept of expected earnings to age-specific productivity, morbidity, and mortality probabilities, the economic theory of the household offers a conceptual framework in which to integrate relevant aspects of household behavior with the basic outcomes of health programs. Thereby, this theory can suggest testable hypotheses concerning program impact, and can help to identify various outcome measures for programs.

Econometrics stresses the empirical aspects of the causal behavioral relationships outlined by the economic theory and, given the social and financial costs of social experiments, can provide a useful and efficient framework for measuring program impact. An econometric approach can, at times, substitute for experimental design, and at other times, complement it, depending on financial and other costs as well as statistical considerations. When experimental design is warranted on statistical grounds because statistical control techniques are insufficient to measure impact, the economic theory of the household may help to minimize the cost of the experiment by suggesting which variables should be controlled. Furthermore, once data from experimental design are available, the use of an econometric approach to explore those data can increase the credibility and generality of the results.

Thus, the combination of theoretical and other *a priori* considerations with econometric estimation techniques and experiments can prove the most efficient way to measure program impact.

ANNEX

A. A simple economic relationship -- say between a household's caloric consumption (Y) and a vector X of household characteristics including, for example, household income -- can be stated by

$$Y = f(X). \hspace{3cm} [1]$$

This is an "exact" relationship in that it does not account for random elements in human behavior. It is also a partial relationship in the sense that it may "ignore" other lines of causality;

a more comprehensive underlying model may also deal, for example, with the effects of caloric consumption on household income. Given a relationship like [1] economic theory is usually concerned with the nature of the changes in Y due to changes in X, within a relevant range.

B.   Assuming that X represents just income and that Y and X are observable, the econometric equivalent of relationship [1] can, for example, be

$$\log_e \ (Y_i) = a + b \log_e \ (X_i) + v_i, \ (i = 1 \ \text{-----} n), \qquad [2]$$

where the index i denotes one of n observations, and v_i is a disturbance, or error, term which is usually assumed to be random, to have a normal distribution with an expected value of zero and a constant variance, and to be uncorrelated with other independent (right-hand) variables and with similar disturbance terms across observations. The term "a" is a shift parameter or "intercept", indicating levels of caloric consumption that are independent of X and v. The term "b" indicates, in this case, the change in log (Y) due to a unit change in log (X). Alternatively, "b" indicates the percent change in Y due to a given percent change in X, or the "elasticity" of Y with respect to X. 22/ Assuming no errors in the specification of [2] , obtaining an unbiased estimate of "b" is possible when X_i is not correlated with v_i. 23/.

C.   The following underlying structure is generally assumed here for discussing measurement of the impact of a program. First, in a given environment where such a program has been implemented, an outcome (Y) is a function of the household's utilization of the program (U) and particular subset of household characteristics (X_1); that is,

$$Y = f \ (U, X_1) \quad , \qquad\qquad\qquad [3]$$

where U and X_1 may be dependent; that is, for biological and behavioral reasons, particular levels of program utilization may have different effects in households of different characteristics; $\frac{\partial^2 Y}{\partial U \partial X_1} \neq 0.$

Second, the utilization of the program is a function of the supply of program inputs (P) indicating the intensity by which the

---

22/ Some other properties of this double-logarithmic function are discussed in Section IV of the text.

23/ When X_1 denotes a vector of variables, any two of those variables should also be uncorrelated.

program reaches different households, and of a subset of household characteristics (X_2);

$$U = g(P, X_2) \quad , \tag{4}$$

where X_1 and X_2 are not necessarily mutually exclusive subsets at least conceptually.

This structure can be reduced by substituting (4) into (3), to

$$Y = f\left[g(P,X_2), X_1\right] = h(P, X_3), \tag{5}$$

where X_3 is a set of household characteristics combining X_1 and X_2.

Estimating relationship (5) may be sufficient to measure program impact. This alone is insufficient, however, for understanding this impact and, thus, for evaluating the program. In particular, such a relationship does not reveal whether variations in impact of given program inputs are due to different levels of utilization, to differences in impact of given inputs on households of different characteristics, or both. The problem can be stated as the researcher's inability to test various hypotheses concerning X_1 and X_2. This problem can be solved by estimating relationship (4), which may be crucial for designing a cost-effective program because this relationship identifies the users and levels of utilization of a particular program. 24/

D. A simple approach to panel data pertaining to a program is to pool baseline and program data, and estimate an explicit function of

$$Y_{it} = g(t, X_{it}, P_i, v_{it}), \quad (i = 1....n, \quad t = 0,1) \tag{6}$$

where: t represents the time period a particular observation was obtained; 25/ Y_{io} and X_{io} represent baseline or preintervention values; $Y_{i1} = Y_{io} + dY_i$ and $X_{i1} = X_{io} + dX_i$ represent postinterven-

---

24/ Although conceptually different, P and U are often interchanged and relationship [3] is estimated instead of [5]. In such a case the researcher should be aware that he may attribute undue failure or success to program services. That is, the program may succeed or fail because of particular household characteristics; some programs may succeed in one setting and fail in another.

25/ t = 0 for preintervention and t = 1 for during or postintervention. This illustration can be generalized to include more than two time periods.

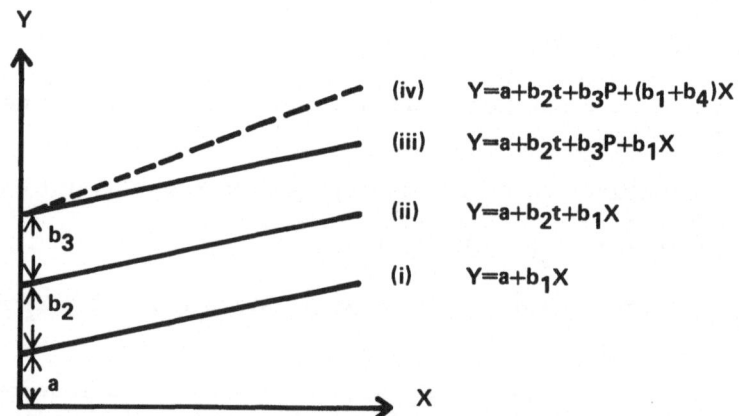

Fig. II. *General Relationship Between Income and Caloric Consumption.*

tion values; and P_i indicates program inputs. 26/ Assuming, without much loss of generality, that the relationship between caloric intakes and the other variables is linear within the relevant range, and that changes in income bring about identical changes in consumption over time, one can estimate this equation as illustrated in Figure II.

$$Y_{it} = a + b_1 X_{it} + b_2 t + b_3 P_i + b_4 P_i X_{it} + v_{it} \qquad [7]$$

First, no interaction is assumed between the program (inputs) and household characteristics, $b_4 = 0$; that is, program impact is independent of the level of household income. Curve (i) in Figure II indicates the general relationship between income and caloric consumption, or the pre-program relationship. Curve (ii) indicates the added effect of time, measured by b_2 that is presumed to be independent of the other effects. For example, it can indicate the effect of child growth on caloric consumption. Curve (iii) depicts the added effect of the intervention measured by b_3.

Second, we assume that Y measures child weight, for given age and sex, and that there is interaction between X and P, or $b_4 \neq 0$;

26/ Alternative, P_i = 1 for participation in, or prevalence of, the program and P_i = 0 otherwise.

that is, for a given level of program utilization the impact of
the program, measured by gain in child weight, differs across
households of different levels of income. For example, children
of better-to-do families may be less exposed to diarrhea than
children of poor families. Consequently, the children of relatively richer families may gain more in weight from a given school
feeding program, *ceteris paribus*. This particular effect is depicted by line (iv) of the figure.

Estimating program impact by using panel data is not feasible
when "p" and "t" are statistically indistinguishable; that is,
when some other events potentially affecting the outcome concur
with the program.

E.   Suppose that the sample underlying relationship [7] and Figure II is drawn from an experimental design which consists of n
observations, m in the control group and (n-m) in the experimental
or program group. That is, $P_i = 0$ for $i = 1....m$, and $P_i = 1$ for
$i = m+1....n$. To measure and test for intervention impact, the
experimental design advocates measuring the difference $dY_e - dY_c$
and testing for its statistical significance, where $dYc = dY_i/m$
is the mean change in the outcome in the control group, and dYe
is the corresponding statistic for the experimental group. This
difference will reflect correctly and fully program impact, only
if the experimental design achieves complete randomization (or
perfect matching) of all other potential effects; that is P_i
does not correlate with any other determinant of the observed
outcome.

To achieve the same goal an econometrician would estimate
relationship [7], by either

$$Y_{it} = G + b_3'' P_i + V_{it} \qquad\qquad\qquad [8]$$

or $$dY_i = E + b_3'' P_i + W_i \qquad\qquad\qquad [9]$$

where W_i is a disturbance term similar to V_i. It can be shown that

$$dY_e - dY_c = b_3 = b_3' = b_3'' \qquad\qquad\qquad [10]$$

when P_i does not correlate with any of the right-hand variables in
equation [7]. Hence, while econometric and experimental approaches
should yield identical statistical results because of the underlying statistical rationale, the econometric approach specifies
particular structural and functional relationships and tries to
account for all relevant determinants of the outcome.

ACKNOWLEDGEMENT

My colleagues A. A. Kielmann, M.D., and D. Coate, as well as
participants in the PAHO conference for which this paper was prepared, should share in any credit for this presentation. However,
neither they nor the World Bank should be held responsible for the
views expressed here.

REFERENCES

1. World Bank. *Health Sector Policy Paper*. Washington, D. C.:
    World Bank, 1975.
2. Becker, G. S. The theory of allocation of time. *Economic
    Journal*, 75:493-517, 1965.
3. Lancaster, K. J. A new approach to consumer theory. *J. Polit-
    ical Econ.* 74:132-57, 1966.
4. Eckholm, E. and F. Record. *The Two Faces of Malnutrition*.
    Washington, D. C.: World Watch Institute, Paper No. 9.
5. Mushkin, S. Health as an investment. *J. Political Econ.*
    70:129-157, 1962.
6. Grossman, M. *The Demand for Health: A Theoretical and Empir-
    ical Investigation*. New York and London: Columbia
    University Press for National Bureau of Economic Research,
    1972.
7. Mincer, J. *Schooling, Experience and Earnings*. New York and
    London: Columbia University Press for National Bureau
    of Economic Research, 1974.
8. Basta, S. S. and A. Churchill. *Iron Deficiency Anemia and
    the Productivity of Adult Males in Indonesia*. Washington,
    D. C.: World Bank, Staff Working Paper No. 175, 1974.
9. Stoch, M. B. and P. M. Smythe. Fifteen-year development study
    on effects of severe undernutrition during infancy on
    subsequent physical growth and intellectual functioning.
    Archives of Disease in Childhood, 51:326-336, 1976.
10. Lechtig, A. Effect of improved nutrition during pregnancy
    and lactation on developmental retardation and infant
    mortality. In: P. L. White and N. Selvey (eds.) p. 117,
    Proceedings of Western Hemisphere Nutrition Congress,
    Massachusetts: Publishing Sciences Group, Inc., 1975.
11. Selowsky, M. A note on preschool-age investment in human
    capital in developing countries. *Economic Development
    and Cultural Change*, 24:707-720, 1976.
12. Selowsky, M. and L. Taylor. The economics of malnourished
    children: An example of disinvestment in human capital.
    Economic Development and Cultural Change, 22:17-36, 1973.
13. Grossman, M. and L. N. Edwards. *An Economic Analysis of Chil-
    dren's Health and Intellectual Development*. New York:
    National Bureau of Economic Research, Working Paper No.
    180, 1977.

14. Duncan, O. D. *Introduction to Structural Equation Models.*
    New York: Academic Press, Inc., 1975.
15. Johnson, J. *Econometric Methods.* Second Edition, New York:
    McGraw-Hill, 1972.
16. Snedecor, G. W. and W. G. Cochran. *Statistical Methods.* Sixth
    Edition, Ames: Iowa State University Press.
17. Chernichovsky, D. The demand for nutrition. Washington, D.C.,
    World Bank, 1977 (Mimeograph).
18. Chernichovsky, D. and D. Coate. *The Choice of Diet for Young
    Children and Its Relation to Children's Growth.* New York:
    National Bureau of Economic Research, Working Paper No.
    219, 1977.
19. Chernichovsky, D. and A. A. Kielmann. Socio-economic status,
    diet and preschool child growth in rural Punjab, India.
    Baltimore: The Johns Hopkins University Press, 1977.
    (Mimeograph).
20. Nasoetion, A. H. Spurious correlation as a result of con-
    straints in randomization. *Research Methodology, Agri-
    cultural Development Teaching Forum Council,* <u>46</u>:
    1975.
21. Taylor, E. C., *et al.* Malnutrition, infection, growth and
    development: The Narangwal experience. Baltimore:
    The World Bank and the Johns Hopkins University Press,
    1978. (Mimeograph).
22. Campbell, D. T. and J. C. Stanley. *Experimental and Quasi-
    Experimental Designs for Research.* Chicago: Rand-
    McNally Publishing Company, 1966.
23. Ross, J. and P. Smith. Orthodox experimental designs. In:
    H. M. Blalock and A. B. Blalock (eds.) p. 339. *Method-
    ology in Social Research.* New York: McGraw-Hill,
    1968.
24. Bennet, C. A. and A. A. Lumsdaine. *Evaluation and Experi-
    ment: Some Critical Issues in Assessing Social Programs.*
    New York: Academic Press, Inc., 1975.
25. Cuca, R. and C. Pierce. *Experiments in Family Planning.*
    Baltimore and London: The Johns Hopkins University
    Press for the World Bank, 1977.
26. United States Department of Health, Education and Welfare.
    *Summary Report: New Jersey Graduated Work Incentive
    Experiment.* Princeton: New Jersey, 1973.
27. Reutlinger, S. and M. Selowsky. *Malnutrition and Poverty.*
    Baltimore and London: The Johns Hopkins University
    Press for the World Bank, 1976.

COMMENTS

Sebastián Piñera, *Comisión Económica para America Latina (ECLA) Santiago, Chile*

Chernichovsky's paper treats two conceptual matters and one methodological matter that have fundamental importance for evaluating the impacts of nutrition and related health programs.

The first conceptual matter is the potential contribution of the "New Home Economics" to understanding the determinants of program impact. The need to evaluate impacts of nutrition and health programs arises from the existence of resource scarcity in face of multiple uses. Therefore, efficiency requires selection of programs with major impacts on the variables one wishes to affect. Moreover, a useful evaluation not only should quantify the aggregate success level of an intervention, but also should locate and identify -- at each stage upon which impact depends -- the leading factors that tend to raise or lower the degree of success. Hence arises the importance and contribution of the "New Home Economics".

This approach regards the household as the basic socio-economic unit whithin which decisions are made about allocation of the household's resources. These decisions include its supply of labor and capital to factor markets as well as its consumption of goods and services. So long as the household is the primary decision-making unit, analyses of the determinants of household behavior seem fundamental for non-experimental statistical evaluations of nutrition and health programs impacts. In the context of this theory, household decisions are made so as to maximize a utility function (or, more fully, a "happiness" function) subject to certain constraints imposed by initial factor endowments, by technical production possibilities for self-consumed goods and services, and by the prevailing prices in different markets. In light of this focus, an intervention program will have an impact only to the extent that it affects the preferences (or the utility functions) of households, or if it affects some of the constraints that shape households' maximizing behavior. In other words, an intervention program will only be able to change the combination of signals, incentives, and stimuli upon which the family unit bases its decisions: income levels, prices, knowledge about the utility of certain goods, and so forth. But without a doubt, it is the household that determines impact by revising its maximizing behavior in light of new conditions introduced by the program. Recognition of this fact is of fundamental importance for correct evaluations.

Some programs may cause such drastic changes in incentives or signals that they leave little or no room for family decisions that might affect impact. Examples of such programs are obligatory vaccination and obligatory or strongly promoted consumption of pills or contraceptives. However, even for these sorts of direct interventions, family members can change behavior so as to make substitutions that modify the intervention's impact. For example, women that get rewards or subsidies for using contraception can simply employ the new methods as substitutes for those used before, perhaps reducing their ages of marriage or the lengths of their lactation periods. The final result is that a program, even though it distributes many contraceptives, may have no impact upon fertility. Likewise, the parents of children that get free milk in school can reduce the amount of milk consumed at home so that their children's total milk intake remains constant. Once again, the program's impact on children's total milk consumption can be zero in spite of the direct milk distribution.

     In less direct programs, family behavior and decisions are even more important in determining success. Examples are programs to improve poor families' nutritional status via income subsidies, food price subsidies, free distribution of food to families, and so forth. With such programs, impacts on the nutritional status of poor families, particularly for members like children and the elderly, depend critically upon family behavior. Income and food price subsidies may have minimal impacts on nutrition when marginal propensities to consume food and price elasticities of demand for food are low. By the same token, under certain conditions, the free distribution of food can be exactly equivalent to an income subsidy and can have an insignificant impact on the nutritional situation it is supposed to affect. Moreover, this sort of program can increase food consumption of certain groups within the nuclear family (adults and men) and either not affect or affect minimally the consumption of others (children and women). In this respect, the few studies of intrafamilial distribution of food consumption show the marginal propensity to consume food varies significantly across members of the family and types of food. In other words, the important thing for measuring program impact is not which resources or what quantity of the food in question was supplied by the program, but rather which of these resources or of this food were actually used by the target population. (One should not forget that powdered milk supplied by a nutrition program may also be used to paint walls, to mark football fields, and so forth!).

     In summary, to guarantee the success of an intervention, it is not enough to create a greater supply of the goods or services one seeks to encourage. As important as supply is, there is also a critical need to induce or generate a demand from the target population for these goods or services. Participation of the target population in all stages of the program can be an indispensible

or very important element for the success of this last objective.
It can succeed through programs of education or incentives for
the target population to participate.

In general, each intervention program tries to produce a
pattern of consumption different from what the program's target
households would have followed if an amount of money equivalent
to the program's resources had simply been made available through
income transfers. Implicit in this attitude is the notion that
the households or people supposed to benefit from the program are
not capable -- due to ignorance, lack of information, or whatever
other reason -- of ordering correctly their wants or the distribution of these wants among different household members. The fact
that the program, in order to be successful, cannot respect
"consumer sovereignty" and must overcome the "erroneous" choice
of wants, underlines the importance of the demand aspects of
intervention programs.

The second crucially important conceptual feature Chernichovsky discusses is the distinction among inputs, intermediate
outcomes, and ultimate outcomes as program impact measurements
variables. In this regard, Reutlinger and Selowsky write:

> *"Just as the educational level of a population should
> ideally be measured by its educational achievements
> and not by its exposure to, and use of, educational
> inputs, so malnutrition should ideally be defined by
> its consequences, such as health status, rather than
> by nutrient intake. In practice, it is difficult to
> define objective indicators of consequences, and it
> is even more difficult to collect and interpret relevant
> data" (1).*

It is exactly this difficulty in defining objective indicators of the intermediate and ultimate outcomes of intervention
programs that has caused most evaluations of program impact to
tend to be based upon program inputs more than upon intermediate
and ultimate outcomes. In light of the discussion with respect
to the role of household behavior as a determinant of program
impact, the difficulties of basing program evaluation upon inputs
shows up clearly. For this reason, Chernichovsky's distinction
among these three types of measurement variables is extremely
important and illustrates the advantage of investigating evaluation approaches based upon programs' intermediate or ultimate
outcomes.

These sorts of approaches can avoid certain circularities
incurred by approaches based upon inputs. For example, traditionally a person's nutritional status is measured by the number of

calories and other nutritive elements consumed daily. Minimum
caloric consumption standards depend among other things upon a
person's weight, which in turn depends upon this person's caloric
intake -- thus introducing an element of circularity.

The third very important item treated by Chernichovsky is
related to methodology. He refers to the advantages and disadvantages of the experimental (or quasi-experimental) methods and of
the statistical control methods as alternatives for evaluating
the impact of intervention programs. This point is particularly
well treated by him. Because of the importance of this matter
to the field of program evaluation, it seems to me helpful to
repeat from the paper a phrase with which I agree fully:

*"In a social setting experimental design may be more
expensive -- financially, politically, and morally --
than measuring impact by means of statistical control".*

The constant progress of econometrics and computation techniques, along with the constant decrease in computation costs,
tend to make the method of statistical control even more attractive as an instrument for evaluation of intervention programs.

REFERENCES

1. Reutlinger, S. and M. Selowsky. *Malnutrition and Poverty*, p. 8,
       Washington, D.C.: World Bank, 1977.

GENERAL DISCUSSION

The Chairman emphasized the dual nature of Chernichovsky's
paper. Its two main themes were (1) the household as a decision
locus; and (2) the use of statistical control, particularly the
methodology developed by econometricians, as an alternative to
experimental evaluations.

Much of the discussion dealt with costs, particularly with
the relative costs and complexities of experimental (or quasi-
experimental) designs as opposed to evaluations via multivariate
statistical control. One speaker emphasized his concern that
expensive evaluations might take funds needed for operational
activities and suggested that no more than three percent of total
project costs be allowed for evaluations (except for projects
clearly labeled as "research" or "pilots"). He noted that China
probably has the largest nutrition program of any developing
country, and yet it spends almost nothing on formal evaluation.
He said the Chinese results are plain to see, in the form of
healthy children, so he thought further "evaluation" there was

unnecessary. He recommended Latin American programs steer a middle
course between the Chinese extreme of no evaluation and the North
American extreme of highly sophisticated and costly evaluations.
But several other speakers disagreed. One said the three percent
target would sometimes be too high, other times too low, all
depending upon the general conditions of health in the project
area, the demands for and use of services, the human and financial
resources available, and the organization and functioning of the
local health system. He said the appropriate level of complexity
and cost for any evaluation would also depend upon what the decision-makers actually want to know (and are willing to act upon)
in any particular situation and upon what information the researchers and evaluators can actually provide. He also suggested there
may be circumstances in developing countries where evaluation and
research are *more* important than for similar projects in the industrialized countries, since the developing countries may not be
able to afford enough "general" development investment (for
higher income and education, for example, as opposed to specific
nutrition and medical interventions) to raise overall nutrition
and health levels. And good evaluations might help developing
countries avoid funding certain very costly programs that would
be likely to fail. The speaker said he knows several past examples
where relatively unsophisticated evaluation techniques helped
Latin American decision-makers avoid such costly errors.

Regarding the relative advantages of experimental evaluation
versus statistical control, one speaker observed that the complexities of many decisions often make it impossible to rely on statistical control, since we simply do not always know all the relevant
variables to measure. Another speaker stressed the need for both
statistical control and experimental design, citing the continuum
and the complementarity between the two. A third speaker noted
Chernichovsky had discussed the differences at the *analytical*
stage between experiments and statistical control, whereas the
most important differences probably arise at the *data gathering*
stage. Therefore, the speaker thought, it is not necessarily true
that statistical control methods are always less costly than experimental control. This speaker also said his own experience
indicated that existing program records are not necessarily less
costly as data sources than surveys, due to the considerable costs
of preparing the records for computer processing.

Several other speakers also discussed possibilities for using
existing non-experimental data in evaluation studies instead of,
or as complements to, new survey data. In Colombia, for example,
a sample drawn from the Census files is large enough to permit
analysis down to the district level of fertility, infant mortality,
income, and education. Using such data for baselines, new evaluations might sometimes be limited to one-shot surveys. It was

observed that in Latin American countries, many of the following existing data categories might also be used in evaluations of health and nutrition projects: price and wage surveys, household budget surveys, agricultural production censuses and surveys, import data, children's weight charts, and research theses in anthropology and sociology by foreign professors and graduate students.

Chernichovsky remarked that he wrote his paper largely as a reaction to experiences working with nutritionists and said he thought economists were more prone than other professionals to work with existing data sources, many of which originally had no connection to economic analysis. He also noted that econometric analysis and statistical control techniques have become much less costly in recent years, due to improvements in computer technologies. And he spoke of the assistance anthropologists could render both in helping "model" family behavior and in improving data sources.

Regarding the analysis of household decision-making and the "new" economic theory of the household, one speaker emphasized that we should not view households' decisions about nutrition and health as "erroneous" simply because they do not necessarily accord with our own preconceived notions. In particular we should realize that simple educational or incentive programs will often not be enough to induce the nutrition or health behavior we want low-income households to follow, and we must be very modest in analyzing the complexities of households' decisions. Another speaker noted not only that target households often fail to respond in the ways programmers want; even worse, program resources may often go mostly to the benefit of unintended households or individuals. (But yet another speaker vigorously defended the milk distribution programs in his country, which he said had achieved an average utilization by intended families of about 60 to 70% since 1925. If there were serious distribution problems, he thought they were mainly intrafamilial).

It was observed that economists have been getting away recently from the concept of "market" or "monetary" income as a measure of the low-income family's welfare. In particular, the family's total available *time* may well be its most important resource. The family's time can be used to generate market income, but it can also be used to generate services (and commodities) like childcare that for many (especially very poor) families may be more valuable than the money income the same amount of worktime can generate (at the margin). Another speaker referred to studies that found health status better predicted by "material style of life" (i.e., various material possessions) than by measured family income.

There was also discussion to the effect that understanding household behavior, although critically important, will not be enough for proper evaluation of large social programs. We also need to do better jobs of analyzing *community* behavior. For example, it may be a social process that determines such things as who cooperates in a program, who comes to present himself for treatment, and why. Such a process may create a "selectivity bias" in household data. Therefore, we might need a large sample of different communities in order for some evaluations to achieve statistical significance. That is, communities receiving different treatments, rather than households, will be the ideal units of analysis in many cases.

There also was extensive discussion of specific outcome measures which could be considered for an evaluation program. These are summarized below.

OUTCOME MEASURES

The group split outcome measures into two levels, household and community.

Household Variables

Income. This serves as a general measure of the flow of resources available for the household to sustain its well-being. Health and nutrition may augment this flow through increases in members' productive capacities. In urban areas, where wages are the main source of income, it is fairly feasible to obtain useful data. In predominantly poor rural areas, income flow can be measured, but it requires careful attention to non-monetary dimensions. In either location, a typical questionnaire instrument might measure money income, in-kind home-produced and consumed goods and services, labor of household members, transfers from outside the household, and financial flows from assets (e.g., long land leases). Concerns were expressed about valuation and aggregation of these components. Given these problems, some expressed preference for stock measurements (see assets) rather than flows.

Assets. These may better reflect total long term resources for sustained well-being. Health and nutrition can improve the capacity to accumulate assets. Measures of major asset stocks seem feasible. Changes in such stocks may, however, be more difficult to detect. Some of the components to be measured were identified.

a. Human capital: educational attainment and activity
    (time of children in school); health status; skill
    accumulations (training, licenses, experience).

b. Land and productive structures: land tenure and
    status; land value; structures; and quality of
    structures. Concern was expressed that through
    knowledge of local conditions plus experience with
    specific level status measurements, an empirical
    estimation should be called upon for details of
    choices and specification of measures. Conversion to
    market values, where feasible, was urged.

c. Productive assets: animals, tools.

d. Consumer facilities or durables: water indoors or out;
    electricity; sewing machines, etc.

Intra-household allocation of resources. The feeling was
expressed that there is a wealth of statistical experience with
components of assets and their aggregation which can be called
upon to enhance data collection and analysis strategies.

Since program interventions are mediated by the household,
effects may appear in the form of reallocations of resources among
household members and, therefore, program impacts may be transformed in unexpected ways. For some areas, measurement of intra-
household allocations appeared feasible and inexpensive, for
others, it appeared feasible but likely to be too expensive, and
for some areas, unfeasible. Measurement and analysis could include
three major areas:

a. Individual activity: both income and asset measures
    call, to some degree, for recording of time alloca-
    tions of household members (e.g., field time, home
    production time, and school activity). Data collection
    concerning approximate time allocations should be
    feasible.

b. Diet and consumption: measurement problems could make
    these outcome measures too costly to be feasible for
    large scale use. Experience suggests that less costly
    methods have questionable value. Whatever measures of
    dietary intake or nutritional status are selected,
    they *should be extended to the entire household,* and
    not be limited just to program participants, since
    reallocation may shift program effects from participants
    to other household members.

c.   Expenditures: household budget studies must be detailed
     in order to capture reliably the expenditures of low
     income people, particularly in rural areas where non-
     local items are liable to be expensive. Therefore,
     their use must be concentrated and specialized for a
     given limited project evaluation, if they are used at
     all.

Community-Level Variables

This topic was given limited attention. Household variables
should be supplemented by community-level variables: electricity;
water supply and sanitation facilities; as well as differences in
distance and access to community facilities. These resources
maintain well-being. To the extent project interventions directly
or indirectly change them, these outcomes are altered and house-
hold-level measures may not capture them adequately.

CONTROL VARIABLES

The group also spent considerable time discussing control
variables and problems in their analysis. Control variables can
be used: (a) to increase precision of outcome effect estimates by
reducing residual variance; (b) in interactions with program variables to detect interactive effects of treatments and non-program
characteristics; and (c) to reduce bias in estimating program
effects in non-experimental evaluations.

Two general topics about control variables were debated at
length. The first was the feasibility and advisability of using
control variables to reduce selection bias in non-experimental
evaluations. Some felt such evaluations may pose more risks than
no evaluation at all. Others felt clear statements of the
assumptions necessary for validity of conclusions under such
conditions would generally reduce the risks of misuse to an
acceptable level. Some urged the pressure for randomization be
increased and maintained with great vigor.

The second centered on the dangers of including endogenous
variables as control variables. As one example, it was noted that
labor force status and health status are endogenously related, so
that to use labor force status as a control in estimating program
effects on health status may seriously bias estimates.

Time Lags and Sustained Effects

The group noted many outcome variables may show impacts only with long lags after intervention. In some cases, short-term changes may not be sustained. Thus, longitudinal analysis is urged where financially and logistically feasible. Changes in household outcome variables outlined above may give some indication of the degree to which any short-term changes in other (e.g., health and nutrition) outcomes may be sustained and transformed into long-term changes in welfare. Lack of changes in the household variables may help explain why short-term gains fail in certain cases to be sustained.

EDUCATIONAL OUTCOMES AND NUTRITION

Selma J. Mushkin
Georgetown University
Washington, D.C.

Educational outcome measurements are a guide to the allocation of resources for formal and nonformal learning. In the developing world they serve as well as input data in assessing the developmental impact of resource commitments to education. In the first instance the outcome measures serve the economist's efficiency purpose; in the second they serve an economic growth purpose.

The present paper addresses the question: What educational outcome data are indicative or representative of adequate nutrition or of malnutrition? What data which are collected by educational authorities would provide information about nutritional status?

In part, to compensate for the narrow focus of the paper, a set of linkages are formulated that can explain symptoms of nutritional deficiencies and relate the hierarchy of input-output relationships from intermediary to final products. Rigorous analytical study would require the formulation of a set of simultaneous equations that would reflect a model of the linkages.

A set of linkages may be formulated that explain symptoms of nutritional deficiencies and relate the hierarchy of input-output relationships from intermediary to final products. These relationships can be stated hypothetically in various ways, including as a set of simultaneous equations, for more rigorous analysis. These relationships include the following segments:

a. Adult population and development

Development is a function of labor skills and physical capital investment (including technology)

Labor skills, in turn, are a function of resources for skill development as well as of personal endowment of the population, its vigor, and "motivation for progress" or "need achievement".

Technological skills also are a function of skill development either for technology transfers, or innovation, or risk taking.

The operational development and implementation of human skills are functions of the health status of the population, the vigor of that population, its personal endowments, and educational resources.

Nutritional status impacts on health and vigor of the working population in two ways: by reducing susceptibility and response to disease, and by providing energy to function, to learn, and to take risks.

Nutritional status, by reducing susceptibility to disease and enhancing curative powers, contributes to a lengthening of life expectancy, encourages postponing today's consumption for tomorrow and thus increases the savings rate, and reduces interest or discount rates on developmental projects. Nutritional status thus is a factor in capital supplies and development as well as in labor skills and technology.

The adult is a product of his genetic qualities and the environment in which he grew, including the nutritional environment and the learning and disease controls to which he had access or was subject.

b.   Child and youth population

Competence of the child and youth -- physical, emotional, and intellectual -- is a product of genetic qualities, community quality, early childhood, and resources for learning and health care.

Genetic qualities are inherited but may be modified by maternal nutrition, and prenatal as well as birth experiences.

Early childhood development is a function of infant environment, health status, learning experiences through parents, preschool activities, community opportunities, health status and nutrition.

Community quality is a product of adult skills, technology, and attitudes toward progress, risk taking, capital, etc.

Learning is a function of quality of preschool population, school characteristics, peer group, parental characteristics, the individual's ability to learn, and his vigor and motivation in learning.

Nutrition is an input into motivation, ability, and vigor to learn.

Nutrition is also an input into physical competence to take up learning by reducing susceptibility to infection and enhancing ability to combat illness.

School feeding motivates school attendance.

The learning of the child is an input to the learning of the adult.

c.   Preschool child and infant

Competence in the preschool child and infancy is a function of genetic qualities, learning experiences, community quality, motivation for learning and need to know, and vigor in learning.

Genetic qualities are a function of genes, nutritional status of the mother, and prenatal environment as well as experiences in infancy.

Learning experiences are a function of parental education, parental motivation, social and economic status, peer group or community qualities and attitudes on learning, and health status including vigor for learning, and ability to learn.

Parental education and parental motivation are a function of a range of factors including nutrition.

Social and economic status of the child is a determinant of nutrition and environmental or community characteristics.

Community quality including education determines the foodstuffs produced and consumed and the existence (or absence) of a supplementary feeding program.

Motivation for learning, circumstances for learning, and vigor in learning are each a function of a range of factors including nutrition.

Nutrition of parents determines a number of characteristics of the infant including physical structure and intellectual ability.

Nutrition of the infant and preschool child is one of the factors affecting learning characteristics.

The learning characteristics of the infant determine the learning characteristics of the preschool child.

The physical and intellectual characteristics of the infant and preschool child determine parental response and motivation for learning.

The segments outlined deal largely with education and economic development, and the roles of nutrition in several dimensions. They do not directly trace still another major segment, namely, the role of nutrition in improving the equality of development, and equality of educational opportunities and learning. If it is the poor children who are undernourished and unresponsive, and the poor children are the ones who cannot benefit from education because of the effect of poor nutrients on ability to learn, then the inequalities among groups in the population become greater even as development takes place.

In the remainder of this paper, we will present the relationships between educational outcomes and nutrition, defined broadly. In the first section we outline measurements of educational outcomes. This summary is followed in the next section by a review of the nutritional literature for guidance on nutrition as an input to education and skill development. In the final section, we discuss the application of what is known for the purpose of policy analysis and evaluation of nutrition programs by taking account of both process variables in education and educational outcomes.

EDUCATIONAL OUTCOMES AND THEIR MEASURES

Our earlier studies suggest that education in the developing world has important multipurpose roles -- economic, social, and political (1,2). In pursuit of these ends education in most countries has claimed a large share of resources.

Resources for education, however, come at sizeable opportunity costs in terms of optional resource use, opportunity costs which underscore the need for careful and detailed analyses and evaluation of educational programs. If, as research at least partially suggests, some of the resources devoted to education are wasted, made ineffective or more costly because of poor nutrition or ill health then nutrition and health care have to be provided as a necessary condition for achievement of the knowledge, skills, and attitudes that are being sought through education. The question is sometimes posed in this way by educators and not without a certain

amount of scorn -- should we, as educators, then ask that the budget
for maternal and child health, or for nutrition programs be increased
at the expense of more funds for the schools? Despite the crossing
of bureaucratic lines the answer becomes plainer if the problem is
stated at its extreme. Suppose all children suffered preventable
mental retardation for lack of adequate nutrition and health care
before reaching school age; would it then be profitable to spend
resources exclusively for conventional schooling?

Measurement of educational outcomes requires initially that the
objectives of education be specified in an output-oriented way.
While educational goals statements are hardly new, the formulation
of such goals in a way that permits the recording of progress generally is.

There does not exist a single metric in education comparable to
the economist's "market price" by which all outputs can be valued
and compared. Because a single satisfactory measure is not available, educational outputs must be defined in other terms. The dimensions of educational outcomes relate initially to the development targets of education -- some development targets are those of
a specific economic project, some are targeted at broader national
educational policies as those policies impact on national development. Outcomes within each developmental target class have different beneficiary groups: the person -- child or adult -- who participates in the learning process; the family; the peer group; and
the broader community -- village, city or nation. Changes in these
groups may be outcomes of education.

Skills and knowledge of learner, family, peers and community are
not only outcomes but at a different stage they are also inputs into
the educational process along with the school and its facilities and
services. Unlike most production processes, however, there is no
single producer of education who controls the full range of inputs
required for a defined product. Instead the sources (inputs) of
individual learning are numerous. The learner comes to formal
schooling with his own personal resources of abilities, acquired
knowledge, skills and physical and emotional energy to learn. He
also devotes resource-time to learning. To measure the changes in
the life of a child who leaves school as if the formal educational
process was the sole learning factor in it would be distorting. A
learner is the output of previous learning experiences, whether formal, nonformal, or informal.

Learning further is a sequential process often captioned "life-
long" learning or recurrent education (3). It is a process that
essentially starts in embryo and continues over the lifetime of
the learner and indeed has impacts into the next generations.

For the purposes of understanding how educational outcomes can
be applied as partial yardsticks of nutrition and other related program inputs, it may be useful to restate the processes in terms of
a series of concepts.

First, we view educational inputs of individual, family, peer
group and school (or educational program) as components of a sequence that produces the learning (or outcome) sought. These are
shown in Figure I as determinants of outcomes. Studies of the variation in educational outcomes among students both in the United
States and in selected nations of the world underscore the importance of the family and its social economic status as a determinant
of a child's learning (4,5). As the figure indicates, there is a
feedback process in which educational outcomes at one state determine, in turn, the characteristics of the person, his peer group,
family relationships and even the response of the schools. Outputs
of the schools when measured and publicized, determine the behavior
of the schools -- the teaching of teachers, the curriculum and so
forth.

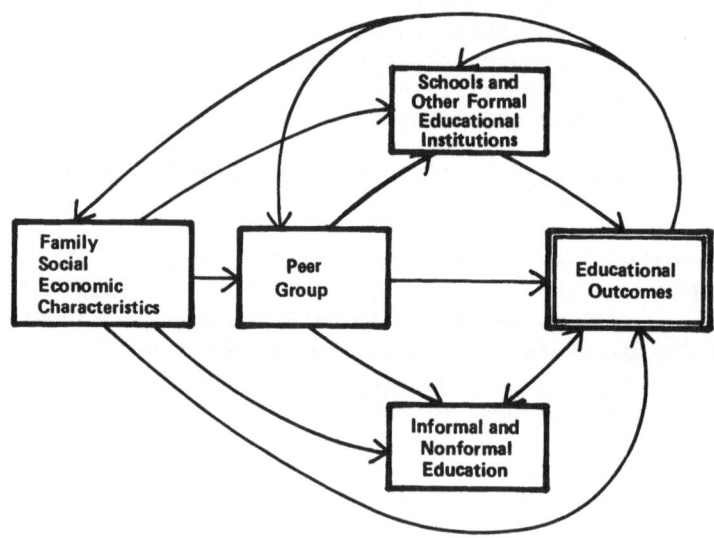

Fig. I. Interaction of Correlates and Educational Outcomes. Source:
A Guide to Educational Outcome Measurements and Their Uses: Seminar
No. 6 Feedback Consequences and Steps Toward Implementation, Public
Services Laboratory, Georgetown University, Washington, D.C., Novem-
ber, 1975.

Second, we examine somewhat more closely the inputs into the
learning responses of individuals. These responses are made up of
the physical, emotional and intellectual characteristics of the individuals combined with factors that contribute to physical, emotional and intellectual vigor and capacity. For the purposes of educational outcome we identify them as the 4A's. These are shown in
Table I.

Underlying each of the inputs and the process by which these
reflect themselves in the 4A's are a range of determinants. In the
case of children, these determinants include: (a) nutrition; (b)
health care; (c) knowledge of parents about personal hygiene; (d)
attitudes of parents toward the child and also toward learning and
other aspects of development; (e) attitudes, competencies and doc-
trines of church, community, and school both in terms of views about
learning and about the child (in general and the particular child).
These are shown in Table II. In the case of adults, the determinants are the product of prior life experience plus education on
the job and in the community. Participation in learning as well
as types and extent of learning are at issue. The characteristics
of the society and its economy determine resources for education
and the consideration of equity as between rich and poor, rural and
urban.

Still an additional model of educational outcomes suggests itself; namely, a model of outcomes of education that divides education's purposes into consumption ends -- the enjoyment of both
process and end results of learning -- and investment ends -- higher
productivity, better jobs, less unemployment, and greater mobility.
Consumption and investment impacts can be assessed on completion of
studies, or during a subsequent period, or into the next generation.
Perhaps it would be well to discuss briefly the content of certain
of these outcomes and achievements.

Educators have traditionally thought of learning outcomes of
the educational process in terms of three broad categories of outcomes -- cognitive, affective, and psychomotor. Cognitive skills
are abilities such as acquiring knowledge, understanding phenomena,
solving problems, creativity, and the art of communicating. Affective skills involve the growth and maturation of aspects of personality. Many of the characteristics labeled "affective" are essentially cognitive. Psychomotor learning is a crucial dimension of
child development affecting strength, flexibility and so forth.
These categories overlap and each is interrelated with the other.

Educational policy officials in Latin America and elsewhere
have come to depend upon two major outcome measures -- knowledge
and skill testing and productivity measures. Knowledge and skill
assessment tends to be of two types: namely, aptitude testing or

measurement of what a student can do, his maximum behavior or ability; and achievement testing or expression of that capacity in terms
of what the student has learned. Productivity is usually assessed
in terms of job and occupation on the one hand, and earnings on the
other. In some studies, however, work productivity is measured in
physical quantities, such as the quantities of rice or sugar cane
produced (6,7).

Achievements

The necessity for assessment of outcomes in terms of achievements in cognitive learning, knowledge, and skill has been relatively clear. Some analysts would allege that the purpose of schooling is plainly achievement and therefore the product of the school
need be tested only by achievements in reading, arithmetic, and so
forth (8).

Achievement measurement necessitates testing; it is a testing
with more rigor than is provided by the usual teacher tests. Viable analysis of outcome requires, moreover, measurement of the
knowledge and skills of individuals inside and outside the formal
education system. It is this type of measurement that has been
very deficient but can be obtained by standardization of testing
instruments. In the past, standardization has been confined to
examination on school leaving for purposes of determining qualifications. These traditional examinations do not serve planning and
analytical purposes.

Tests for planning purposes at earlier grades of schooling
have been developed in some places. Some of these tests are adaptations of tests developed in other countries. At present, the instruments developed by the International Association for the Evaluation of Education (IEA) are available and these, in fact, were
designed for cross national use and have been administered in Chile.
The advantage of IEA tests is that they were painstakingly constructed and extensively validated. But the IEA effort was initiated to
analyze across nations the effect of various in-school and out-of-
school variables on learning. The research orientation on international comparisons of these tests may not coincide with the outcome
informational needs of planning in a particular country.

Indeed despite the many decades if not centuries of giving
tests, the use of standardized testing programs to provide systematic data on the outcomes of schooling is a relatively new concept,
but one that is becoming increasingly important in systemwide planning for evaluation. It is important to underscore that measuring
the effects of instruction is far from an exact science, but it can
yield useful information on the quality of formal and nonformal educational systems.

Aptitudes

For purposes of this paper, we have defined aptitude to include what a person can do intellectually or physically as a result of native ability or inheritance. Ability or IQ testing would be included by definition. Instrumentation for such measurement has been developed over many decades with increasing awareness of the limitations of IQ scaling as an indicator of "native ability"; studies have shown ability to be subject to environmental change. Standardized measures for aptitude testing have such a long history that they are fully familiar. For present purposes of exploring the relation of nutrition and health programs such aptitude measurement is especially important. As will soon become plain, most of the empirical work on nutrition and human development has centered on ability, both intellectual and physical.

Attitudes and Attributes

Attitudes and values affect learning and are altered by it. They function both as inputs and outputs of education. In fact more attention has been given to personal-social attributes as inputs into the learning process than as outputs of that process. Research has been oriented toward discovering relationships or correlations between personality variables and achievements, with the idea that psychological tests might be used as predictors of academic success. Some of the personality factors that have been found to have a positive relationship to achievement include independence, impulse control, achievement motivation, ability to make consistent judgments, persistence, order, endurance and stability. But the research results have not been entirely consistent with respect to the achievement implications of most personality variables.

There are several possible explanations for the lack of clear-cut findings. One is that personality factors interact in ways we do not wholly understand, and therefore studying characteristics in isolation is likely to be misleading. Another problem is that many of the instruments used in this research were developed by clinical psychologists for the diagnostic identification of maladjusted individuals. These tests tend to be slanted toward negative personality traits or neurotic disorders; they often are quite inappropriate for educational assessment. Only in the last decade or so have educational psychologists developed instruments to measure particular attributes in a school setting but these have not been subjected to the extensive and rigorous procedures necessary to produce somewhat more reliable achievement and aptitude tests. In general affective outcomes have largely been neglected.

   To implement measurement of attitudes and attributes as outcomes of education it is necessary: (a) to choose the significant
variables or particular variables from the vast array of psychological and social attributes that have been identified and measured;
and (b) to locate good instruments to measure these variables.

   Table III shows a range of cognitive and personal-social style
dimensions and personality expressions of concern with varying emphasis in different countries and contexts.

   Two constructs in particular -- self-concept and locus of control -- are seen by many investigators as central variables. These
two characteristics encompass the individual's view of himself and
his view of the world in relation to him. It has been found that
a generalized high self-concept has a positive but weak relation to
intelligence, and a stronger positive relationship to specific self-
concept of school ability and reported school grades (9). The importance of the opinions of "significant others" to self-concept
has been noted. Investigators have found a high correlation between the child's self-concept and the teacher's reports of perceptions of them, and also between the child's self-perceptions and
his parents' perceptions.

   Researchers have also found a positive relation between self-
esteem and academic success. Coopersmith found that a high discrepancy between goals and performance or a high discrepancy between
self and teacher evaluation led to repeated failure in the 5th and
6th grades (10).

   There remain many unanswered questions about the meaning of
personality variables and learning in different societies. For example, what is the relationship between self-concept and locus of
control within different status groups? One hypothesis is that in
a highly traditional society members of lower classes may have a
high level of self-esteem (derived from the security of a class
structure with clearly defined roles and expectation for individuals) combined with an external locus of control orientation that
breeds fatalism. This configuration might be reversed for upper
class members, who have greater mobility but higher self-expecta-
tions. Another problem to be more fully investigated is the effect
of modernization, and the requirements of modernization, in relation to these variables. Generally it can be said that high self-
esteem and internal locus of control are desirable outcomes; but
much remains to be learned about the dynamics of these characteristics for different groups -- that is, rural people, farmers, urban
workers, women, shopkeepers within the developing nations.

Social and Political Change

Studies which have undertaken to explore the processes of political and social development have identified those which relate to changes in the attitudes and behavior of individuals and those which relate to changes in the broad patterns of social conditions.

Modernity has, among other traits, been subjected to much measurement. The following have been listed as behavioral consequences of modern attitudes: voting often, discussing politics with wife, contacting officials about a public issue, reading newspapers daily, scoring high on geographic, political and consumer information scales. Other measures of modernity have been suggested; these include:

a.   risk-taking
b.   trust
c.   flexibility as opposed to rigidity
d.   tolerance
e.   rationality
f.   attitudes toward government
g.   attitudes toward work

A risk-taking scale measure, for example, is:

Which would you prefer?

A job where I am almost certain of my ability to perform well.

A job where I am usually pressed to the limit of my capabilities.

Among the political outcome measurements of modernity are migration, urbanization, voting practices, attitudes toward clan and nation, and toward justice.

Economic Outcomes

A substantial amount of research has been done on education and its contribution to economic growth and development. In recognition of the need for balance in economic development, much emphasis is placed on education for rural development and on work skill development in addition to the more general approaches to education as a factor contributing to overall national growth.

Measurement of education's role in economic development more generally calls for several different outcome assessments, the most familiar of which is the present value of future earnings.

A partial listing follows:

a. increased earnings for the individual;
b. consumption benefits for the individual;
c. increased capacity of individuals to adjust to new
   circumstances, jobs, job opportunities; and to take
   risks;
d. provision of manpower for economic growth;
e. increased productivity for society;
f. better citizenship;
g. intergenerational effects on learning and
   motivation;
h. external effects on other individuals, family, employees,
   and employer.

Education importantly can affect the distribution of income
as well as its size. It can do this in two separate ways. The
first is measured directly through increased productivity and output of goods and services as a result of specific educational experiences. The second is an indirect measure of productivity based
on increases in income associated with increasing years of education.

In the first instance, the key to relating changes in the distribution of income to education is to measure the opportunity of
acquiring an education according to income class of families, and/
or to the educational dropout rate by income. The degree to which
family income relates to an individual's opportunity to enjoy the
rewards of education serves as a measure of anticipated changes in
income profiles.

Economic purposes have been pursued principally by nonformal
education and work skill development. Educational programs of a
nonformal type are designed to provide rural families with ancil-
lary skills for home improvement, better farming methods and the
use of fertilizer, and improved nutrition, personal hygiene and
sanitation; the outcomes must be assessed in these terms. Some
programs provide rural young persons with skills for off-farm employment -- for example, to upgrade and broaden skills of practic-
ing artisans, craftsmen and small entrepreneurs. Health education as a component of such rural education aims to improve nutrition,increase life expectancy, increase productivity, decrease absenteeism, and accidents, and increase the use of family planning
methods. Again the educational outcome is best assessed by indicators that determine the extent to which the objectives are being
reached.

We have outlined several models that relate inputs into education and outcomes of education and suggested in a cursory way meas-

urements of educational outcomes. We ask now which of these measurements of outcomes are relevant to understanding nutrition status.

We can examine this question from the perspective of quantity
of education on the one hand, and quality of education on the other.
Each of the outcomes is subject to measurement given current instrumentation. None of the outcomes can be measured precisely and the
degree of precision varies markedly.

On the quantity side there are the number and percent of children and of adults who are enrolled in school at different levels
and its converse, namely, dropout rates and school absenteeism.
On the quality side there are:

a.   Improved aptitudes and achievements of children and
     adults;

b.   Improved attitudes such as reduction of fatalism and
     the encouragement of risk-taking, entrepreneurship,
     need to achieve and motivation for progress;

c.   Favorable parental attitudes toward the child,
     support of child's learning, and parental enthusi-
     asm for intellectual and cultural pursuits;

d.   Improved physical vigor and health including greater
     height and weight, physical dexterity and competence,
     and a reduction of absenteeism from school, training,
     and work. Included here would be school or teacher
     responses toward the student.

With this summary of outcome measures as a background we now
inquire about what is known about the relation of nutrition programs to these components.

NUTRITION AND EDUCATIONAL OUTCOMES

We now review the literature on nutrition and related health
services and ask what is known about nutrition and educational outcomes of the multiple types identified.

Nutrition and Numbers Identified

A major impact of nutrition on educational outcomes lies in
the numbers and proportion at each age group attending educational
offerings, and the number and percentage who continue their education through successive levels of schooling rather than dropping

out. Especially important to progress are number and percentage
of those who are (a) from rural areas, or (b) poor families who
participate in education and continue their education through
successive levels (11).

Nutrition studies do not generally deal with the question of
numbers attending except as they measure school absences. While
absenteeism in school plays a not inconsequential role in leading
to grade repetition and to discouragement on the part of the child,
school absences are only one facet of enrollments and enrollment ratios. It is not difficult to document high rates of absenteeism
from school on the part of children who have a history of malnourishment and weakened resistence to infection and disease. Berg
cites the experience of four Latin American countries where illness
caused children to miss more than fifty days of school per year,
representing as much as one-third of the school year (12,p.11).
Mönckeberg notes that one of the main problems in Latin America during school age is the high percentage of dropouts. Of every 100
children who enter primary school, only 20 finish it. He believes
that such a high dropout rate is due at least in part to learning
difficulties and low mental performance of malnourished children
(13). This high dropout rate may very well have a prior long history of absenteeism due to infection and disease as a contributing
factor.

Nutrition versus Aptitudes and Intellectual Achievement

Perhaps the logical place to start in a review of the research
on links between nutrition and quality measures of educational outcomes is the effect of varying degrees of malnutrition on aptitudes
and intellectual achievement. The first finding of our review of
the nutrition research as it relates to educational aptitude and
achievement is that the studies of linkages are mostly made about
"gross" conditions of malnutrition that are not necessarily representative of nutritional status variations of most children in the
population. It becomes important, accordingly, to understand the
condition of nourishment in the population of low income rural families in order to understand the potential impact of nutrition policies on educational outcomes.

To date numerous studies involving laboratory animals have
been undertaken to determine a causal link, if any, between inadequate nutrition and the capacity to learn. These studies have included comparative follow-up studies of laboratory animals in which
malnutrition had been experimentally induced to determine the animals' "behavioral competence", as well as studies of the cumulative
effects of malnutrition through generations of malnourished laboratory animals.

Human studies have been more varied and complex and yet, for ethical reasons, have at the same time been more limited than the experiments on laboratory animals. Human studies have generally taken the following shapes: a) comparative studies of well and poorly nourished children as far as cognitive achievement is concerned; b) retrospective follow up studies of the nutritional histories of well and poorly functioning children; c) intervention studies in which children living in communities where the risk of malnutrition was high were selectively nutritionally supplemented or not supplemented during infancy and evaluated in terms of learning ability; d) follow up studies of the intellectual performance of clinical cases hospitalized for severe malnutrition in childhood; and e) intergenerational studies to determine the degree to which the conditions of risk of malnutrition in the present generation may have derived from maternal histories of inadequate nutrition. What has clearly emerged again and again from these various studies is that a history of severe malnutrition during pregnancy and/or infancy, in both animal and human subjects, is associated with a whole range of deficient cognitive and intellectual abilities and performance, together with altered patterns of social behavior (14).

However, just what constitutes the causal likage? How does malnutrition affect the learning process in both animals and man? Several hypotheses have been advanced, notably that malnutrition directly affects the intellect by inflicting damage on the central nervous system, the extent of which depends upon the timing and severity of the nutritional "insult". In animal studies where moderate to severe malnutrition was induced at the developmental stage of the central nervous system, clearly reduced brain sizes in the experimental animals emerged. Winick cites an actual reduction in numbers and size of brain cells in such animals (15). Similar reductions in brain cell number and size have been recorded in cases of human infants who have died as a result of severe malnutrition (16). Alan Berg has discussed a 15-20% numerical reduction of brain cells in severely malnourished humans (12, p.9).

It would seem then that a history of malnutrition may inflict primary damage on the central nervous system. However, the extent and severity of the damage will depend to a very large extent on the timing and severity of the nutritional insult (17). If the insult occurs and continues without rehabilitation during the crucial period of central nervous system development in either the human or animal infant, damage to the central nervous system will occur and may not be susceptible to rehabilitation. Whether such primary damage to the central nervous system is permanent or not remains a moot question. Winick has demostrated that if nutritional rehabilitation commences during the crucial central nervous system developmental stage in previously malnourished laboratory

rats, damage can be reversed (15, p.93). This has yet to be proven
in human cases, and various optimistic and pessimistic outlooks
based on observation and experimentation can be found in the literature (18-21).

Quantifiable lags in learning performance have been noted between the malnourished and the adequately nourished child (e.g.,
retardation of language development and poorer performance on standardized tests of cognitive learning, intellectual ability and aptitude (21)). Survivors of severe infant malnutrition have been observed to have both interference with reading and writing abilities
and "to run higher risks of failing to profit from the cumulative
knowledge available to the human species in general and to their
socio-economic group in particular" (22, p. 64).

Behavioral outcomes in both laboratory animals and in humans
with a history of malnutrition have been documented. Experiments
have been conducted on both nutritionally deprived and well nourished rats with regard to such abilities as maze learning, avoid-
ance conditioning, and so forth. While defects in the design of
such experiments have been noted in terms of such factors as differing handling and caging of animals, the emerging conclusion is that
the malnourished animals have a tendency to be disadvantaged learn-
ers (14). In human studies, again and again what is termed "defective information processing" has been recorded in children who
have been subject to malnutrition in infancy.

A key question worth raising here is one formulated by Klein
and co-workers: Does the condition of mild to moderate malnutrition, a condition affecting the majority of growing children in
developing countries, affect the mental development of these children? (23). From evidence accumulated in the Guatemala intervention
study, Klein argues that there is a strong, substantial case for
the association of inadequate nutrition with lower cognitive performance. Klein's "reasonably clear association" between nutritional status and cognitive performance is supported by findings
of numerous other studies as well (24). While not strictly comparable on all points, these various studies involved testing of
previously malnourished children for language development, inter-
sensory integration, intelligence quotient for chronological age,
and psychomotor behavior as well as adaptive social-personal behavior; the conclusion is that such children evidenced markedly
deficient performances in all tested areas, the degree of deficiency usually depending upon the severity, timing and duration
of the nutritional insult. In evaluating these results, the Guatemala investigators in particular raised the question of reduced
levels of attention and awareness of the environment on the part of
the child acting as important "mediating mechanisms" in these poor
test performances. Also noted was a tendency toward impulsive test

response where some reflection was required, often completed with a general lack of motivation and interest (23,27,28). It should be noted here that at this point these tests have been administered to children only so that any longer-range association of malnutrition and cognitive development and performance in adults is not yet known (21).

The experience in developing countries has strongly suggested that adults who had been subjected to malnutrition during childhood perform intellectually more poorly than their peers who were well nourished in childhood (29). This has implications for training and development of a populace in national efforts of modernization and economic/social development.

Does good nutrition make for job skill development? Nutrition of adults has been shown to improve adult productivity on the job but the studies have not dealt with learning for job skills (30). Little formal education is required of jobs for which productivity gains are reported. The tasks and occupations that more typically require learning and skill development as educational outcomes are not among those studied.

Essentially the studies reported to date have concerned nutritional variables and the output of workers in road construction, sugar cane fields and rubber plantations (30, pp. 282-285).

In Indonesia an iron supplementation intervention program to correct anemia among 300 rubber plantation tappers and weeders indicated a gain in output. Some question, however, has been raised as to the reliability of the tests of the experimentation. Studies in the Philippines examined the relationship between anemia and road construction productivity for soil loaders, unloaders and tampers Anemic workers in all three groups were found to have lower productivity than those who were not anemic. Both in the Indonesia study and in the Philippines, worker absenteeism was lowered with iron intervention. A study of U.S. pre-school children by Pollitt, et al. (31) showed that deficits in learning and memory tasks by iron deficient children disappeared following four months of oral therapy.

Spurr and others have shown that productivity of sugar cane cutters was related to height and body fat (6). Cupo's studies indicate that work performed among field workers on an estate farm in Jamaica varied with diet (32). Viteri and his colleagues have shown the relation of anemia to reduced physical work capacity among peasants in Guatemala (33). Also Guatemala studies indicate that sugarcane cutters on higher caloric intake increase their work and energy output (6).

While for the present purposes it is important to understand
the relation of nutrition to creation of work skills and to related
motivation, creativity and modernity, studies of the link of nutrition and worker productivity do not provide the information needed.

Nutrition and Attitudinal Change

The research on nutrition has not focused on the full range
of attitudinal behavior that the educator is concerned about. Mc-
Clelland has shown that economic development rests on the motivation for achievement of individuals and changes in self-image (34).

Attitudes associated with malnourishement may be behaviors and
attitudes developed by the child as a direct result of his undernourished state (e.g., apathy, lack of attention and response), and
also the attitudes and modes of behavior that the adult has acquired
that are barriers to learning and developing competence.

Nutrition study findings underscore the relation between nutrition and responsiveness or apathy. We have extended these findings
into those psychological and sociological contexts vital to development and labeled earlier as educational outcomes in furtherance of
a development objective, namely, removal of attitudes of fatalism
on the one hand and encouragement of attitudes of risk-taking, entre-
preneurship, and achievement on the other.

Malnutrition in children has been found in nutrition studies
to produce clinical manifestations of apathy and irritability, together with what has been termed as "gross unresponsiveness" to the
environment. At this point, cause and effect of malnourishment
tend to become inextricably intertwined with the child and his environment, with the result that the worst aspects of the situation
reinforce one another, and continue to inflict substantial effects
on learning abilities.

It has been noted many times over that malnutrition does not
occur in a vacuum (35). In fact, malnutrition tends to occur in a
context of family malnourishment, low socio-economic class, inadequate or wholly lacking concepts of personal hygiene and health,
defective methods of childrearing, and a host of other factors which
have the effect of compounding the more easily quantifiable nutritional insult.

Greater social interaction on the part of a well nourished,
active, stimulated and in turn stimulating child has been documented repeatedly, notably in recent studies in Colombia and Mexico
(36,37). It is not difficult to project the malnourished child's
pattern of low social interaction and hindered development into the

child's future performance at school. A less than adequate school performance in turn may elicit less and less attention, encouragement of, and interest in the child on the part of both parents and teachers, resulting in further isolation of the child from stimulus. A pattern of school failure might then become inescapable.

Attitudes and behaviors evident in malnourished children include apathy, and a lack of interest ranging from inability to pay specific attention in testing situations, for example, to "gross unresponsiveness" to the surrounding environment. In terms of the family and school environment, the implications of such attitudes and behaviors are clear.

Parental Attitudes

Educational outcomes have been repeatedly linked with attitudes of the parents to the child. The immediate behavioral effects of malnutrition in infants, in addition to apathy, irritability and gross unresponsiveness, have been found to affect the quantity and quality of maternal response to the child (38, 39). Cravioto and DeLicardie have established a strong association between the environmental stimulation available to the child and the presence or absence of severe malnutrition (39). This lack of stimulus has a strong influence on the course of the child's social learning. Recent studies of malnourished children and their families in Bogotá, Colombia, have shown that mothers of malnourished children had reduced educational and occupational expectations for their children, generally gave less attention and "verbal reinforcement", and tended to teach the children less. Beyond this, there was noted a greater tendency to assigning an older sibling to direct care of the child (36).

The connection between malnutrition and parent-child interaction has been further researched by Chavez through observations of nutritionally supplemented and unsupplemented children. In contrast to the unsupplemented, the supplemented children were markedly more exploratory, active and expressive. In addition, growing as they did more rapidly and visibly, the supplemented children elicited greater attention and care from all family members concerned. As Chavez explains, "...it may be said that the supplemented group had a different level of stimuli than the non-supplemented group. The majority of these differences can be attributed to the greater weight and physical activity of the children" (37, pp. 219-20). The point to be made here as far as educational outcomes is concerned is that the physically active child tends to be a stimulated child, eliciting attention and stimulus from his surroundings and developing into an active, inquiring human being.

Klein and coworkers' studies support these findings. They have suggested that adults and older children treat a better nourished and
therefore physically larger child as a more mature individual and
so increase his "social learning opportunities" (24, p.239). Such
was not the case with the unsupplemented children.

The effects of lack of stimulus and inability to respond to
such stimulus on the part of the malnourished child has been found
to retard severely his social learning and adaptability. It has
been speculated that the unsupplemented, non-active child does not
elicit maternal or family interest and stimulation and, in fact,
may be grossly unresponsive to his environment. Other performance
differences between the supplemented, vigorous child and his unsupplemented counterpart include the latter's shortened attention
span, lack of persistence, and impulsive behavior (29,41). This
pattern of decreased interaction with family and environment is
believed to have significant effects on the child's further behavior development. As Klein and coworkers have put it: "The implications of reduced levels of attention to novel stimuli for intellectual development during infancy are potentially very important.
Much of early intellectual development proceeds by attention to and
incorporation of novel sensory and motor stimuli. To the extent
that early and severe malnutrition limits the infant's sensory and
cognitive intercourse with his environment, the normal course of
early cognitive development may be altered. However, whether alterations in the normal course of infant cognitive development due
to malnutrition are permanent, or have any long-term significance,
is still an open question (29, p.319). In terms of the educational
process, it is abundantly clear that the unsupplemented, undernourished child is operating under substantial handicaps and that the
supplemented child would, on the face of it, derive far greater
benefits from education than his malnourished counterpart.

Favorable parental attitude is often lacking for the malnourished child. Among the attitudes present in the child's family and
socio-economic environment which may present obstacles to any significant formal education may be discouragement of learning as a
result of economic pressures to go out and support the family unit.
Since malnutrition tends to occur in the context of an inadequate
income to secure enough food for the family unit, the economic pressures to abandon school for labor are not insignificant. The pressures may be even more powerful if the child's poor school performance is an issue. Finally, a certain degree of fatalism, of passive acceptance and an otherwise non-risk orientation may prompt
further disengagement from education and the effort which the education process requires of the child (42).

Improved Physical Vigor

One of the basic physical associations with malnutrition documented in the literature is reduced anthropometric measurements.
In fact, time and time again the samples selected for retrospective
studies of human experiences of malnutrition are selected on the
basis of reduced height, weight, head circumferences, and other
body dimensions in comparison with well-nourished peers. Reduced
anthropometric measurements are inherently regarded as indicators
of nutritional status (43).

The results of various intervention studies undertaken over
the past 10 to 20 years clearly indicated that nutritional supplementation of mothers during pregnancy and infants through the critical early years of life in populations running a risk of malnutrition produced increased birthweights, and larger, more active babies throughout that early growing period. In comparison, similar
babies in such risk-prone malnourished populations whose mothers
did not receive supplementation and who did not themselves receive
enough nutritional sustenance during the early critical developmental period, exhibited deficits in physical development, including smaller height, lower weight levels, and reduced anthropometric dimensions. A number of studies have shown the adverse
association between malnourishment and hindered physical development on the one hand and the positive association between adequate
levels of nutrition through nutritional supplementation programs
and physical development to normal limits on the other.

Adequate nutrition through supplementation programs has been
productive of greater physical vigor and activity on the part of
the children involved. In an intervention study conducted by Chavez, Martinez and Yaschine in Mexico, activity levels of 17 supplemented children (supplemented from the 45th day of pregnancy
through lactation and weaning) and 17 unsupplemented children
were monitored. As a group the supplemented children evidenced
higher activity levels than the non-supplemented group, with as
much as a six-fold difference in level of physical activity by age
2, as a demonstrated association between adequate nutrition and
level of physical activity (37).

The documented relationship between inadequate levels of nutrition and weakened resistence to disease is not new, though it is
worth noting once again here. Inadequate nourishment has been
clearly associated with lack of physical vigor and lowered resistance to infections. The snowballing implications of inadequate
nutrition and lowered resistance to infections are not difficult
to imagine -- a progression of disease and illness, reduced intake of nutrients and/or interference with the body's processes
of nutrient absorption (e.g., through diarrhea conditions), sub-

sequent weakening of vigor and resistance to disease and infections, and ensuing physical growth deficits (45). Many studies have shown the significant associations between nutrition and increased physical dimensions and increased levels of physical activity of adequately nourished children.

What are the implications of these physical condition factors for educational outcomes? A question posed by Klein and his colleagues in the Guatemala intervention study is worth mentioning here: "Is big smart?" they asked. Based on their studies of 3 to 6 year old high-protein, high-calorie and low-calorie supplemented children, the group made the preliminary conclusion that the children who received the high-protein - high-calorie supplement and who were the larger children scored better in terms of cognitive performance than the smaller, low-calorie supplemented group of children. This preliminary conclusion is based on limited experience and the study is continuing (46). However, on the basis of these preliminary findings that there is indeed a tendency for big to be smart, the group suggested that such nutritional intervention programs do have value in terms of educational outcomes in developing countries.

Joaquin Cravioto and Elsa DeLicardie showed a direct association between deficits in height and weight of malnourished children and retardation in psychomotor, adaptive, language and social-personal behavior, as measured by Gesell, Cattell, or Bayley techniques. They report that available knowledge leaves no doubts about the strong association between the antecedent of severe malnutrition in infancy and suboptimal performance at school age (26).

The nature and extent of the suboptimal performance would seem to vary according to the severity, timing and duration of the child's nutritional insult. Longitudinal studies are proceeding and seek to document the long range effects, if any, of such nutritional insults.

Students of malnutrition further point to another aspect in the environment of the malnourished child -- that is, the synergism of infection and malnutrition. The malnourished child runs clearly greater risks of infection, has a lowered immunity to diseases, and is subject to more generalized and severe illnesses and physical debility which may impact on his physical prowess, energy level and psychomotor competence.

Episodes of illness have the effect of disrupting the child's acquisition of knowledge and course of intellectual growth. This has implications both for the pre-schooler as well as the in-school child, although academic ability and performance deficiencies resulting from absence from school as a result of illness may be more easily perceived.

The net effect of such absenteeism is further disruptions and lags in educational and intellectual performance. The resulting poor school performance on the part of these malnourished and recurrently ill children thwarts teacher expectations in much the same way as unresponsive behavior in malnourished babies diminishes maternal attention, stimulation and interest. While the evaluative data are hardly complete, the attitudes of teachers to a child may impact on his learning. The child whose stature is impaired by poor nutrition, who is subject to illnesses, may well have a hard time gaining recognition in the classroom that would give added support to his studies. Withdrawal of teachers' interest in the poorly performing child plus the child's obvious inability to keep up with his classmates has enormous implications for the child's (and subsequent adult's) feelings of self-worth and esteem.

What emerges from this brief and cursory discussion of research on malnutrition is its damaging effects on the malnourished child's nervous system, social and learning behavior, and subsequent intellectual deficits and lags -- all of which may or may not be permanent. It is not surprising that malnutrition produced such multifaceted and overlapping effects since malnutrition itself is such an all-enveloping condition which usually occurs in an environment of poverty, disease, and lack of stimulation. Thus a cycle is created in which a poor environment leads to malnutrition, which in turn to a large extent determines behavior, thus perpetuating poverty, intellectual handicaps and malnutrition.

THE ROLE OF NUTRITION PROGRAMS IN THE APPLICATION OF EDUCATIONAL INDICATORS

In the first section of this report we have outlined a range of educational outcomes that in some combination are criteria that capture the objectives of education and have identified those outcomes that hypothetically have nutritional inputs. In the second we have summarized the literature of nutrition research to determine what is known about nutrition and nutritional deficiencies as they impact on those educational outcomes that in concept are nutritionally related.

The research evidence we have thus far reported suggests primarily that the nutrition of mother and infant is important to learning and to size of the child into adulthood. And big has been associated with smarter. Nutrition in childhood and later life can perhaps overcome early deficits to some degree. Lack of nutrition in later childhood and adult life for those who had good nutrition

in infancy is debilitating and can reduce vigor and also resistance
to diseases. It can impact unfavorably on learning, but basic cognitive abilities may remain largely unaffected.

Additionally, the review suggests:

a.   Many of the conceptual linkages between nutrition and edu-
     cational outcomes identified at the outset of this paper
     are neither supported nor refuted by research evidence;

b.   While the important educational outcome link between nu-
     trition and productivity of workers has been examined,
     with the finding that nutrition makes a difference, the
     studies that have been carried out have been done precise-
     ly in those unskilled manual employments where educational
     inputs are low;

c.   The yardsticks applied in assessing nutritional status,
     physical, biochemical and psychological, are generally
     different from those used in assessing educational prog-
     ress;

d.   Mental deficiencies through aptitude measurements may be
     used as symptomatic of diet deficits as well as a guide
     to school policy decisions;

e.   Psychometric measurements and changes in such measurements
     as part of aptitude measurement may be expected to signal
     dietary differences and also are outcomes of school per-
     formance;

f.   Nutrition is not likely to impact on achievements despite
     the importance of cognitive learning except when gross
     changes in nutrition are involved;

g.   Tests of nutrition intervention on attitudes have not been
     sufficient to indicate whether or not change impacts on
     education;

h.   Major inputs that account for much of the variation in
     achievement levels in education appear to be affected by
     nutrition. Among these are parental and teacher attitudes
     toward the child and the child's vision in turn of himself.

We now turn the question around and ask, given those research
findings, what measurements made by the educational community may
be used to identify nutritional deficiencies. We elaborate on certain educational outcome measurements that may be symptomatic of
nutritional deficiencies and query whether quantification can be

carried out so that changes in those educational outcomes as reported by school officials, and by community leaders concerned with non-
formal education, can record changes in nutrition.

Quantity of Education

Differences between geographic areas or income groups in the
percentage of children participating in education beyond compulsory
school age, drop out rates, and school absenteeism rates provide
measures that can be applied to raise questions about nutritional
status. It could turn out on investigation that nutrition is an
important input whose neglect contributed to the variations. Data
on such quantities can be expected to signal possible nutritional
problems and may be used to evaluate nutritional interventions.

IQ and Aptitude Scales

An obvious measurement often used in education is the measurement of aptitude (defined here to include physical and mental ability). Such measurement can be expected to identify possible nutritional problems and to provide yardsticks by which to evaluate nutrition intervention programs.

For intellectual development measures such as Stanford Binet
IQ test, the Wechsler Intelligence Scale and many others have become standard. Research on IQ or ability testing demonstrates the
possibilities of raising IQ levels within significant limits by intervention programs that deal with the "whole child". Nutrition
research certainly points to intervention through maternity care and
infant feeding.

Physical measures such as height and weight of the children are
often components of school programs. In a rural community observers
or instructors associated with nonformal educational programs certainly could be called upon to report approximate information that
would yield data relevant for signaling nutritional problems, including information on general levels of height and weight conditions in the community and approximate uniformity or disparities
among groups or individual families within a community.

Nutritional research points to early intervention. Accordingly, what needs to be identified are the communities that are particularly subject to deficiencies that may be diet deficiencies.
School records on IQ or physical measurements could pinpoint for
national authorities possible geographic regions calling for special targeted nutrition intervention. It could be on the production of foods, the use of foods, a feeding program for mothers, and

so forth. Similarly, uniform findings for a number of localities
of wide disparities in symptoms of nutritional deficiency among
families point to different interventions more directly targeted
to the special families at risk.

Achievement Testing

Achievement tests can serve much the same purpose as aptitude
testing, namely, identifying either geographic areas or groups within the population of a community that give evidence of slow intellectual responses. They can also be applied as evaluation yardsticks in measuring the effect of intervention programs.

Achievement tests, however, are a crude method of assessment.
Measurement of achievement difficulties in school children becomes
a way mainly to identify geographically or for identified groups
in the population possible diet deficiencies in mothers and infants.
The importance of such tracking back arises out of the findings
about nutrition and both intellectual and physical development in
infancy and early years of life. As indicated earlier, nutrition
studies do not verify a direct relationship between school learning
and school feeding programs.

In less formal settings it may be possible to identify what is
learned as a consequence of education and training inputs and to use
the responses to educational inputs as a possible signal of nutritional deficits. Nutrition has been found to contribute to productivity in farming type skills for which formal education often is
not a prerequisite. But there are other skills in the rural community. Traditional training for community skills often has some
type of screening of individuals and of families implicit in the
mores of the community. To break from the traditional both in terms
of who is trained, method of training, and what the training is to
achieve essentially requires a different screening method, one aspect of which may signal nutritional status. We found no studies
directly relating nutrition and screening for access to nonformal
or rural community education. If inputs of educational services
do not produce results then certainly the question of nutritional
deficits arises. Are those who are not learning or are not motivated to learn suffering from poor nutrition? New approaches are
being taken to educational outcome measurements, especially
modernity, and an individual's perception of self and society.

Modernity and Need Achievement

A range of measurements have been formulated for the purposes of assessing education's developmental objective. Among these are measures of aspects of modernity including risk taking, flexibility rather than rigidity, trust, attitudes toward government, work attitudes, and the need to achieve. Instruments have been developed for these types of conceptual constructs. However, nutrition research has not produced a clean set of findings on the relation of nutrition to such educational outcomes.

The current emphasis on social equity and rural development requires certain personal characteristics including motivation to advance. However, this need to achieve is tempered by the close relation between self-progress and community progress. A spirit of community concern and attitudes of societal improvement and of cooperation are also parts of "rural modernity", along with the belief in the virtues of betterment. Vigor and motivation are important to these attitudes as they are to still other qualities such as a spirit of innovation and creativity.

Rural modernity, when defined as a goal of nonformal education, requires that the construct be clearly formulated and that appropriate instruments be developed to measure it and to relate it to nutritional status in the rural community.

Measures of Self-Esteem and Control

Still an additional item on the agenda for measurement concerns measures of self-esteem and control as a basis to learning. A great deal of work has been done on these two variables both in defining the constructs and in instrument development. There are perhaps 200 measures of self-concept and additional measures of locus of control. This presents opportunities as well as selection problems. Presently, no norms are available for assessing self-concept or locus of control. Such measures of self-concept and locus of control as we have, moreover, are dependent on the place and circumstance under which they would have been developed.

The present situation of measurement of self-esteem and control in the context of the developing nations is highly unsatifactory for educational measurement purposes. Measurements are not available to signal nutritional deficits. However, it may be expected that over time the current unsatisfying state of the art in measurement of these variables will be overcome. It is urgent that relatively extensive and thorough steps be taken to develop and validate measures of self-concept and control for use in educational assessment programs. Such steps will involve collaborative efforts of differ-

Table I. DETERMINANTS OF EDUCATIONAL OUTCOMES: THE FOUR A's

Attributes of the individual, including his in-
    tellectual and physical vigor, and capaci-
    ty, vitality, and appearance;

Aptitudes of the individual for special aspects
    of living, including his native abilities,
    his artistic or special physical prowess;

Attitudes of the individual, including attitudes
    toward achievement; risk-taking; motivation
    for progress; self-esteem; and his view of
    society, clan, nation, and their mores; and

Achievements of the individual, including psycho-
    motor and cognitive learning.

Table II. FACTORS CONTRIBUTING TO LEARNING FOR COMPETENCE

	Nutrition	Health	Parental Competencies-Attitudes	School-Church Competencies-Attitudes	National Mores-Policies
Prebirth	X	X	X	X	X
Birth	X	X	X	X	X
Preschool	X	X	X	X	
School	X	X	X		
Length of Schooling	X	X	X	X	X
Education-Job Training					
ex ante	X	X	X	X	
post	X	X		X	

Table III. *COGNITIVE AND PERSONAL-SOCIAL STYLE*

I   Basic Drives, e.g.,

self assertion, fear, gregariousness, succorance, curiosity

II General Dimensions of Personality, e.g.,

withdrawn vs. involved	active vs. passive
masculine vs. feminine	apathetic vs. energetic
rebellious vs. compliant	solitary vs. social
expressive vs. restrained	assertive vs. timid
tense vs. relaxed	aimless vs. purposeful
sensitive to others vs.	rigid vs. flexible
self-centered	happy vs. unhappy
submissive vs. dominant	academically motivated vs.
	otherwise motivated

III Areas of Personality Expression, e.g.,

A. Personal-Social Characteristics B. Controlling Mechanisms

achievement	scanning-focusing
affiliation	field articulation
aggression	conceptual differentiation
anxiety	tolerance for delay of
autonomy/independence	reward
curiosity	internal vs. external locus
deference	of control
dependency	risk-taking strategy
dominance	impulsivity-reflectivity
nurturance	conceptual style
creativity	cognitive complexity
	distractability
	coping styles

C. Values, Attitudes and Interests

Interests: attitudes toward manipulative cognitive aesthetic

1. family	6. important beliefs and acts
2. groups (political, ethnic)	7. national and international
3. community	8. nature
4. self	9. the future/posterity
5. tasks (physical)	

Source: Reference (1).

ent investigators focusing on similar aspects of the measurement
problem. At each step, items will need to be selected and validated
for individuals of differing age, sex, socio-economic status levels,
and national problems. Once available the measurements will become
available and identify attitudinal problems that may be characteristic of poor diets.

    In summary, educational officials concerned with improved edu-
cational outcomes may assist in identifying symptoms of possible
nutritional deficiencies and in judging nutritional input modifications and their consequences for development of competence.

    Tracking of the status of infant and maternal nutrition is sig-
naled as part of education. The tracking programs can be projects
either for communities or nationwide; that is, a tracking program can
be set up for a particular school or it can be tracking for a national
education program. Tracking can take the form of project monitoring, large-scale statistical data collection, or an experimental
study. The purpose would be to analyze educational outcomes for
their nutritional inputs where nutritional intervention is known
to make a difference.

    By tracing back from educational outcomes in their several di-
mensions to symptoms of malnutrition, and possible nutritional deficiencies as a causative factor, it becomes possible to more appropriately design nutrition interventions at the right time and in the
right proportions.

REFERENCES

1. Public Services Laboratory, Georgetown University, U.S.A., and the Institute of Development Research, Ethiopia. *Educational Outcome Measurement in Developing Countries*. Washington, D.C.: Public Services Laboratory, Georgetown University, 1975.

2. Mushkin, S. J., and B. R. Billings. *A Guide to Educational Outcome Measurements and Their Uses, Seminars 1-6*. Washington, D.C., and Costa Rica: Public Services Laboratory and CEMIE, November, 1975.

3. Mushkin, S.J. (ed.). *Recurrent Education*. Washington, D.C.: National Institute of Education, DHEW, U.S. Government Printing Office, 1974.

4. Mosteller, F., and D. P. Moynihan (eds.). *On Equality of Educational Opportunity*. New York: Vintage Books, 1972.

5. Coleman, J. S., E. Q. Campbell, C. J. Hobson, *et al*. *Equality of Educational Opportunity*. Washington, D.C.: DHEW, U.S. Government Printing Office, 1966.

6. Spurr, G. B., N. M. Barac, and M. G. Maksud. Productivity and maximal oxygen consumption in sugar cane cutters. *Am. J. Clin. Nutr.* 30:316-321, 1977.

7. Gardner, G. W., J. R. Eagerton, E. J. Barnard, and B. Seneuivatne. Physical working capacity and iron deficiency anemia. Paper presented at the *10th International Congress of Nutrition,* Kyoto, Japan, August 1975.

8. Levine, D. M. *Performance Contracting in Education: An Appraisal*. Englewood Cliffs, N.J.: Educational Technology Publications, 1971.

9. Bachman, J. G. *Youth in Transition*. Vols. I and II. Ann Arbor, Michigan, Institute for Social Research, University of Michigan, 1969 and 1970.

10. Coopersmith, S. *The Antecedents of Self-Esteem*. San Francisco: W. H. Freeman, 1967.

11. Selowsky, M. A note on preschool-age investment in human capital in developing countries. In: *Economic Development and Cultural Change,* 24:707-720, July 1976; and Selowsky, M., and L. Taylor. The economics of malnourished children: an example of disinvestment in human capital. *Economic Development and Cultural Change,* 22(1):17-30, 1973.

12. Berg, A. *The Nutrition Factor: Its Role in National Development*. Washington: Brookings, 1973.

13. Mönckeberg, F. Malnutrition and mental capacity. pp. 48-51. In: *Nutrition, the Nervous System, and Behavior*. PAHO Scientific Publication No. 251, Washington, D.C., 1972.

14. Birch, H. G. Malnutrition, learning and intelligence. *Am. J. Publ. Hlth.* 62:773-784, 1972.

15. Winick, M. *Malnutrition and Brain Development*. New York: Oxford University Press, 1976, p. 91.

16. Winick, M., and P. Rossi. The effect of severe early malnutrition in cellular growth of the human brain. *Pediatr. Res.* 3:181-184, 1969.

17. Klein, R. E. Some considerations in the measurement of the effects of food supplements on intellectual development and social adequacy. Paper presented at the *International Conference of Amino Acid Fortification of Protein Foods*, MIT, September 1969; Frisch, R. E. Present status of the supposition that malnutrition causes permanent mental retardation. *Am. J. Clin. Nutr.* 23:189-195, 1970.

18. Mönckeberg, F. E. Effect of early marasmic malnutrition on subsequent physical and psychological development. pp. 269-278. In: N. S. Scrimshaw and J. E. Gordon (eds.). *Malnutrition, Learning and Behavior*. Cambridge: MIT Press, 1968.

19. Yatkin, U. S., and D. S. McLaren. The behavioral development of infants recovering from severe malnutrition. *J. Mental Deficiency Res.* 14(1):25-32, 1970.

20. Brockman, L. M., and H. N. Riccutti. Severe protein calorie malnutrition and cognitive development in infancy and early childhood. *Dev. Psychol.* 4(3):312-319, 1971.

21. Klein, R. E., and A. A. Adinolfi. Measurement of the behavioral correlates of malnutrition. pp. 73-82. In: J. W. Prescott, M. S. Read and D. B. Coursin (eds.). *Brain Function and Malnutrition: Neuropsychological Methods of Assessment*. New York: John Wiley and Sons, 1975.

22. Cravioto, J., and E. DeLicardie. Neurointegrative development and intelligence in children. pp. 53-72. In: J.W. Prescott, M. S. Read and D. B. Coursin (eds.). *Brain Function and Malnutrition: Neuropsychological Methods of Assessment*. New York: John Wiley and Sons, 1975.

23. Klein, R. E., M. Irwin, P. L. Engle, *et al*. Malnutrition, child health and behavioral development: data from an intervention study. Presented at the *4th International Congress of the International Association for the Scientific Study of Mental Deficiency*. Washington, D.C., August 1976.

24. Freeman, H. E., R. E. Klein, J. Kagan, and C. Yarbrough. Relations between nutrition and cognition in rural Guatemala. *Am. J. Publ. Hlth.* 67(3):233-239, 1977.

25. Chase, H. P., and H. P. Martin. Undernutrition and child development. *N. Engl. J. Med.* 282(7):933-939, 1970.

26. Cravioto, J., and E. DeLicardie. The effect of malnutrition on the individual. pp. 3-21. In: A. Berg, N. S. Scrimshaw and D. L. Call (eds.). *Nutrition, National Development, and Planning*. Cambridge: MIT Press, 1973.

27. Canosa, C. A., J. B. Salomon, and R. E. Klein. The intervention approach: the Guatemala study. pp. 185-189. In: W. M. Moore, M. M. Silverberg and M. S. Read (eds.). *Nutrition, Growth and Development of North American Indian Children*. DHEW Publication No. (NIH) 72-26. Washington, D. C.: U. S. Government Printing Office, 1972.

28. Klein, R. E., B. M. Lester, C. Yarbrough, and J. P. Habicht. On malnutrition and mental development: some preliminary findings. p. 319. In: A. Chávez, H. Bourges, and S. Basta (eds.). *Nutrition*. Basel, S. Karger, 1975.

29. Scrimshaw, N. S., and J. E. Gordon (eds.). *Malnutrition, Learning, and Behavior*. p.11. Cambridge: MIT Press, 1968.

30. Popkin, B. M. Human resource development and productivity: the role of nutrition. In: *Economics and Finance in Indonesia (EKI)*, Vol. 24, No. 3, September 1976.

31. Pollitt, E., D. B. Greenfield, and R. Leibel. Behavioral effects of iron deficiency in a U.S. pre-school population. Presented at the *Conference of the International Society for the Study of Behavioral Development*, University of Pavia, September 1977.

32. Cupo, G. *Variations in Work Performed Among Field Workers on an Estate Farm*. Jamaica, University of West Indies.

33. Viteri, F. Considerations on the effect of nutrition on the body composition and physical working capacity of young Guatemalan adults. pp. 350-375. In: N. S. Scrimshaw and A. M. Altschul (eds.). *Amino Acid Fortification of Protein Foods*. Cambridge: MIT Press, 1971.

34. McClelland, D. C., and D. G. Winter. *Motivating Economic Achievement*. New York: The Free Press, 1969.

35. Cravioto, J., and E. DeLicardie. Nutrition and behavior in learning. pp. 96-97. In: M. Rechcigl (ed.). *Food, Nutrition and Health*. Basel, S. Karger, 1973.

36. Christiansen, N., L. Vouri, and M. Wagner. Social environment as it relates to malnutrition and mental development. pp. 186-199. In: J. Cravioto, L. Hambraeus and B. Vahlquist (eds.). *Early Malnutrition and Mental Development*. Uppsala: Almqvist & Wiksell International, 1974.

37. Chávez, A., C. Martínez, and T. Yaschine. The importance of nutrition and stimulation in child mental and social development. pp. 233-239. In: J. Cravioto, L. Hambraeus and B. Vahlquist (eds.). *Early Malnutrition and Mental Development*. Uppsala: Almqvist & Wiksell International, 1974.

38. Cravioto, J., E. DeLicardie, and H. Birch. Nutrition growth and neuro-integrative development: an experimental and ecological study. *Pediatrics*, 38 (Supplement 2, Pt. II): 319-372, 1966.

39. Moss, H. A. Sex, age and state as determinants of mother-in-
     fant interaction. *Merrill-Palmer Quarterly,* 13:34, 1967.
40. Cravioto, J., and E. DeLicardie. Ecology of malnutrition -
     environmental variables associated with clinical severe
     malnutrition. pp. 157-166. In: C. A. Canosa (ed.).
     Nutrition, Growth and Development. Modern Problems in
     Pediatrics, Vol. 14. Basel: S. Karger, 1975.
41. Klein, R. E., O. Gilbert, C. A. Canosa, and R. DeLeón. Per-
     formance of malnourished in comparison with adequately
     nourished children on selected cognitive tasks (Guatema-
     la). Presented at the *Annual Meeting of the Association
     for the Advancement of Science,* Boston, December 1969.
42. Adinolfi, A. A., and R. E. Klein. The value orientations of
     Guatemalan subsistence farmers: measurement and implica-
     tions. *J. Social. Psychol.* 87:13-20, 1972.
43. Klein, R. E., J. P. Habicht, and C. Yarbrough. Effects of
     protein calorie malnutrition on mental development. pp.
     75-91. In: I. Schulman (ed.). *Advances in Pediatrics,*
     Vol. 18. Chicago: Year Book Medical Publishers, Inc.
     1971.
44. Chávez, A., and C. Martínez. Nutrition and development of in-
     fants from poor rural areas: 2. Nutritional level and
     physical activity. *Nutr. Rep. Intern.* 5(2):139-144,
     1972.
45. Lechtig, A., J-P. Habicht, C. Yarbrough, *et al.* Morbidity and
     physical growth in children from rural Guatemala. pp. 177-
     186. In: *Pediatría XIV: Crecimiento y Desarrollo Endocri-
     nológico.* Buenos Aires: Editorial Médica Panamericana,
     1974.
46. Klein, R. E., H. E. Freeman, J. Kagan, *et al.* Is big smart?
     The relation of growth to cognition. *J. Hlth. Social.
     Behavior.* 13:219-225, 1972.

COMMENTS

Ernesto Pollitt*, *Massachusetts Institute of Technology, Cambridge,
Massachusetts*

This discussion of Educational Outcomes and Nutrition focuses
on methodological issues stemming from the different modes in which
nutrition may offset the educational process. A differentiation of
these modes is pertinent to a selection of outcome measures and
study designs. Different evaluative approaches may be required
according to different modes or conditions. For example, if the focus
of these evaluations were limited exclusively to long term educa-

---

*Mailing adress: Dept. of Population Studies, School of Public Health,
 University of Texas, P.O.B. 20186 Houston, Texas

tional goals such as achievement measures, useful information would
be lost regarding the dynamics of the nutrition factor and the ways
to establish effective priorities in treatment programs.

However, before discussing the modes in which nutrition may
interfere with education, it will be useful to outline two propositions related to the effects of malnutrition on learning and behavior. The purpose here is to set limits to expectations regarding evaluations of the nutrition-education relationship.

Proposition one is a probablistic linkage between malnutrition
and any form of behavioral deviation. Available data show that even
severe forms of protein calorie malnutrition may, but do not necessarily have to result in cognitive impairment. Moreover, in those
cases where there is impairment it is generally not severe but mild
to moderate in degree (1). The existence of impairment associated
with malnutrition seems to depend in part on the social and familial circumstances of the child. Early intellectual deficits associated with early trauma may be ameliorated by favorable environmental characteristics. Conversely, a stressful environment may exacerbate the behavioral or cognitive disturbances caused by malnutrition.

It follows from proposition one that evaluations of effects of
nutrition on education must rely on strong study designs that permit
assessment of the complex interactions between nutrition and social
environmental variables. Moreover, the educational outcome measures
to be chosen must have discriminatory power. The issue at hand is
to differentiate among subjects whose educational process is dis-
turbed by a nutritional deficiency from those whose educational
problems result primarily from other factors. At issue here is the
validity of the evaluation measures.

Proposition two is that the state of knowledge of the nutrition-
behavior relationship is such that presently we have only a crude
estimate of its nature and scope. Thus, although there is now a
basis to conclude that there is a probablistic linkage between malnutrition and cognitive impairment it is not yet possible to identify the biological basis of the impairment or the cognitive abilities which are likely to be altered. Thus, for example, we are
unable to say whether nutritional deficiencies cause impairment in
short or long term memory, or whether vocabulary acquisition or
comprehension suffers more than perceptual organization. This means
that the selection of measurement instruments to assess behavioral
or cognitive areas in an evaluation paradigm must depend on educated
guesses. It is obviously important to develop theoretical models
from which specific hypotheses may be derived and tested.

Turning now to the main issue of this discussion, the different
modes in which nutrition may offset the educational process, I will

try to use the two propositions outlined above as an umbrella for
the following suggestions.

It is useful to distinguish between short and long term nutritional effects. Short term effects refer to temporary food deprivation or hunger conditions. This state may affect learning through
specific and transient metabolic or neurohormonal changes. Long
term interference, on the other hand, refers to modifications of
body tissue due to nutritional deficits which may affect learning
through neural alterations.

A reasonable assumption concerning the role of short term food
deprivation is that hunger over a few hours is not likely to affect
structural changes in central nervous system tissue. Metabolic or
neurohormonal changes will probably affect process variables such
as attention and concentration. This assumption, which I think
rests on strong grounds, provides us with an opportunity to take
advantage of available theoretical models which separate process
from structural variables. As an example of one such model one can
refer to Atkinson and Shiffrin (2). In this model, a structural
feature, like the hardware of a computer, is a built-in aspect of
the system. The actual size of the memory system (its total capacity) is a structural feature. Although such features may be modified (increased in size through maturation; decreased in size
through insult), these modifications are considered permanent and
not relevant to the assessment of short term effects. Control processes, on the other hand, like the software of a computer (e.g.,
programs) are short term and modifiable. Deciding on how to organize or rehearse information or paying attention to specific aspects of the stimulus information are examples of control processes.
Such processes have a relevance to school learning and seem likely
to be affected by psychological symptoms associated with short term
hunger. Accordingly, an evaluation of the effects of short term
food deprivation in school related behaviors may include aspects of
selective attention, rehearsal strategies in memory function, or
aspects of reflective-impulsive behaviors.

Let us now return to the case of long term interference. Here,
in contrast to the case just discussed, it may seem obvious that
the most appropriate targets for evaluation are results of education such as achievement test scores. This may be even more apparent in those situations where the objective is an assessment
of the impact of a program such as school feeding. Improvement in
standardized test scores would point in the direction of a beneficial effect on the nutrition intervention.

However, covariations among standardized tests of achievement
and changes in school feeding conditions are insufficient evidence

to conclude that the nutrition factor is responsible for improvements in achievement scores. From the experience of previous experiments on the efforts of intervention programs, "Hawthorne-type"
effects should be expected on an initial evaluation following the
implementation of the treatment. Moreover, in the long run, other
non-nutritional variables which correlate with the nutritional supplement, such as greater interest on the part of the teachers,
could well produce beneficial changes in achievement test scores.
This is particularly true if the recipients are severely deprived
children whose behavior is highly sensitive to factors that improve their environment -- for example, village children in the
high Andes or urban slum youngsters in Lima, Bogotá or Santiago.

On the basis of the above discussion, it follows that long term
measures of educational outcomes such as aptitude or achievement
tests do not meet the prerequisites of test sensitivity derived from
proposition one. Measures of behavior or of psychological constructs associated with the learning process in the school setting
will come much closer to meeting this requirement.

The issue in terms of evaluation is to define the cognitive
processes which are important in the classroom setting. This definition requires at the level of cognition, for example, an identification of the cognitive elements that play a salient role in
the acquisition of information. These elements may vary substantially from setting to setting according to curriculum and educational organization, among other factors. In the Altiplano in Bolivia, for example, the education of an Aymara child exposed to a
Spanish curriculum is not likely to depend, in the same form or
degree, on the learning of cognitive skills used by an urban child
in a school in La Paz.

Evaluations aimed at cognitive variables in the learning process may have to face the complex problem of measurement construction. This is a difficult task and for this reason this strategy
is frequently side-stepped in favor of methodologically less costly
and time consuming approaches.

I have tried to describe some of the methodological issues and
complexities associated with the evaluation of nutritional effects
on variables related to education. It is apparent that, although
research in this area is not an easy endeavor, it is within our
reach given adequate funding and institutional support. Thus, it
is to be expected -- for example -- that we will soon see evaluations of the educational benefits of school breakfast programs in
the United States.

I find it very difficult to conceptualize, however, a situation

in Latin America, with possibly two or three exceptions, where these
types of evaluations can be carried out with the currently available
administrative infrastructure and national resources for program
funding. Moreover, new large scale nutrition-education programs
in a few South American countries could be jeopardized with the
inclusion of evaluation components. Their infrastructure as they
now stand is too weak. Finally, such evaluations may even be unnecessary if they are conducted elsewhere under highly controlled
experimental conditions and the data obtained in these settings
is adapted to Latin American conditions. Useful generalizations
can come from valid evaluations -- and that is what is needed.

ACKNOWLEDGMENT

The author wishes to thank Daryl Greenfield for the description of the model presented in this paper.

REFERENCES

1.   Pollitt, E., and C. Thomson. Protein calorie malnutrition and
        behavior: a review from psychology. In: R. J. Wurtman
        and J. J. Wurtman (eds). *Nutrition and the Brain*. Vol.
        2. New York: Raven Press, 1977.
2.   Atkinson, R. C., and R. M. Shiffrin. Human memory: a pro-
        posal system and its control processes. In: R. W.
        Spence and J. T. Spence (eds.). *The Psychology of Learn-
        ing and Motivation*. Vol. 2. New York: Academic Press,
        1968.

GENERAL DISCUSSION

The discussion began with questions posed by the conferees
about the relative utility of various outcome measures of educational attainment. It was generally agreed that outcome measures must
relate directly to the original aims of the program, and that multiple outcome measures should display a pattern or mosaic of results which the evaluation can interpret.

Following this exchange, sharp disagreement was expressed with
Pollitt's contention that the administrative infrastructure of many
Latin American nutrition education programs was too weak to support
evaluation components without jeopardizing these programs. Those
disagreeing with Pollitt insisted that evaluation must be an integral part of the entire program and that any division between
program implementation and evaluation was artificial. Pollitt

reiterated that in his opinion the organizational barriers to the evaluation of educational outcomes of nutrition programs represented a serious problem.

The discussion then turned to the complexity of the relationship between education and nutritional status. The fact that illness and a variety of other socio-economic factors complicate the nutrition-education relationship makes definitive evaluation results extremely difficult to obtain. In this context, the importance of experimental controls to rule out alternative explanations for observed changes in educational outcome variables following program implementation was stressed. Specific examples from income maintenance experiments were presented to illustrate these points.

There was general agreement that planners and evaluators must examine the critical assumptions related to the goals of applied programs and the probability of seeing the hypothesized effects of the intervention. Specifically, this demands an awareness of previous research establishing a relationship between the program intervention and the hoped-for outcome. Secondly, given this evidence from the published literature, it is important to estimate the probability of seeing such effects in the particular study setting. For example, does the published research literature provide evidence for a nutritional impact upon grade repeat rates in primary schools. Once a possible relationship is demonstrated, what further evidence exists that reduced grade repetition rates represent a positive outcome in the particular applied setting. For example, if the availability of school grades is limited, a high repeat rate may be an expression of student efforts to maximize their exposure to the school environment.

If planners have not accomplished this critical examination in preliminary project planning phases, the evaluator should recommend that this analysis be conducted. Not only would it eliminate the appearance of program failure under conditions which make program goal attainment impossible, but it would also reduce the cost of the evaluation by eliminating measurements which lack applied utility. There was general agreement that a greater degree of coordination in the nutrition/health area between policy research and process-impact evaluation is sorely needed.

The discussions produced a list of simple indicators of educational outcomes which, given certain assumptions, might be affected by nutrition and health interventions, either directly or indirectly through non-nutritional mechanisms.

Educational Performance and Outcome Measures

This list may be supplemented by referring to recent works by Mushkin (1,2) on measurement of educational outcomes in developing countries.

1. Long term measures which are easily obtainable and susceptible to surveillance:

    a. Grade repetition rates
    b. Enrollment rates
    c. Absenteeism rates
    d. Dropout rates
    e. Length of schooling
    f. Progress to higher education
    g. Standardized achievement scores in reading, mathematics and vocabulary
    h. Aptitude test scores
    i. Access to higher paid jobs

2. Short term measures which tend to be more research related:

    a. Content measures: composite scores on intelligence tests; tests of memory capacity; tests of perceptual organization.

    b. Process measures: tests of attention maintenance; tests of vigilance; tests of concentration; rehearsal strategies of memory.

REFERENCES

1. Public Services Laboratory, Georgetown University, U.S.A., and the Institute of Development Research, Ethiopia. *Educational Outcome Measurement in Developing Countries*. Washington, D. C.: Public Services Laboratory, Georgetown University, 1975.
2. Mushkin, S. J. and B. R. Billings. *A Guide to Educational Outcome Measurements and Their Uses, Seminars 1-6*. Washington, D. C., and Costa Rica: Public Services Laboratory and CEMIE, November, 1975.

POLITICAL AND ORGANIZATIONAL ISSUES IN ASSESSING HEALTH AND NUTRITION INTERVENTIONS

Antonio Ugalde
    University of Texas
    Austin, Texas

and

Robert Emrey
    Association of University Programs in Health
      Administration
    Washington, D. C.

The issues we wish to discuss are fundamental to establishing a successful program evaluation in Latin America. Technical and computational problems will certainly impede development of evaluation methods under current circumstances in Latin America, and one may add in most developing countries in the world. Compared to them, however, we contend that political and organizational factors will prove to be even more difficult to overcome, will require the longest time to change, and will demand the greatest investment of intelectual and official energy to find adequate solutions in the development process. Without attention to these issues, no model of impact assessment -- whether imported or developed within Latin America -- can hope to survive and take root. In brief form, the issues are of four types:

a.   Purposes for program evaluation differ greatly among designers and users of impact measurement techniques in Latin America;

b.   Data handling methods and organizations are not adequate to collect, transmit, and present the complex variables required in studying the causes and effects of health and nutrition program impacts in Latin America;

c.   People having both sufficient technical knowledge and
     political influence either cannot or will not participate
     in program evaluation efforts in Latin America; and

d.   Bureaucratic processes are not understood well enough to
     ensure implementation of programs. Knowledge of bureau-
     cratic decision making is a requirement for the establish-
     ment of evaluation procedures. Similarly, there is lim-
     ited reliable information about the functioning of the
     political systems in these nations.

Each of these issues will be discussed in turn, concluding with
some proposals for ways to make progress in development of Latin
American program evaluation arrangements. Before entering into this
discussion, however, it might be useful to present an organizational
frame of reference within which the evaluation process can be placed.

The focus of attention in program evaluation is assumed to be
on a particular organization and a particular population served.
These organizational units of analysis may be international, national, or local agencies and may come under public or private control. A view of that organization as a living system would reveal
certain more or less permanent features such as money provided to
operate it, people employed, services produced, and a variety of
other less tangible phenomena which influence the ways the organization operates over time. These latter would include enacted policies, worker attitudes, political support, and economic conditions.

The organization viewed from this perspective contains a variety of complex, interacting elements. In the simplified form shown
in Figure 1, the organization consists of certain elements which
are within the organizational boundaries, but where many significant
parts are in the environment outside. 1/ The administrative and
political characteristics of the organization will influence the
policies adopted and services provided just as do policies and funds
from agencies outside the organization.

As programs are implemented, various changes occur within the
organization, including effects on services provided and the working conditions of employees. These changes we will call "program
impacts". As services are provided, various changes will occur
also in the outside community. These changes we will call "programs outcomes", meaning those changes in the population served

---

1/   This model draws on systems theory notions. Applications of
similar models to organizational processes in local government agencies are found in Kraemer, et. al., (1) and to the United States Department of State in Warwick (2).

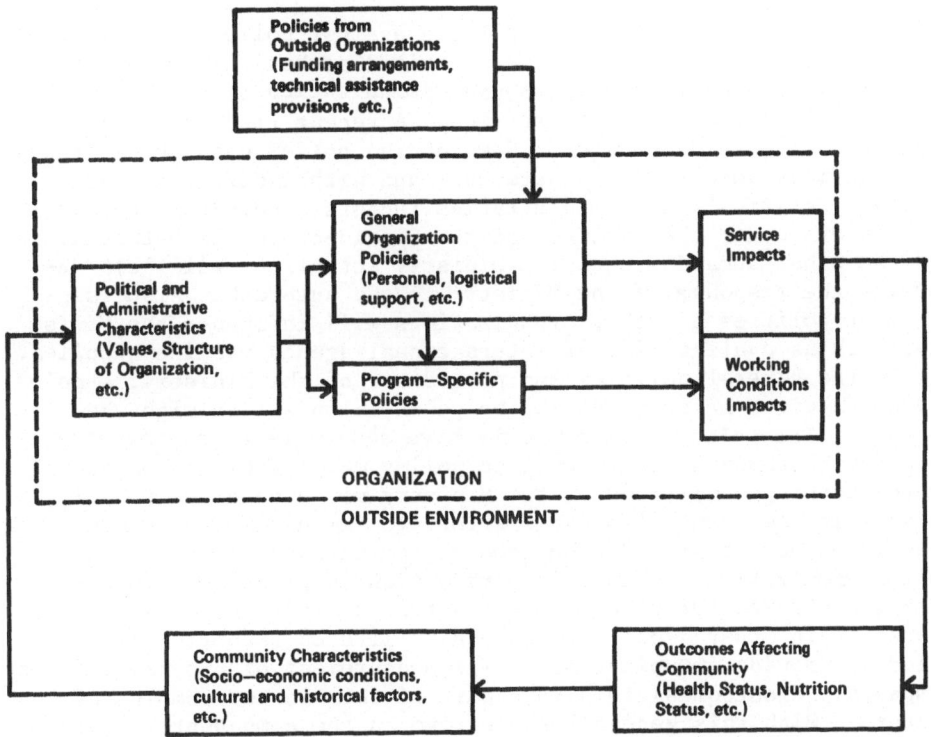

FIG. I. *Program Evaluation Model of Organization and Environment in Procedures.*

which are being discussed in this volume. These outcomes occur in the larger context of a country's social and economic conditions, cultural patterns, and historical experiences which consistently influence the manner in which the organization operates. Program evaluation is usually defined as the systematic comparison of the goals of a social intervention policy with the resulting impacts and outcomes. 2/

A brief description of how the model may be applied will illustrate these features. An imaginary Ministry of Health operates

---

2/   The literature of program evaluation is voluminous. The relationships discussed here are explored at length in Suchman (3), Van Maanen (4), Caro (5), and Bernstein & Freeman (6).

a limited program to immunize children against polio. The people
served by this agency may be characterized as having low incomes
and not being experienced in seeking immunization services. As a
result, not many utilize the service. A recent rise in the incidence of polio is discovered. News of the polio outbreak is viewed
with alarm by some Ministry personnel and with indifference by
others. Political and administrative factors, including the availability of funds, the interest of the President in the outbreak,
and the other demands requiring Ministry attention, will help determine the response of the Ministry to the outbreak. Also, significant policies of other organizations will influence the Ministry, such as availability of international agency vaccine supplies.
Within the general policies and procedures of the Ministry, a policy which gives major attention to polio immunization might be
adopted. The policy will probably have some effect in providing
people with immunizations, but the policy may not be implemented,
or the working conditions of the Ministry may change drastically,
such as in the event of a rapid effort to immunize many communities in a short time. The outcome of the changed policy toward
polio immunization may include a reduction in polio incidence, a
rise in requests for other medical services, and perhaps a deterioration in other aspects of community life as resources are devoted to provide immunizations. The measurement of program effects
(impacts and outcomes) is always part of this larger complex of
factors. With this general perspective on the components of program evaluation and measurements of program effects, let us turn
to the purposes of such evaluations.

PURPOSES OF PROGRAM EVALUATION

The ultimate purpose of program evaluation is to confront program effects with the manifest intent of the policy maker or, in
the case of pilot projects, with the manifest goals of the projects.
For evaluation purposes the difference between a public program and
a pilot project is important because evaluation generally has secondary purposes which tend to be different in the case of public
programs or pilot projects.

In public programs evaluation serves as a means of control and
accountability of the bureaucracy. Through its discretionary power,
which as will be seen later is large in most Latin American countries, the bureaucracy makes important decisions affecting program
effects. For example, if a program calls for the establishment of
rural health posts, program evaluation can scrutinize the bureaucracy rationale for the choice of locations, types and quality
of services rendered, populations served, utilization of services,
cost-efficiency of the services, etc. In other words, the purpose

of the evaluation is to verify (which is a way of control) that the
program has been implemented according to the design, and furthermore, that the design is consistent with the policy goal. It can
be suggested that in Latin America the purpose of control and accountability can be linked with the ultimate purpose of evaluation
(the measurement of program effects) by making the assumption that
if a program is properly implemented according to the design, then
the intended effects will follow. Of course, it can be argued that
to make this assumption is to take a risk, and we concur that this
is so in the case of complex social programs in developed nations.
However, health and nutritional status in most Latin American countries can be dramatically altered with very simple programs such as
immunization, potable water, or primary health care. In these cases
it can be safely assumed that proper program implementation will be
followed by the anticipated program effects. In fact, as will be
discussed later, one of the main problems in Latin America is lack
of implementation of social programs and limited knowledge to explain implementation failures.

By making the above assumption the evaluation circumvents complex social measurements by substituting simple proxy indicators
such as utilization, population served, types of services, etc.,
which should be readily available in any administrative system although it is acknowledged that frequently they are not. We call
this type of evaluation *administrative evaluation*. For example,
the effects of a rural potable water supply program can be measured by verifying the number of aqueducts or wells in use, assessing
water utilization (in some rural communities potable water is not
used for drinking), determining the quality of water consumed (the
water could be potable at the source but contaminated in the haul-
ing or storage process), and showing that other possible indicators
are in accordance with the design of the program. We can then assume that health conditions will improve.

Pilot projects are experimental interventions and are not national in scope. Consequently, control and accountability are seldom considered to be purposes of evaluation. However, frequently
the research teams or the managers of the projects need to demonstrate to the funding agencies that the impact effects are worth
additional funding for the project or future projects. The tendency is to use impact measurements which are quantifiable since
it is believed that they are more rigorous. As a result only those
aspects of the project which are amenable to quantification are
evaluated, while equally important dimensions of the project are left
outside of the evaluation because of political, administrative and/
or technical difficulties. Pilot projects are particularly useful
to test hypotheses of cause-effect relations in complex social problems where control of variables needs to be rigorous and impact

measurements need to be quantifiable. As a result, only those aspects of the project which are amenable to quantification are evaluated while equally important dimensions of the project are left outside of the evaluation because of political, administrative and/or technical difficulties. Pilot projects are particularly useful to test hypotheses of cause-effect relations in complex social problems where controls of variables need to be rigorous, impact measurements are difficult to operationalize, and the evaluations exercise is relatively costly. The utility of pilot projects in Latin America is beginning to be seriously questioned because they are too expensive and therefore they cannot be extended to the national scene or because they function in a political-administrative vacuum under experimental conditions which do not exist in the "real" world. Some other critics also attack pilot projects because in their opinion they represent strategies to postpone long overdue structural transformations. Alford (7) illustrated in his study of health care in the state of New York that the inconclusiveness of research is utilized by political interests to postpone decisions which are contrary to the wishes of the decision-makers.

Two recent contrasting nutrition evaluation research projects are illustrative of the above discussion and of the varying purposes which evaluation studies may pursue. The cases are particularly interesting because the two were conducted in the same area in rural communities in the vicinity of a major center of nutrition and health research in Latin America.

In one case, a highly competent research team assumed that the causes of malnutrition were within the rural communities to be studied, an assumption which could be considred ideological or based on the perception of the nature of a problem by the researchers. Political views, professional orientations, and cultural values separately or in some degree of interaction could have led the researchers to formulate this assumption. The researchers made a logical deduction from the assumption: *if* the causes of malnutrition are to be found in the communities, *then* the implementation of solutions will require changes in the behavior of the communities. As the report issued by the project indicated: "....the implementation of the remedies for malnutrition will depend to some extent in their acceptability by the community as well as *in the community's willingness to adapt itself to the required changes*" (emphasis added). Once this frame of reference was established, the research design followed two logical steps: first, the preparation of survey instruments (nine in all) to identify within the community the causes of malnutrition and to determine the habits and customs of the population; and second, the identification of required changes and the design of mechanisms to insure the implementation of changes. Quantitative techniques were justified to evaluate "the accuracy of the diagnostic procedure in order to predict the outcome of the solutions".

In the other research project, a social anthropologist did intensive field work in the same region. His point of departure was quite different from that of the other study. The researcher assumed that the causes of malnutrition were outside the community. As could be expected, his research topic and design also were different. Instead of looking at the value system of the community, at its organization and internal dynamics, he considered it more appropriate to identify the causes of malnutrition through an "... historical analysis of the politico-economic development of agriculture in the region". Within this frame of reference sample survey techniques were considered inappropriate. The study could only be done at the macro level without control groups because according to his original assumption malnutrition was not the result of some behavioral traits of the population but of certain structural conditions in the social system. The researcher utilized for his research project non-quantitative techniques such as participant-observation, indepth nonstructured interviews, and analysis of archival materials and records. For him, as for many other social scientists, measurement of success or failure of social interventions in pilot projects defies quantification because laboratory testing conditions of the physical sciences are not present in the field. According to this line of thought efforts to quantify social interventions frequently respond more to the political needs to justify pilot projects than to the present possibility of scientific rigor in the social sciences.

We are faced, then with a set of different purposes and approaches to program evaluation. Depending on the purpose involved, the data collection, communication and presentation processes must change. The following question needs to be raised: For what purposes of program evaluation should the research tools of the physical sciences be adapted to these social institutions? It is precisely for the purposes of measurement and evaluation that researchers have for some time attempted to borrow the more precise tools of the physical sciences, but this in itself -- as it will be seen -- reflects a conceptualization of reality according to which the physical and the social world can be manipulated in similar ways.

In the following section we consider the implications of this question by exploring the problems of assembling data for program evaluation.

DATA HANDLING METHODS AND ORGANIZATIONS

Data handling is a major cost for many evaluation efforts. In deciding the approach to be taken, the relative cost of evaluation procedures to the cost of the services provided must always be borne in mind. In the United States, health and nutrition services may be expensive and evaluation procedures relatively cheap on a per capita basis. In Latin America, an opposite situation often occurs where the services are relatively cheap but evaluation procedures require a relatively high investment, particularly if social measurements are to be developed for assessing effects of experimental or quasi-experimental projects. Given the tentative nature of mathematical models in the social sciences, the difficulties of controls, and the scarce financial resources in Latin America it is understandable that the payoffs of having impact evaluation information are seen as relatively low, and that the support for devoting resources to such efforts may also be quite low (at least for non-administrative evaluation). Even in the United States, the limited experience to date is that program evaluation does not produce much of an effect on public programming. Some authors go as far as affirming that evaluation research has a negative impact in the adminstrative process of an agency and at best is wasteful of "money, time and people" (8). In fact, the legislative mandate for evaluation responded more to the Congressional need to control the bureaucracy than to attempts to measure program impact. Thus, according to Suchman recent proliferation of evaluation research responds to " . . . pressures upon public agencies for greater accountability"   (3, p. 5).

Another dimension of data handling, perhaps more important than the financial dimension, is a philosophical one that has plagued social science since its beginnings and continues to be unresolved. We have touched on this issue earlier and we will return to it later: data collection techniques and analytical procedures are themselves a reflection of the conceptualization that social scientists have of the social reality. 3/   For example, the traditional conflict between soft and hard techniques goes deeper than the researchers' own preference and likes. Methodologies reflect theoretical constructs which in turn reflect philosophical and political views of reality. Many social scientists now agree that theory influences the choice of methodologies and that different methodologies are instrumental in the development of different theoretical approaches (9, 10).

3/   This point heavily reflects the influence of Sjoberg and Nett (9).

Technologies required to handle evaluation data must be organized to take these political and economic realities into account. Experiments with sampling techniques, for example, offer much promise for reducing costs of impact data gathering but on the other hand may distort social reality by imposing the researchers' categories on the respondents' minds. This is particularly the case when researchers belong to different social or ethnic groups than those of the interviewees, a frequent situation in rural research by urban scientists.

Data regarding the functioning of public bureaucracies are indispensable for any administrative evaluation, and the political constraints for the gathering of these sensitive data are obvious. Confronted by the difficulty, evaluators may be tempted to relegate the analysis of these data to a marginal position. Similarly, the difficulties of quantifying organizational information could exclude some important dimensions in an evaluation effort.

Given these practical and political limitations the following questions need to be asked: is it possible that incomplete data (a situation which probably occurs in most evaluation exercises) permit interpretation of findings by criteria other than scientific, by conjecture or by intelligent guesses, and then values and ideologies might exercise a hidden influence? What are the consequences when evaluation research follows verification procedures and measurements which do not adhere strictly to the principles of scientific experimentation, as is the situation in practically all social science research? Is it possible that the professional and financial interests of the researchers, or the political interests of the dominant groups, bias the interpretation of findings? It is perhaps in this sense that Myrdal (11) calls all social science opportunistic. It is in this context that the issue of who should participate in data collection, analysis and use for program evaluation becomes of paramount importance.

PARTICIPANTS IN PROGRAM EVALUATION

In every facet of nutrition and health evaluation, the program evaluator encounters dimensions of social behavior. It is known, for example, that the utilization of health care facilities responds to social norms, that it differs from one social class to another and from culture to culture (12). Similarly, modalities of purchasing health care are related to each society's understanding of the role of the state, the dignity of life and human rights, and of the nature of the economic system. As Hamilton (13) put it: "Wants are social phenomena, the product of cultural conditioning". The anthropological literature contains a myriad of examples des-

cribing food taboos, eating habits, symbolic and ritual uses of food
in different cultural settings which health professionals and nutritionists have decried as inimical to normal physical growth, and
western economists from their cultural vantage point have considered highly irrational.

    Latin American health evaluators and planners have been drawn
predominantly from the medical profession, and medical training has
not prepared its professionals with a solid background in the behavioral sciences. As a result, an important dimension of health
and nutrition evaluation has been left out, and only after trial
and error have evaluators "rediscovered" that values, norms, and
ideologies condition human and social behavior. It should be acknowledged that health planners are now aware of the social dimensions of planning and various social sciences are being incorporated -- albeit in secondary roles -- into the health and nutrition
planning efforts. In this context it may be worth noting also that
decision-making in most health ministries is still in the hands of
medical doctors rather than health administrators. The same applies
to health related international agencies.

    Following this reasoning, two logical conclusions can be made:
(a) *if* social planning, within which health and nutrition should
be placed, includes an important social science component, *then*
social planning will be influenced by the values, ideologies and
conceptualizations of reality held by the planners. For example,
whether a social plan is based on structural-functional or on conflict theory depends on the understanding of social reality of the
planners. 4/ *If* program evaluation is part of social planning and
social planning is part of the policy process, *then* program evaluation will be influenced by the values, ideologies and the conceptua-

---

4/   "Structural-functional analysis presumes that social units
(groups, institutions, etc.) that are in interaction mutually influence and adjust to each other, so that through the various social
processes, including cooperation, competition, conflict, and accommodation, the various groups and segments of a society form a relatively unified social system" (15, p. 442). Structural-functional-
ists perceive social reality the same way biologists perceive living
organisms. The possibilities of value-loaded orientation of struc-
tural-functionalism is stated by Mayntz and Scharpf (16, p. vii):
".......this approach permits to stipulate normative reference points
for an empirical analysis, whether these are derived from the values
of system members or some value standard of the analyst". Conflict
theory on the other hand views social process not "in terms of the
cooperation of social groups but in terms of man's aggressiveness.
Emphasis is placed on conflict as a creative or at least an inevitable fact of social life....." (15, p. 71).

lization of reality of evaluators. For example, in his interesting study of contemporary politics of public health in the People's Republic of China, Lampton (14, p. 202) shows that evaluation procedures responded to the perception of the nature of sanctions held by subordinates. Since perception is influenced by socio-cultural factors and sanction is a concept defined by cultural and political norms it is easy to understand the subjective and political foundations of evaluation.

It can be hypothesized that in Latin America, as elsewhere in the world, the researchers and evaluators are by and large members of the middle and upper classes who tend to see the nature of the social problem (in this case poor health status and malnutrition) from their own social class perspective and from their own cultural vantage point. To avoid incrimination of one's own social, cultural, or professional group the best course of action is to study the poor, among whom social problems exist and whose value and cultural system can be changed with the least expected resistance. Their poverty is integral and includes political powerlessness. 5/ Social scientists who attempt to look at social problems outside their physical habitat, who prepare proposals to study the overfed (decision-makers) instead of the undernourished, or the superparticipant (political and economic elites) instead of the *marginados*, will encounter difficulties in financing the research. Funding agencies are also controlled by middle and upper classes who do not see much promise and at times for obvious reasons do not have much interest in promoting changes of their own values and cultural norms or to alter the present power arrangements. 6/

The above considerations together with those presented in the previous section have important practical ramifications. For example, it can be suggested that the selection of projects and the techniques for their evaluation correspond to: (a) the researcher's and evaluator's understanding of the nature of the social problem; (b) his expectation of the funding agency's response to some orientations and issues, a subtle but real political constraint to objective inquiry; (c) accessibility to data and information, a

---

5/   See example in Alford (17) for critical study of poor people in the U.S.A.

6/   A provocative discussion of this political and ethical problem can be read in Glazer (18)

practical but also a political constraint since data could exist
but not be made available, or data would not be collected or processed because some interest groups or decision-makers prefer not
to do so; 7/ (d) support or authorization from the government which
is heavily influenced on political-ideological grounds.

The selection of participants in program evaluation and the
roles they are permitted to play can strongly affect evaluations of
health and nutrition programs. Administrative evaluations in Latin
America -- the few that exist -- are mostly an in-house exercise.
It is understandable that it will be difficult for a minister of
public health to self-evaluate without biases. Even in some cases
in which it might be possible, the outside reader of the evaluation
will always entertain the doubt of its validity. International
lending institutions could request outside administrative evaluations of government agencies. The development of methods for drawing a wider group of expert teams, community members and program
clients into evaluation efforts is an immediate need for most
evaluation exercises. Well-established universities and research
centers could be called in from within the country or from other
Latin American countries. In this context, it is worth mentioning
the work of the PRIDES group in Cali under the sponsorship of WHO/
PAHO and the goverment of Colombia; their 1976 administrative evaluation of health services of the Colombian Institute of Social
Security is one of the most rigorous efforts in administrative
evaluation. Also, the AID health assessments in some Latin American
countries have provided stimulus for some administrative evaluation.
What could be in our opinion most promising for the innovation of
evaluation methodology is the organization of mixed evaluation teams
of experts, community members and program clients. We believe that
careful experimentation in this area could lead to some breakthroughs
in evaluation.

INSTITUTIONALIZATION OF ADMINISTRATIVE EVALUATION

Up to the present, the rate of implementation of health and
nutrition plans in Latin America, has been very low. There are
several dozen national health plans, but very few have been carried
out to any appreciable extent. A former Venezuelan Minister of
Public Health suggested that if only a fraction of the health plans
would have been implemented, health conditions in Latin America
would be different (20).

7/   For an enlightened discussion of political and ideological influences of data selection, analysis, and utilization, see the "Introduction" of Littrell and Sjoberg (19).

Several explanations have been advanced for the dismal rate
of implementation: (a) lack of planning experience -- health planning is relatively new in Latin America, and very few published
plans existed before 1960; (b) health planning, like planning in
general, was imposed from abroad, and success is problematic without
internal impetus; (c) developing countries are confronted with serious administrative deficiencies, such as shortage of qualified personnel, limited financial resources, poor physical facilities, and
little administrative know-how. These limitations are real, and
as we will see later, they affect the quality of planning and programming which in turn makes implementation and evaluation difficult.
Obviously, it will be useless to attempt impact evaluation of a program which has not been implemented.

But perhaps the main reason for implementation failure is to be
found elsewhere, for decision-makers in many countries do not adequately utilize available data. In some cases, well trained nationals have successfully adapted PERT programming techniques only
to find that these techniques did not facilitate implementation.
In the words of a health agency administrator who promoted PERT
programming, "It had to be discontinued because it did not fit the
political realities of our society". Our respondent touched the
core of the problem. Soon after the planning epidemic had spread
over Latin America, Waterston in his monumental work made the observation that most technical planning problems had been solved and
what remained unresolved were the political dimensions of planning
(21). Unfortunately, health planners paid little attention to his
warning. It can be suggested that implementation failures are to
a great extent the result of health planners' misunderstandings of
the policy process and their attempts to plan in a political vacuum.

Improvements in this area require a better understanding of
the policy process and a more accurate knowledge of how bureaucracies function in Latin America. Recent studies of health systems by social scientists are beginning to provide useful methodological and theoretical insights which we believe are applicable
to Latin America (7, 14, 22, 23). Certainly, the paucity of reliable studies of Latin American political systems is a formidable
constraint for the rapid growth of knowledge of bureaucratic behavior.

Administrative evaluation could become a most useful tool for
the understanding of bureaucratic dynamics which in turn could lead
to more realistic planning. Furthermore, for reasons explained
earlier, administrative evaluation through the development of proxy
indicators can provide a relatively accurate and inexpensive instrument for measuring program effects. In the pages that follow

we will limit ourselves to outlining a few political and organizational guides which should be helpful in efforts to institutionalize
administrative evaluation.

A first task is to develop evaluation guidelines for political,
economic, technical and organizational viability of policies and
plans. At the outset it should be recognized that a policy should
have certain characteristics such as clarity, specificity, and internal and external consistency. It should be recognized that many
health and nutrition plans are weak in each one of these characteristics so that it is important that evaluators examine them according to some simple criteria. An example might clarify our point.
A recent program in one Latin American country calls for centraliza-
tion of decision-making and at the same time increased community
participation. A careful evaluation of this program should point
out the internal inconsistency and alert policy makers of the possibility that implementation may fail as implementors were not given
a consistent program.

Political Viability

The formulation of a policy and the preparation of a plan or
program could be relatively easy and rapid when activities are designed by a small inner group of a centralized ministry without
inputs from groups whose interests and lives are affected by them.
These latter groups include: labor unions, peasant leagues, professional associations, community organizations, business concerns,
political parties or factions, and bureaucratic cliques. The Latin
American experience has been characterized by an outpouring of hastily conceived policies, plans and programs to satisfy immediate political needs or the will of international lending agencies. However, what was gained at this phase of the policy process was lost
during the implementation phase. It is not possible to avoid a
political debate, and if the parliamentary forum does not exist or
is not a functioning one, the decision-makers need to provide the
mechanism for debate in order to achieve a minimum of consensus
among the future recipients of services and those whose interests
are affected.

It should be clear that we are not advocating necessarily the
incorporation of interest groups in health policy formulation or
planning; in some cases, it might be desirable, in others less so.
We use the term "interest group" to refer generally to any formally
or informally organized group which attempts to influence the policy process. We are aware that interest group has a defensive con-
notation toward economic interests and as such might not exist in
socialist economies. Our definition is broader and encompasses

bureaucratic cliques which might attempt to influence the policy
process for other than economic self-interest. In some countries
some interest groups are well organized and extremely powerful, and
the health planner needs to make a political decision to incorporate them or not to incorporate them in the policy process. A
decision has to be made also in regard to the modality of incorporation and the selection of the groups to be incorporated. All
these are political decisions, and in Latin America the bureaucrat
makes many political decisions in the absence of influential parliamentary forms. His political acumen is as important as his technical abilities.

An understanding of the degree of consensus achieved through
mechanisms of accommodation may help to anticipate:

   a.   Authority leakages in the implementation process and lack
        of compliance within the bureaucracy itself. For example,
        failures may occur among the physicians or nurses or
        among the bureaucrats at the provincial level, which is
        almost impossible to correct by supervision alone. 8/

   b.   Poor utilization or misuse of health and nutrition serv-
        ices for lack of interest, knowledge, and at times indig-
        nation by clients. This has frequently been the case in
        some rural health and nutrition programs or in social
        security systems.

   c.   Lukewarm cooperation and eventual withdrawal of other
        public agencies whose participation was necessary for
        the successful completion of a plan.

   d.   Opposition and eventual destruction of parts of a plan or
        program by interest groups. 9/

8/   Downs (24) has documented well this phenomenon in the Pentagon
and Lampton (14) for the health system of China during the Cultural
Revolution. Allison (25) has shown that such processes may be
viewed from several points of view: rational actors; organizational
routines; and bureaucratic politics.

9/   As examples of the last point, programs of government drug manu-
facturing and distribution frequently come under the attack of the
pharmaceutical industry, and environmental health plans face opposition from multinational firms. Conversations with an employee of an
international agency reported that in Brazil the multinational pharmaceutical firms destroyed a government attempt to manufacture ge-

In Latin America the need to achieve some degree of consensus
is particularly important in view of the political instability that
characterizes the continent. Obviously, the implementation of a
plan or program prepared under one government will have no viability
if the new government represents a complete ideological break with
the past, as for example in the case of Cuba or the more recent
coup in Chile. However, the political instability in Latin America
frequently is manifest only by a change of guard or of political
groups with similar ideologies. The political crisis which characterizes political instability produces ministerial shuffles or
changes of ministers whose life expectancy is low (a two-year term
would be a good average in many countries). It should be noticed
that it is not so much the change as the unpredictability of the
change, its nature and timing which makes implementation uncertain.
Each minister, even in cases in which the new appointment does not
represent an ideological break with the past, comes to the ministry
with his own ideas, projects and personnel. How much the health
bureaucracy changes with changes of ministers differs from country
to country and according to the political factors which forced the
change. In Colombia, one of the few countries with a relatively
high constitutional continuity in the last twenty years, every minister brought his own planning director to the ministry. As a former director general of a Ministry of Health once commented: "Our
problem is that in our society the first thing that a person does
when he comes to office is to undo whatever his predecessor has
done." Frequently, the undoing is not an aggressive attack but rather letting the plan or program die of natural causes while efforts
of the bureaucracy are steered in other directions. 10/ Furthermore, in health and nutrition a great majority of plans and programs

---

neric drugs. In Colombia, the Association of Pharmaceutical Industries (AFIDRO) influenced the government of President Pastrana, who
had been its head, to dismantle a timid attempt to manufacture non-
patent drugs. In another country, a knowledgeable person at the
Ministry of Public Health indicated that any attempt by the Minister
to tangle with the pharmaceutical industries would cost him the job.
In Mexico major opposition to CONASUPO low price distribution of
drugs come from the pharmaceutical industry (26). The policy of
moving polluting industries from developed nations to the developing countries is advocated in one of the industry's main journals
(27). Many multinationals are politically and economically more
powerful than most Latin American national governments.

10/ This phenomenon was documented in Wilkie for Mexico (28) and
Bolivia (29).

require the participation of other public agencies in which similar continuity characteristics are present; under these conditions implementation will be problematic unless a minimal consensus is achieved.   In sum, and contrary to what is found in some other Western democracies where policy is formulated at the lower bureaucratic units and flows upward for approval (16, p. 71ff) in Latin America the flow is often from the top down.   Low stability of top personnel produces discontinuities in programming and implementation.

In some societies in which some historical events have produced an ideological homogeneity, the necessary consensus might be easy to achieve; in others with great social problems and profound ideological cleavages, a minimum understanding might not be possible. In the latter cases planning might be a futile exercise.   What seems clear is that expanding the participation of persons and groups with conflicting interests will probably increase the time and energies to prepare an implementable plan.   *According to this criterion, the quality of a health plan can be evaluated by the consensus given to the plan or identification of conflicting interests by groups.   The degree and the nature of participation in policy formulation and planning might also be a good measure of quality.*   It might be useful to begin developing operationable indicators of consensus.

In the same way that one should be suspicious of a plan hastily put together with few inputs, the timing of a policy and plan might also be good determinants of its implementation capabilities.   Policies issued hurriedly during a political campaign might not survive election day.

Economic and Technical Viability

Another dimension which has not been given adequate attention by Latin American health policy makers is the economic viability of a policy or plan.   Zschock and Robertson (30), in their study of health finances in Latin America, have shown that plans and programs frequently are prepared without securing the funding for operation and maintenance.   Similarly, plans are approved without consideration of the manpower or other technical needs for operation and maintenance.   Thus, it is not unusual to see rural health clinics without medical or paramedical personnel, or if they have the personnel, the equipment may not be available.   At times these deficiencies are the result of the lack of adequate financing.   It is well known that policymakers often have a preference for the construction of physical facilities.   Hospitals are inaugurated only to be closed down a few months later because of insufficient funding for their operation.   Health surveys are designed and executed without securing the funds and the technical know-how for processing

and analyzing data. A recent Latin American national health survey
was carried out at the cost of $80,000 before preparing the design
and obtaining funds for its analysis. It took three years to get
the first crosstabs.

If funding for a plan or part of a plan is to be financed and/
or disbursed by one or several other agencies, then a firm commitment needs to be previously reached before beginning plan implementation. In one country, for example, a well designed multimil-
lion dollar immunization campaign failed half way through when the
ministry of finance stopped salary payments of campaign workers,
who finally decided to find employment elsewhere. In other cases,
immunization campaigns have been launched without firm financial
commitments for maintaining immunization levels.

We can conclude by saying that there are two basic principles
which could be used to evaluate the quality of a plan in reference
to its economic viability: (a) whether it has secured funding for
maintenance and operation of new facilities and the degree of commitment by the funding agency; and (b) whether the funding agencies
have or have not guaranteed the smooth flow of fund disbursement,
and the degree of commitment. 11/

Administrative Viability

It is not possible within the limits of this paper to discuss
the multiple dimensions that make a plan more likely to be implemented from an administrative point of view. We will concentrate
on the area of policy coordination, some aspects of which have already emerged in the two previous discussions. Health and nutrition plans are particularly multisectorial. It will be impossible
to prepare a nutrition plan without the participation of the agricultural, the educational and the economic sectors in each of
which several agencies and divisions participate. The problem of
policy coordination in nutrition plans has recently been underlined
by a group of PAHO experts (36). Three modalities have been advanced to facilitate horizontal and vertical coordination: (a)
reducing the number of agencies responsible for health and nutrition, for example, by merging social security with the health ministry; (b) organizing an interministerial council or board, for
example, the national health council which is presided by the health
minister or by the director of national planning; and (c) the organ-

---

11/ For further discussion and examples, see Hinrichs (31), Bird
(32), Musgrave (33), Wilkie (34), and Caiden and Wildavsky (35).

ization of a superministry with decision-making power in one field.
12/ A plan in which the coordination mechanisms are clearly defined
will tend to have more possibilities for successful implementation
than one which leaves the inter and intra coordination to the good
will of individual participants.

The establishment of coordination mechanisms does not by itself insure coordination (22, p.119ff). The PAHO discussion on
national nutrition policies observed:

"One of the major obstacles to formulation and execution of
national food and nutrition plans has been a lack of political decision on the part of governments to establish the necessary inter-
sectoral coordination" (36, p.12). Thus, the coordination mechanism might exist, but without the political support it may be in-
operative. The PAHO comment is illustrative of the political dimensions of coordination; it will be difficult for a plan or program to be administratively viable unless first it is politically
viable. In other words, when the implementation of a plan fails,
the apparent causes might be administrative flaws, but the real
causes are in many cases political. Besides the existence of coordination mechanisms the evaluation of viability should consider
the institutionalization of the interaction among agencies, the
frequency of interaction, the approval of formal agreements by heads
of agencies to abide by the decisions taken by the coordinating councils or boards, and the existence of legal mechanisms for bureaucratic compliance.

Relationship Between Policymaking and the Administrative Process: The Discretionary Power of the Bureaucracy

In most Latin American countries, health policies and plans
are prepared by small groups in ministries of public health or
national planning agencies. An important part of the policy process
is the translation of policies and plans into programs, and the
translation of these programs into outputs through the implementation process. It is in these translations where the discretionary
power of the bureaucracy is exercised. For example, a national

---

12/ In many countries national planning has with more or less success attempted to carry out the role of a superministry. In some
countries one ministry has been assigned the job of superministry.
Such is the case of the ministry of rural development in Malaysia.
For the advantages and limitations of the idea of a superministry,
see Ness (37).

health plan calls for the development of preventive health activities, with a technical council of the ministry to make the budgetary decisions. A technical council having a majority of medical
doctors might interpret mother and child care programs as the ones
to be promoted while a technical council controlled by sanitary en-
gineers could decide that aqueducts are the first priority. The relation between professional background and decisions in Latin American public health systems has yet to be explored. Our limited
studies suggest that selection of programs and allocation of funds
represent the career background and professional ideologies of decision-makers, mostly medical doctors. Thus, in spite of the over-
whelming evidence against the need for highly specialized hospitals
many countries continue to build expensive hospitals. In Colombia,
for example, university and specialized hospitals spent 29 percent
of the public health budget. 13/   Studies of one university hospital in the same country showed that normal delivery continued to
be attended there in spite of the established regionalization and
referral system.

The evaluation of the discretionary power of the bureaucracy
implies the monitoring of decisions along with the programming and
implementation phases of the policy process. Who makes what decisions, the understanding of his/her rationale might be difficult to
assess but it is a fundamental component of administrative evaluation.

CONCLUSIONS

Program evaluation has a multiplicity of purposes: verification
that program effects match the original policy goals; satisfaction
of lending agencies requirements; control and accountability of
bureaucracies; and testing hypotheses in experimental or quasi-experimental programs.

One of the highest priorities in Latin America should be to increase program implementation because in the past very few health
and nutrition plans have been carried out, and a precondition for
evaluation is implementation. Social measurements and the control
of social variables are extremely difficult to operationalize and
may be particularly expensive in Latin America where the data base
is weak. In developed nations solutions to social problems might
require complex programs whose evaluations could frequently demand

---

13/ The first study of public health expenditures in Colombia was
published in 1975 at the initiative of a group of industrial en-
gineers (38).

complex social measurements. However, in these nations, evaluation costs on a per capita basis might be low relative to the total cost of the program. In Latin America basic health and nutrition demands can be satisfied with very simple interventions which should be evaluated by low cost measurements. Under these conditions adminis- trative evaluation might be the most desirable approach to satisfy evaluation requirements. It is important to develop simple indica- tors of implementation of interventions which could be used as prox- ies for social measurements.

Given the nature of the social sciences and the tentative basis of mathematical models, data collection, analysis and interpretation allows for subjectivity and biases. Under these circumstances selec- tion of evaluators becomes an issue of strategic importance. If we take into consideration the additional facts that administrative evaluation should be carried out by persons from outside the agency to be evaluated and that in Latin America experts tend to belong to social classes and ethnic groups different from the majority of the population, then the importance of organizing evaluation teams with representation from community groups, program clients and experts is more readily understood. Lending and international agencies could provide valuable assistance to governments and ministries of public health in experimenting with mixed evaluation teams.

Administrative evaluation in Latin America is handicapped by the limited knowledge about bureaucratic behavior and the scarcity of reliable information about Latin American political systems. It is our suggestion that administrative evaluation should start by de- veloping indicators to evaluate policy viability and the uses of discretionary power of the bureaucracy. In this way, evaluation and administrative controls can be served by the same activities.

REFERENCES

1.   Kraemer, K. L., J. D. Danziger, W. H. Dutton, *et al*. A future cities survey research design for policy analysis. *Socio- Economic Planning Sciences*. 10:199-211, 1976.
2.   Warwick, D. *A Theory of Public Bureaucracy, Politics, Person- ality and Organization in the State Department*. Cambridge: Harvard University Press, 1975.
3.   Suchman, E.A. *Evaluation Research: Principles and Practice in Public Service and Social Action Program*. New York: Rus- sel Sage Foundation, 1967.
4.   Van Maanen, J. *The Process of Program Evaluation*. Washington: National Training and Development Service Press, 1973.
5.   Caro, F.G. (ed.) *Readings in Evaluation Research*. New York: Russell Sage Foundation, 1971.

6.   Bernstein, I.N., and H. E. Freeman. *Academic and Entrepreneur-
      ial Research: The Consequences of Diversity in Federal
      Evaluation Studies*. New York: Russel Sage Foundation,
      1975.
7.   Alford, R.R. *Health Care Politics. Ideologies and Interest
      Group Barriers to Reform*. Chicago: University of Chicago
      Press, 1975.
8.   Bissonette, R., and J. Zusman. The case against evaluation.
      Int. J. Mental Health. 2:111-125, 1973.
9.   Sjoberg, G. and R. Nett. *A Methodology for Social Research*.
      New York: Harper and Row, 1968.
10.   Olson, S.R. *Ideas and Data. The Process and Practice of So-
      cial Research*. Homewood, Ill.: Dorsey Press, 1976.
11.   Myrdal, G. *The Asian Drama. An Inquiry into the Poverty of
      Nations*. Abridged edition. New York: Random House, 1972.
12.   Glaser, W.A. *Social Settings and Medical Organization. A
      Cross-National Study of the Hospital*. New York: Atherton
      Press, 1970.
13.   Hamilton, D. *The Consumer in Our Economy*. Boston: Houghton
      Mifflin, p. 64, 1962.
14.   Lampton, D.M. *The Politics of Public Health in China: 1949-
      1969*. Unpublished Ph.D. Dissertation, Stanford University,
      1973.
15.   Theodorson, G.A. and A.G. Theodorson. *Modern Dictionary of
      Sociology*, New York: Thomas Y. Crowell Co., 1970.
16.   Mayntz, R. and R.W. Scharpf. *Policy-Making in the German Fed-
      eral Bureaucracy*. Amsterdam: Elsevier, 1975.
17.   Alford, R.R. Political participation and public policy. pp.
      429-479. In: *Annual Review of Sociology*. Palo Alto:
      Annual Reviews Inc., 1975.
18.   Glazer, M. *The Research Adventure: Promise and Problems of
      Field Work*. New York: Knopf, 1972.
19.   Littrell, W.B. and G. Sjoberg (eds.) *Current Issues in Social
      Policy*. Beverly Hills: Sage Publications Inc., 1976.
20.   Gabaldon, A. *Una Política Sanitaria*. 2 vol. Caracas: Mi-
      nisterio de Sanidad y Asistencia Social, 1965.
21.   Waterston, A. *Development Planning: Lessons of Experience*.
      Baltimore: Johns Hopkins University Press, p. 3, 1965.
22.   Krause, E.A. *Power and Illness. The Political Sociology of
      Health and Medical Care*. New York: Elsevier, 1977.
23.   Ugalde, A. Los procesos de toma de decisiones en el sector
      sanitario y sus implicaciones políticas. *Rev. Sociolo-
      gía*. 5;101-124, 1976.
24.   Downs, A. *Inside Bureaucracy*. Boston: Little, Brown, 1967.
25.   Allison, G.T. *The Essence of Decision: Explaining the Cuban
      Missile Crisis*. Boston: Little, Brown & Co., 1971.
26.   Grindle, M.S. *Bureaucrats, Politicians and Peasants in Mexico*.
      Berkeley: University of California Press, 1977.

27. Ross, S. Third world commodity power is a costly illusion. *Fortune* (November): 147-162, 1976.
28. Wilkie, J.W. *The Mexican Revolution: Federal Expenditure and Social Change Since 1910*. Berkeley: University of California Press, 1967.
29. Wilkie, J.W. *The Bolivian and U.S. Aid since 1952*. Latin American Center, University of California at Los Angeles, 1969.
30. Zschock, D.K., and R.L. Robertson. Health sector financing in Latin America: Conceptual framework and case studies. Unpublished report prepared for the Office of International Health, U.S.D.H.E.W., Washington, D.C., 1976.
31. Hinrichs, H.H. Tax reform constrained by fiscal harmonization within common markets: growth without development in Guatemala. D.T. Geithman (ed.). Chapter 4. In: *Fiscal Policy for Industrialization and Development in Latin America*. Gainsville: University of Florida Press, 1974.
32. Bird, R.M. Agricultural taxation in developing countries: theory and Latin American practice. Chapter 5. In: D.T. Geithman (ed.). *Fiscal Policy for Industrialization and Development in Latin America*. Gainsville: University of Florida Press, 1974.
33. Musgrave, R.A. Expenditure policy for development. Chapter 6. In: D. T. Geithman (ed.). *Fiscal Policy for Industrialization and Development in Latin America*. Gainsville: University of Florida Press, 1974.
34. Wilkie, J.W. Recentralization: the budgetary dilemma in the economic development of Mexico, Bolivia, and Costa Rica. Chapter 7. In: D.T. Geithman (ed.). *Fiscal Policy for Industrialization and Development in Latin America*. Gainsville: University of Florida Press, 1974.
35. Caiden, N., and A. Wildavsky. *Planning and Budgeting in Poor Countries*. New York: John Wiley, 1974.
36. Organización Panamericana de la Salud. *Políticas Nacionales de Alimentación y Nutrición. Discusiones Técnicas de la XXIII Reunión del Consejo Directivo de la OPS*. Publicación Científica No. 328. Washington, D.C.: OPS, 1976.
37. Ness, G. *Bureaucracy and Rural Development in Malaysia*. Berkeley: University of California Press, 1967.
38. Ministerio de Salud Pública de la República de Colombia. *Gasto Institucional en Salud 1973*. Bogotá: Imprenta del Instituto Nacional de Salud, 1975.

COMMENTS

Dr. Adolfo Chávez, *National Institute of Nutrition, Mexico 22, D.F., Mexico*

The purpose of these comments is to evaluate some of the characteristics of the socio-political structure of underdeveloped
countries which are closely related to the course they follow and,
consequently, to the achieved results of the basic nutrition and
health programs. This is important so as to better implement the
programs and interpret correctly the real needs which they will
help solve. Not to do this would be like trying to find out why an
automobile does not perform at top capacity by studying only the
automobile without taking into account road conditions, existing
obstacles, and the route it will take.

It is well known that in underdeveloped countries it is unusual for fundamental nutrition and health programs to deeply affect the communities and really modify the living conditions of the
majority of the population. Frequently, these so-called health programs are stereotyped copies of those of developed nations and have
no impact on social welfare even though they utilize a large amount
of material and human resources.

Often, the causes of program weakness are not the programs themselves, but the socio-political atmosphere which surrounds them.
The meaning of underdevelopment is not just poverty and ignorance,
as many would believe. Basically underdevelopment means lack of
capacity and resources for the organization and resolution of community problems, social injustice, human exploitation, and many
other things which are rarely mentioned but which are very obvious
in the majority of the underdeveloped countries.

To interpret the reasons for the very little political interest
placed on these important problems, which not only affect the welfare of the majorities but whose presence thwarts all possibilities
of achieving a real socio-economic development, it must be kept in
mind that the essence of underdevelopment itself probably resides
in a social structure based on important class or social differences. This orientation is recognized in few underdeveloped countries
such as India, where castes and the different rights among them are
officially and legally recognized, but not so in other countries
where the problem is thought not to exist simply because it is not
articulated nor legitimized. Traditionally, the same rights claimed
by the upper social classes are not recognized for the lower ones;
thus, they do not have the same political weight (influence), a
most important factor in effecting change. Unfortunately, the populations in remote areas do not complain of their children's whooping cough, simply because they are used to its presence and do not
know that it can be prevented with a vaccine which costs only a few
pennies, while in some countries the high-income sector could really pressure the Government to improve an inefficient garbage collection service. This explains why many millions are spent on sumptu-

ary (incidental) expenses in underdeveloped countries while there
is a constant lack of funds for basic feeding programs for the rural
population.

There is nothing more important than food and health for a person's well-being; without them everything else loses significance.
When food and health cannot be enjoyed, neither can life be enjoyed
and it becomes, instead, a struggle to survive. We all know of the
relation between poor nutrition and illness and the relation of both
to the poor physical, mental and social development of the individual.

In most underdeveloped societies it is surprising how little
importance is placed on the nutrition and health conditions of the
majority population. What is done will habitually take a form directly proportional to the permitted social inequality and inversely proportional to need; paradoxically, this means that less is done
for those who need it the most. As a consequence this tends to maintain individual and collective incapacity which, in essence, perpet-
uates socio-economic underdevelopment, thus closing a vicious circle
which the underdeveloped countries cannot break.

It can be said that the isolation suffered by some sectors of
the population in regard to nutrition and health services can only
be explained as the remains of colonial and pro-slavery structures
which, although they are not part of actual political systems, are
rooted in behavior patterns not only of those who govern but also
those who are governed. Similar thought patterns underlie the working philosophy of the majority of institutions in charge of solving
these problems.

The real bottleneck in nutrition and primary health care programs in poor countries lies in the lack of firm decision-making
on the part of leaders and authorities concerning the resolution
of these problems. That is, what is really lacking is the establishment of priorities, endorsed jointly by authorities and societies,
to allot sufficient funds and political support to actions required
to solve nutrition and health problems.

I have always insisted that there is no country that is too
poor to feed its people, nor so ignorant that does not know it;
what really happens is that society does not put forth enough effort.
By really trying, it would not be difficult to eradicate malnutrition as well as a series of infectious diseases for which the control is known. One example among others which demonstrates this
is China. After World War II it was the poorest and most complex
country in the world.and yet, even at the height of an economic
crisis, it could in a few years solve the serious nutrition and
health problems of its great rural population.

What is needed in underdeveloped countries is to give nutrition all the attention it needs, applying all the necessary economic and social resources to solving the problem. Underdevelopment is the cause of undernutrition -- not as it deals with poverty, as most believe, but as it deals with a social structure which condones marginal settlements, allows its population to maintain a very low level of education and economic resources, and ultimately keeps them susceptible to malnutrition and poor health.

Another important obstacle in the realization of effective programs lies in the strength of their execution. When some nutrition programs for the marginal populations finally are instituted, it is common that they are incompletely implemented and lack impact, allowing them to exist more at an abstract level in their organization and structure where their performance in the field fails to really help solve the problems. The failure is attributed to bureaucracy, a word defining the attitude taken by officials, but which does not actually explain the real reasons for the lack of dedication and effort. Definitely the problem is more complex than simple interventions, although basically failure is just one more proof of the lack of interest, reaching open discrimination of the most needy sectors of the populations.

It is also quite common that programs be planned which are disproportionate in their assignment of personnel and services. That is, there is an excess of technicians and administrators having a very limited radius of action and intensely covering a small population area as if what has to be done were not known. This perhaps is the principal cause of their poor impact on the population.

This type of program has two apparent roots. One is the imitation of programs originated in developed countries, where there is always a lot of investigation and an administration which must be justified by the magnitude of its functions. The other is the interest on the part of the executing sector in bettering their economic and social condition by justifying larger budgets, ultimately coming from taxation. It is not unusual that in underdeveloped countries more than 50% of the program's budget be allotted for administrative or technical expenses at a central level. What happens in this case is that a program is planned; an excessive number of technicians are hired; fancy offices are installed; vehicles are bought; secretaries, chauffeurs, etc. are hired; and later, as it frequently happens in underdeveloped countries, not all of the promised funds arrive, thus making it necessary to cut expenses. In this case the easiest and most expedient way is to do it at field level by reducing or eliminating specific actions.

I have always insisted that nutrition and basic health programs in underdeveloped countries are very different when described at a

central level than when evaluated from the receiving population's
point of view. At the central level there is always reference to
impressive figures -- millions of vaccines, thousands of services,
tons of food, etc. But when these same programs are evaluated from
the beneficiaries' point of view, considering the size of the population and how spread out it is (to which should be added possible
corruption), it is easy to see how few vaccines are provided compared to those really needed, how weak the services actually are,
and how small the amount of food is that finally reaches those who
need it.

In underdeveloped countries it is also important to comment
that the distinction between technicians and politicians is not as
clear as in developed countries. It is not unusual for politicians
to make technical decisions without consulting with the specialists,
believing themselves capable of doing it. Also, the so-called technicians really may be poorly trained and, therefore, unable to make
appropriate decisions.

Results of evaluations in underdeveloped countries are frequently used more for establishing socio-political pressure to obtain
greater support for new programs than to improve the quality of the
present techniques. In fact, in developing countries the results
of evaluations are not always used to modify a program since generally a program, once started, is hardly ever changed due to vested
interests.

It is unjust to blame only the politicians for the programmatic
deficiencies, a situation which at present is less true in many of
the Latin American countries. Many politicians, convinced of the
necessity for action, are changing their ways even though it may
sometimes be for their own benefit and under their own terms. Frequently it is us, the technicians, who are behind, proposing reduced
programs with little capacity to solve the problems. We keep proposing and backing what can be called experimental programs instead
of applied programs, which shows that technicians are more interested in attractive rather than useful work. This is the reason why
complicated evaluation schemes are disproportionate regarding programmatic actions.

I believe that at present it would be absurd to design projects
having extensive and expensive experimental components instead of
truly effective applied programs. There is enough existing information on various activities. For instance, it is already known that
the whooping cough vaccine is effective and we also know how to apply it. Consequently, there is no reason for designing weak regional programs providing for few vaccinations and lots of experts. The
majority of such activities may be left at present in the hands of
auxiliary or intermediate personnel.

To understand the execution of a program we must plan a comprehensive and integral study of the situation and the intervention that
is planned. From the beginning it is important to distinguish between those programs which are real and those which look like programs but that are barely a structure, without real impact, since it
would be absurd to invest heavily in the latter type of program.

Furthermore, experimental programs are costly and should only
be carried out by very specialized personnel for teaching purposes
but, above all, to look for better ways for solving techniques directed especially to those problems for which there is no present
answer.

Thus, when the evaluation of programs is discussed in this socio-political ambience so common in developing countries, care must
be taken in selecting evaluative criteria, in the application of
techniques, and in determining how indicators are to be used. In
general, evaluations must examine the program itself, its action
process, its impact and effect, taking into account the socio-political situation in which it will be developed.

In general there is no specific evaluating technique or methodology to be used by developing nations, although undoubtedly emphasis must be placed on certain aspects according to unique conditions
found in specific situations. As a first step, simple technologies
must be found that lead to more easily managed data. In developing
countries it is difficult to control large samples of a whole universe. Therefore, it frequently is better to select evaluation areas or to stratify according to the different social groups or different action levels of the program. External evaluations are also
convenient since the lack of scientific background on the part of
most of the program personnel influences many phases of the results
that would be obtained. Within the evaluation of administrative
processes it is important to pay special attention to studies related to the real impact of the action on the target populations.

The purpose of the above comments has not been to discourage
evaluations but rather to recognize the obstacles to be cleared
so that these programs will have greater impact and ultimately
change the existing situation. I have tried to mention the few
possibilities which underdeveloped countries have for implementing
really effective nutrition and basic health programs. By acting
only according to technical and scientific norms, without awareness of these limitations, little is truly gained -- just as little
has to date been achieved in most of the programs being carried out
in the majority of the underdeveloped countries. But better results
can be obtained. In many places in the world results of really

effective and efficient programs are becoming known as a result of honest and realistic attitudes directed toward decreasing hunger and disease. To promote this type of program, and to do it better and obtain effective results, we as technicians have to recognize and work with the socio-political factors involving each one of our activities.

SOME SUGGESTIONS FOR IMPROVING THE APPLICABILITY AND UTILIZATION OF EVALUATION ASSESSMENTS

Jerome S. Stromberg
World Health Organization
Geneva, Switzerland

INTRODUCTION

Evaluation studies have frequently been conducted in a technically competent manner, written up in an understandable way, and distributed to the relevant decision-makers, only to have the results literally collect dust on the shelves. Other chapters in this volume have focused attention on various technical aspects of impact evaluation. I will raise some basic questions at this point about why the results of evaluation studies are not more broadly used in action programs, and to briefly propose some approaches for improving and broadening the utilization of evaluation results.

In speaking of "evaluation studies", I have not limited my comments to the assessment of impact, *per se*, although some observations are specifically relevant to that particular type of evaluation study. Rather, I have tried to look at the broader range of evaluation research activities which especially include attempts to assess the effects -- not necessarily measured in terms of impact-- of an action program on a particular problem or set of problems.

Let me not mask my major argument in subtlety or indirection. There *is* a very general problem of well-executed evaluation studies whose *potential* for broader applicability or utilization by implementation is not realized. I believe the *central* problem is one of relevance or salience of the evaluation itself to the potential users. While there are many measures which may be used to increase awareness and interest in any particular evaluation result, the major improvement in utilization will come in assuring -- before the evaluation is actually carried out -- that the questions *are*, in fact, of practical interest to the potential users.

Having stated my major thesis, I should like to review a few examples of use and non-use of evaluation studies in an attempt to identify some of the more common problems in this area. Next, I shall try to describe a type of evaluation strategy which might as- sure a higher level of utilization of the results of evaluation studies, especially in the area of health and nutrition. Lastly, I should like to suggest a number of mechanisms which might be used to more broadly disseminate evaluation results and increase their utilization by potential implementors. Illustrations will be drawn from a variety of country situations, and are not specially weighted towards Latin American countries. There is, however, an emphasis on rural situations in developing countries.

ILLUSTRATIONS OF USE AND NON-USE OF EVALUATION RESULTS

Evaluation results are all too frequently ignored or not ap- plied by those potential utilizers who might have adapted the re- sults. Moreover, such findings are frequently not even acted upon by those for whom the evaluation study was ostensibly carried out. This is by no means limited to any particular subject or geograph- ical area, but the following examples briefly illustrate some of the more common reasons for both use and, especially, non-use of evaluation results. They are drawn primarily from the health area, and are representative of various types of action programs, that is, organized efforts to effectively apply appropriate knowledge to a particular problem or set of problems.

Changes in Program Priorities and Objectives

There are often shifts or changes which occur during the life- time of an evaluation study which alter the applicability of the eventual results. In one case in South East Asia, careful studies were made of local traditions, health care practices, and means of mobilizing resources to meet common problems, so that proposals could be made for a new form of primary health care largely depen- dent on local priorities, initiative, resources and administrative control. Before pilot studies which were to test these proposals could be carried out, political changes occurred in the country which radically altered both national policies as well as opportu- nities (or maybe even the need) to test the original proposals.

In a less dramatic case in Africa, an action research program to test the relative effectiveness of various forms of delivery of family planning services had one of its major scientific goals al- tered when other external findings strongly suggested that the re- search question no longer had the importance it once had, i.e., it had already become sufficiently clear that family planning services should be delivered as an integral part of maternal and child health services.

In the above cases, the evaluation studies cannot hope to have the audience once anticipated for the results, largely because the original question is no longer as relevant as it may have been. While some of these shifts may be unexpected and unpredicted, they certainly are not rare, and experience suggests that great care is needed in determining the appropriateness to the potential users of the questions being addressed in the evaluation.

Evaluation Priorities Determined Externally

Sometimes, and for a variety of reasons, local collaborators will participate in international or comparative studies which have a high degree of technical, methodological, or even financial appeal. Results of such studies may vary greatly in their applicability if for no other reason than that standardization almost certainly leads to a reduction in the specifically applicable nature of the questions and the results. Participation in such studies has sometimes led to disinterest, rather than an open and accepting stance towards the results, because the study is identified with "foreign interests". Clearly, the justification for such studies must lie in the generation of meaningful and applicable cross-national or cross-situational comparisons and similarities, and not merely in the suggested methodological accomplishments which such studies might entail.

Potential for Direct Application of Results

Another example can be given in which the particular relevance of a problem led to immediate application of evaluation findings in a West African country. As a part of a nutrition rehabilitation program, a "food and health house" was established which featured a three-to-four-week residential rehabilitation and training program for malnourished children and their mothers. Many of the well-known components were present, but special emphasis was given to training of the mothers so that they could become "village nutrition agents" and demonstrate nutritional practices to other village women on return to their own villages.

While the nutritional rehabilitation program was quite successful, evaluation studies revealed that the mothers of malnourished children were *not* effective teachers or nutrition agents when they returned to their villages. Perhaps they suffered some loss of respect because of the malnourishment experience, or perhaps their disadvantaged educational background or economic situation or other factors were common to both the malnourishment experience and their lack of effectiveness as change agents. Whatever the reason, these women did not receive sufficient respect to enable them to serve effectively as nutrition agents.

Another action program in the same country, anticipating its own local nutrition education program, very readily accepted the evaluation results of the above program, and, as a result, took quite a different approach in identifying potential local nutrition workers. In the latter case, government nutrition workers and community development staff went to the villages and worked with women there who were selected by the villagers themselves as meeting local standards of respect, leadership, and practical knowledge and thus were more suitable to be local nutrition agents.

The above examples illustrate a simple but essential principle relevant to the utilization of evaluation results; that is, those evaluation results are more likely to be applied which are directly applicable to the needs of problems of potential users.

Relationship of Evaluation Activities to Action Program

Another factor influencing the use of evaluation results is the structural relationship of evaluation activities to action programs. At a recent workshop on evaluation and monitoring of rural development and other programs, evaluation of rural development activities in one or two projects in East Africa, were described as isolated or at least overly separated from the implementation program activities. In order to assure proper objectivity and control of the evaluation activities, a separate unit had been established which was related to, but operationally quite separate from the implementation staff. The evaluation personnel found it overly difficult to communicate results, to have the continuous feedback arrangement that had been anticipated, and even felt cut off from information about and relationships with the implementation activities Obviously, the acceptance and application of evaluation findings in such a situation are severely hampered.

While this description may be extreme or unrepresentative of many evaluation experiences, it typifies an important issue. Evaluation is sometimes thought of as a necessarily *objective* activity which should remain neutral and essentially separate from the activity which is being studied. But both empirical results and good sense show that this is not really attainable. In the first place, the fact that something is important enough to warrant study is

already an introduction of values. Moreover, measurement *is* a form
of intervention and has quite important effects on what is being
measured (1-3). Therefore, it is important to understand and make
explicit the nature of one's non-objectivity or bias, to recognize
the effects of measurement or evaluation, and to attempt to determine just how it is affecting the activity being evaluated, and
even to use this influence to make both the implementation and evaluation more effective (4). Therefore, the practice of having separate evaluation structures and personnel seems not only difficult
methodologically, but also may prejudice the potential utilization
of the results thus generated.

Other Factors

Certainly many other factors influence the acceptance and utilization of evaluation results. Results may not reach the appropriate
person(s) in a timely manner; the implication may not be sufficiently
clear to allow proper application of the results; conflicting results
may not be reconciled and so neither are used; or the results may not
be compatible with current beliefs or commitments, so that contrary
or non-conventional findings may meet inordinate resistance (5).

All of these factors can and do influence the use of evaluation findings, but I have emphasized problems which relate to the
appropriateness of the questions being asked and the structure or
relationships of the evaluation activities to action programs, since
it is in these areas that I believe the most useful improvements can
be made.

Evaluation for Whom?

Many of the problems of utilization of evaluation results parallel the problems of utilization of health services. It is common
in both cases to point to the need for more education of the potential clients to show them how to use the (supposedly) adequate services or information properly. Jaffe and Polgar demonstrated the
error of such conclusions when applied to the utilization of family
planning services (6). They saw the critical need to revise the
services to meet the identifiable needs of the potential clients,
rather than blaming the non-users for their inability to comprehend
or avail themselves of the services. The Executive Board of the
World Health Organization (WHO) more recently applied the same kind
of criticism to conventional explanations for low utilization of
general health services (7). Too often they are designed for the
providers and not the utilizers; the services do not fit the life
styles and requirements of those in need, but rather of those who

are the supposed providers. In a sense, these health services do
not belong to the population, but rather to the health professionals.

At the risk of carrying the analogy a bit too far, I have suggested the appropriateness of the above kind of criticism because I
think there *are* problems of a similar nature when we take a hard
look at evaluation strategies. For the most part, evaluation strategies have been devised and designed to serve the needs of program
directors, funding agencies, and others whose questions often concern the relative merit and worthwhileness of several or even a
great number of projects or programs. Major changes in styles of
evaluation strategies are quite common, and these changes, in turn,
have their effects as they are introduced throughtout whole systems
of program activities. These changes usually are introduced at the
"top" of the system, and then are more or less imposed on the other
levels of the system as varying types of targets, indicators, time
frames, and reporting schemes are called for. In fact, the World
Bank and USAID have recognized the tremendous reverberations which
result when new evaluation schemes are introduced within the life
span of existing, planned projects. This is a reflection of the
basic reason many evaluation results are not used in action programs;
they are not used in these programs because the evaluation questions
asked are really for other purposes. No measure of education or
training of potential utilizers can overcome this fundamental problem.

COMMON PROBLEMS IN UTILIZING. EVALUATION RESULTS

Discrepancies in Evaluation Requirements

One of the enduring problems is the frequent discrepancy between, on the one hand, the needs or requirements of funding or
other agencies in a position to make certain demands of the structure or content of evaluation and, on the other hand, the needs and
interests of those responsible for the action program itself. Sometimes actual targets and timetables are set by outside agencies.
Even if they are not imposed, then the *necessity* of having targets
and timetables will almost certainly be required.

I recall, for example, an African government director saying
with respect to outside assistance, that his government's problem
was not really in knowing *what* to do, but in having the resources
to do it, while the assistance received was largely in terms of
planning and management. Recently, an evaluator in a country project complained of "over-consultation" by parent agency officials
from the bureau's main office. Those of us from "headquarters" can
not avoid the many references to the different way we view field

staff colleagues. Since, no doubt, there is much truth in these observations, it is not difficult to visualize the discrepancies which often arise between the goals and priorities of evaluators responding to external directions and the goals of action program implementors.

Appropriateness of Evaluation Methods and Data

Sophistication of evaluation techniques is another potential barrier between evaluation and action elements of a program. Whatever the methodological justification may be, implementors are often dissatisfied by their inability to get data that are easy to comprehend and that are available in sufficient time to be acted upon. I was recently impressed by the simplicity of data collected in some nutrition rehabilitation programs which had no "external" evaluation components, (e.g. number of admissions of mothers and children, length of stay, total number of acres planted and harvested by women while resident and in the following growing season, etc.). At the same time, other programs which included external evaluation activities were having difficulty obtaining the results because, for example, one investigator was "still writing up the results" and, in another case, there were problems of cleaning the data file adequately to enable computer analyses. Often these less sophisticated methods serve evaluation purposes as well, or even better, than more sophisticated techniques. Parallel with the need for "appropriate health technology" is the need for appropriate and usable measurements and techniques for evaluation, a field which is now attracting the attention of the United Nations Research Institute for Social Development and others (8).

STRATEGIES FOR ASSURING UTILIZATION OF EVALUATION RESULTS

Having said some critical things about the purpose of much evaluation that is done, let us look at how the conduct of evaluation might be more closely related to the needs and problems of potential utilizers. Here we can be guided by some of the more effective evaluation experiences and we can especially look at several of the more prominent models relating evaluation activities to potential users.

Davis and Salasin (9) describe a number of models of the research-development-dissemination-utilization process, of which three will be briefly discussed here. These may be called the "research, development, and difussion model", the "problem-solving model", and the "action research model".

The Research, Development and Diffusion Model

This model assumes that there is a relatively passive target
audience of consumers which will accept an innovation (evaluation
result), if it is delivered through a suitable medium, in the right
way, at the right time (9, p.628). Clearly, the "passive target
audience" characteristic of this model is not consistent with our
intent to have evaluation carried out so that it reflects the salient concerns and interests of the potential users. Nonetheless,
there are many evaluations which may be relevant to audiences which
have not participated in shaping the evaluation design, but which
may be interested in the results. This may be especially true of
more basic scientific research and less true of applied or action
programs where the application of knowledge within a specific local
social situation renders the results less generally applicable.

Where evaluations of this nature are of potential interest to
users, the process of communication in the diffusion process is of
considerable importance. A large and increasingly specialized number of journals and publications exist to communicate scientific
evaluation results. In addition, specialized and tailored means
of communicating evaluation results, especially for potential users
in action programs, have been developed. Numerous action programs
have developed newsletters or other means of providing rather continuous information on their program activities.

A practice-oriented summary of the large WHO International Collaborative Study of Medical Care Utilization is one example of a
communication especially designed to be more accessible to potential
consumers (10), and the practice of including "executive summaries"
or other ways of highlighting study findings are becoming more common.

Meetings to review program results constitute another method
of bringing together both personnel from a particular action program and those potentially interested in the evaluation results (11,
12). A recent study tour in Iran, brought together people actively
engaged in innovative health care projects in which they jointly
visited three of four projects and compared results and experiences,
the net effect in an educational sense being much more than individual visits or a group visit to only one project (13).

Registries of projects and bibliographies have become more common, with the United States Public Health Association "State of the
Art Study" and the WHO Register of Health Services Development Projects being just two examples (14, 15).

Contact (16), provides almost monthly descriptions of primary
health care activities, and Alternative Approaches to Meeting Basic

Health Needs in Developing Countries and *Health by the People* are
two examples of efforts by WHO and UNICEF to make information on
innovative health care programs more widely available (17, 18).

There is a growing literature on evaluation itself, and numerous publications focus on evaluation issues of special relevance to
health and development (8, 19-24).

The papers in this volume should serve to communicate additional information and viewpoints about evaluation in the health and
nutrition fields to potential utilizers beyond the particular group
assembled for the conference. But that greater potential audience
is not easily identifiable, and to be effective, the communication
process must be quite assertive.

The Problem-Solving Model

This latter problem is somewhat reduced in the problem-solving
model, which "starts with the user's needs as a beginning point for
research, with diagnosis as an essential first step in the search
for solutions. The outsider helper, or change agent, in this model,
is largely non-directive, mainly guiding the potential user through
his own problem-solving processes and encouraging him to utilize internal resources" (9, p.628). This resembles the conventional con-
sultant relationship to the user, and assures a high interest on
the part of the user in the results of the particular evaluation.
Generating interest in the results for a broader audience tends to
be difficult, since the results are rather specifically applicable
to the particular client's situation. The type of "problem-solving
model" described is of limited use for situations in which the potential user is unable to identify or formulate a specific problem
calling for external problem-solving assistance, which might frequently be the case with respect to health and nutrition problems
for many underserved populations.

While both of the above models are discussed briefly, they both
present problems of separation or lack of interaction between the
user or potential user and the research-development or evaluation
activities. In the one model, the target audience is more or less
passive and the researcher frames the questions; in the second case,
the user frames the questions (if he is able) while the researcher
or evaluator plays a more or less non-directive or passive role,
and the results are limited in broader applicability.

The Action Research Model

A third model mentioned by Davis and Salasin is the action-research model (9, pp.628-629). It is most distinctive in emphasizing

the development of research within the organization (client situation). As noted by these authors, the model assumes the action research to be a continuous process of research, action, evaluation, and more research. Action research, in the context of this presentation, refers to research on the application of appropriate scientific knowledge to particular problem situations, with the objective of studying and evaluating this application in order to modify, adapt or otherwise improve on the application of this knowledge. Examples could include determination of the most effective nutrition-related activities to be carried out by village health workers; or, given various alternatives for agricultural development in a rural area, which one(s) will result in the most beneficial availability of foods for local diets; or, which method(s) of education result in the most enduring form of dietary change among village women, etc.

Because of the continuous and vital relationship between the research and evaluative activity on the one hand and the user on the other, I would prefer to call this an "interactive action research model". This model, I believe, comes closest to the kind of evaluation strategy which both assures that program activities will be evaluated and that the evaluation questions asked are meaningful to and can be used by the potential consumer.

Action research has become not only acceptable, but the preferable style in many scientific circles. There is now a theoretical acceptance of action research which allows or even encourages an integration of scientific and activist tendencies. In fact, anyone who becomes involved in an action program has a responsibility to engage in evaluation, not simply to meet a donor or other agency's requirements, but as a fundamental aspect of program designs and the determination of the effect of program activities.

In the context of this particular presentation, the interactive action-research model is an especially effective way of addressing the problem of utilization of evaluation findings. It is, in fact, a form of research and evaluation which attempts to assure that the questions being asked are relevant to the actual or potential users by specifically shaping the evaluation around the user's needs in applied or action settings. To do so with an acceptable measure of success requires a continuous, and therefore interactive, strategy bringing the evaluation and action elements into a close relationship. Initial questions become modified by experience, and the evaluation strategy must be flexible enough to follow new directions in the action approach which may, in turn, be the response to previous evaluation results.

This is, of course, much easier said than done. It would probably be hard to find, today, an evaluation proposal which did not

describe an intention to relate to (monitor, evaluate in an on-going
manner, etc.) implementation activities or which did not have feedback loops in a systematic decision chart or project progress diagram. Thus, what is being said is not new, but it might be worthwhile to reflect on some of the practical problems of carrying out
these intentions.

A Practical Illustration: Ghana

Perhaps I could illustrate some of the practical problems more
concretely by referring to a program in Ghana with which I have some
familiarity (25). This is a primary health care program for which
the Government of Ghana has responsibility for all implementation
activities, with WHO participating in and financially supporting
the evaluation activities. The program emphasizes the community involvement component of primary health care and is broad in its approach to general rural development. WHO is participating in the
evaluation of this program in the sense that the Organization not
only wishes to assist in the development of primary health care programs, but specifically wants to study the process of implementing
such a program so that these lessons might be adapted to benefit
other countries. There is also the practical desire to limit financial input so that the implementation activities could be carried
out with the level of resources which could be replicated on a wider
basis.

Even though this program may not be familiar, the above situation is probably similar to one or more situations which are familiar, so that it is possible to identify with the action-evaluation
context. My comments are not on the program *per se*, or on what the
evaluation process has learned about the implementation activities,
but rather on what we have learned so far about the evaluation process itself.

In the early stage of the program, surveys were carried out as
a baseline against which to assess program development. Although
it proved difficult to obtain questions from some technical depart-
ments in order to include these questions in the survey, for the
most part there was an interest in developing the baseline survey.
Information was collected about expressed needs or priorities of
communities in the program area, and the rapid tabulation of these
results met with interest and provided a basis for formulation of
the Government's plans to assist the communities in various technical areas. There was occasional cause for disappointment on the
part of the evaluation staff when a survey result was regarded by
implementors as "something they already knew". However, this knowledge may have come to them through the process of the evaluation

team asking about and collecting the information, so that the information was generated by the evaluation team but not "credited" to their efforts.

The question of roles and responsibilities has been a rather persistent one. Not only has there been room for confusion and misunderstanding about technical and administrative areas or responsibility, but the evaluation-implementation distinction has been impossible and impractical to maintain. Evaluators have wanted to *act* when their responsibilities have been to observe and describe. Government personnel and the population sometimes expected to see WHO provide more direct financial and material support. Similarly, evaluators who know and understand what the program intends to implement have been seen as critical of implementation efforts when they describe activities as falling short of what they think could be accomplished. Oftentimes, evaluators and implementors are close enough to benefit from frequent interaction, which leads to greater sharing of goals but also highlights human differences.

Over the past two years there has been a shift in evaluation activities which has brought the evaluation component into closer harmony with the implementation goals. Proposals to evaluate at fixed times or according to a specific plan of work have been modified to place greater emphasis on *ad-hoc* evaluations (or monitoring) of specific field activities, such as training sessions of traditional birth attendants, logistical arrangements for providing assistance to community farms, conduct of seminars arranged by Government personnel for community development committee members, first aid training courses for primary school teachers in the area, etc. These evaluation reports are prepared quickly and provided to the implementation personnel so that specific activities can be modified, if necessary. In principle, the reports are to be discussed in regular joint meetings, but these have not always materialized.

Specific developments in the program have given rise to requests by the program director for more detailed evaluation of particular activities. For example, a village health worker (called a "community clinic attendant" or CCA) program has been developed and the first group of trainees has been working in their villages for almost one year. These CCAs are selected by their villages, trained by the Government for about four months at nearby health centers or health posts (during which time their communities provide financial support for food and housing), and then return to work in their villages. The villages (village development committees) are responsible for financial support and determine the fees to be paid by patients. The Government provides technical supervision and drugs. The project director wishes an evaluation of various technical areas of CCA's performance as well as an in-depth account of the experiences and problems encountered in this program to date. While such

an evaluation was anticipated in general terms, the specific request
and the elaboration of the areas to be evaluated go a long way towards assuring that the evaluation results will find a responsive
audience.

The above example is given to show that while problems are not
prevented by developing an interactive action-research strategy for
conducting evaluation, there are definite benefits in terms of the
salience of the evaluation questions for the users.

IMPLICATIONS FOR TRAINING

In this final section, I shall not attempt to give specific
proposals for training programs, but rather to suggest some general
guidelines for the way in which training for evaluation might be
shaped, based on the above suggestions for improving the utilization of evaluation assessments.

Having strongly endorsed an interactive action-research strategy for evaluation activities as a most meaningful way to attain a
high level of utilization of evaluation results, allow me to suggest
some areas in which the above research strategy may *not* be the most
appropriate. This suggestion especially applies to those cases of
basic scientific study in which it is necessary to obtain a certain
body of knowledge before applied research and action programs can
be launched. This does not mean that these scientific studies will
be free of bias or that evaluation will have no effect on the outcome of the study. However, in various types of studies it is important to determine, with a high degree of assurance, the impact
of a particular intervention on health status or other areas of interest. For example, suppose that in a certain area, vegetable
storage entails considerable spoilage with adverse effects on the
nutritional status of the population. If intensified solar drying
is introduced with the potential of reducing spoilage and consequently increasing the retention of nutritional value of the vegetables, it is important to carefully establish the relationships
between amount of drying required and the retention of nutritional
content of the vegetables. Or, suppose that a local herbal preparation is believed to be useful to reduce nausea. Such a potential
aid for oral rehydration could prove to be most valuable and careful study might be undertaken to determine if the herb did, in fact,
possess such useful properties.

In these cases of basic research, evaluation studies should be
conducted with careful attention to impact and the necessary accompanying measures and indicators. Training for this type of evaluation will probably entail training in the relevant technical areas
as well as training in evaluation methodology and statistics.

However, the implications for training for interactive action research evaluation are quite different. Here the nature of the dominant health and development problems suggests quite a different approach to evaluation, and, consequently, to training for evaluation. The major need facing those responsible for health programs today is not for more basic knowledge about diseases or about effective therapeutic interventions (as useful as this information will always be); rather, the primary need is for effective means to apply the knowledge we already have. The major evaluation studies, therefore, should not be on the part of the spectrum of questions which asks *if* a particular health action -- which is known to be effective in improving health status -- actually *does* have a positive effect on the health status of a given population group when applied as part of an action program. Rather, we should be evaluating the process of applying this health action to a population in order to improve our ability to make this health action accessible.

By way of amplification, and using the illustrations mentioned earlier, if solar-dried vegetables *do* retain sufficient nutritional content to provide a valuable foodstuff for a considerable period after normal harvest, then evaluation should focus on the process of implementing this solar-drying method. Such evaluation would be different than overall evaluation of the *impact* of such a preservation process on a population's health status, but the evaluation would focus, I believe, on the part of the problem which would be of greatest interest and hence the results would be more likely to be used. Similarly, once the relationship between the traditional herbal preparation and rehydration is established, evaluation should properly focus on elements of the process which contribute to use of the rehydration fluid, rather than on its health status impact.

I emphasize the point here because it seems to me that too often impact assessments are required as the only true test of the value of a particular action program. In addition to the practical requirement described above, the conceptual and methodological difficulties are rather substantial. For example, we argue considerably and convincingly about the multiplicity of factors which influence health, from specific disease agents through various physical environmental factors and general socio-economic development, not to mention hereditary factors. The problems, therefore, of identifying the contributions of a particular intervention to changes in, for example, the health status of a population group, become extremely complex, and have resulted in proposals for highly complex control methodologies. While some people no longer can justify the tremendous cost necessary to approximate these control conditions, others continue to develop even more sophisticated methods which often have little relevance to the problems towards which they were first directed.

I am convinced that evaluation of an *appropriate* level of sophistication should be an integral part of action programs, that
this evaluation should be planned for, and should be structured so
that the evaluation process continuously interacts with the action
program.

Thus, I would strongly urge that preparation and training for
evaluation be primarily directed towards the strengthening of abilities to function in an interactive, action-research setting. The
evaluation questions will vary, but a large proportion of them will
relate to the performance of people within various action programs,
and thus training in the social sciences should be encouraged. Implementors in health and nutrition programs should be given basic
skills in shaping and refining critical questions relevant to their
particular areas, and in giving direction to evaluation activities.
The development of specialized cadres of evaluators, if at all warranted, is secondary to developing the skills of implementors so
that they can shape appropriate evaluative questions, carry out
evaluation, and apply the evaluation assessments.

It is currently popular to mention the community's role in evaluation. While I am convinced of the importance of this perspective,
some have argued that it is unrealistic to assume that the community
can do much in the way of evaluation. I prefer not to be so pessimistic. As was said earlier, insistence that the evaluation questions are relevant to the potential user is the best way to ensure
that the results of the evaluation will be used. And having the
community identify its own problems and evaluate the progress of its
own action programs is a very basic example of the interactive action-
research model.

The methods should be very practical, of course, and might be
phrased as simply as: "What is our most serious problem?" "What
can we do about it?" and, later: "How serious is the problem now?"
"Is our project to improve the problem going well or not?" "What
could we do to make it go better?" There is a growing number of
practical examples of such approaches that have been worked out in
various country situations (26-28).

However positive these limited examples may be, usually the
specific evaluation tools or techniques have been developed with the
assistance of someone (from outside the community) with a knowledge
of evaluation methods and an ability to extract basic principles
and adapt quite simple tools so that they could be used in an unsophisticated way. There is a real need for people with the training
and perspective to accomplish this kind of task, and for the preparation of an "appropriate evaluation technology" in the health field.
This appears to be a most necessary and more specialized area of
evaluation training.

SUMMARY

In this presentation I have briefly described some of the common problems which affect the utilization of evaluation results.
It has been suggested that the appropriateness of evaluation to potential users is central to any attempt to improve the applicability of evaluation studies. Moreover, the planning of action programs to include a structurally-integrated evaluation component which continuously interacts with the implementation activities is a strategy which has been shown to be most useful in enhancing the applicability and utilization of evaluation assessments. Finally, some general guidelines have been proposed concerning training necessary and appropriate for those who will be involved with evaluation activities.

REFERENCES

1.   Gouldner, A.W. Explorations in applied social science. In:
        A. W. Gouldner, and S. M. Miller (eds.). *Applied Sociology: Opportunities and Problems*, pp. 5-22. New York:
        The Free Press, 1965.
2.   Hoethlisberger, F.J., and W.J. Dickson. *Management and the Worker*. Cambridge, Mass.: Harvard University Press,
        1939.
3.   Glasunov, I.S. *et al.* Repetitive Health Examinations as an Intervention Measure. *Bulletin WHO* __49__: 423-432, 1973.
4.   Yancey, W.L. Intervention as a strategy of social inquiry: an exploratory study with unemployed negro men. In: L.A.
        Zurcher, and C.M. Bonjean (eds.), *Planned Social Intervention: An Interdisciplinary Anthology*. pp.460-466.
        Scranton: Chandler Publishing Company, 1970.
5.   Velikovsky, I. *Worlds in Collision*. New York: Dell Publishing Company, 1965.
6.   Jaffe, F.S., and S. Polgar. Family Planning and Public Policy:
        Is the " Culture of Poverty " the New Cop - Out ?
        J. of Marriage and the Family. __30__: 228-235,
        1968.
7.   World Health Organization: Official Records of the World Health
        Organization, Number 206. *Organizational Study on Methods of Promoting the Development of Basic Health Service*.
        Geneva, 1973.
8.   Scott, W. *The Measurement of Real Progress at the Local Level*.
        Geneva: UNRISD, 1973.
9.   Davis, H.R., and S.E. Salasin. The utilization of evaluation.
        In: E.L. Struening, and M. Guttentag (eds.). *Handbook of Evaluation Research*. pp. 621-666. London: Sage Publications, 1975.

10. White, K.L. *et al.* *Health Services: Concepts and Information for National Planning and Management.* Geneva: WHO Public Health Papers No. 67., 1977.

11. *Proceedings of the Seventh Annual Review Meeting. Danfa Comprehensive Rural Health and Family Planning Project, Ghana.* Accra, Ghana: University of Ghana Medical School, 1976.

12. *Programa para la Investigacion y Desarrollo de Sistemas de Salud (PRIDES).* Cali, Colombia, April 1976.

13. Andreano, R. *et al.* *Assignment Report: Evaluation of Primary Health Care Projects in Iran.* Alexandria, Egypt: World Health Organization, Regional Office for the Eastern Mediterranean. EM/RH/33. June, 1976.

14. Karlin, B. *The State of the Art of Delivering Low Cost Health Services in Less Developed Countries: A Summary Study of 180 Health Projects.* Washington, D.C.: American Public Health Association, 1977.

15. Register of Health Services Development Projects. Compiled to date by the Division of Strengthening of Health Services. Geneva: WHO, 1975.

16. *Contact.* Geneva, Switzerland: Christian Medical Commission. World Council of Churches.

17. Djukanovic, V., and E.P. Mach (eds.). *Alternative Approaches to Meeting Basic Health Needs in Developing Countries: A Joint UNICEF/WHO Study.* Geneva: World Health Organization, 1975.

18. Newell, K.W. (ed.). *Health by the People.* Geneva: World Health Organization, 1975.

19. United States Agency for International Development, *Project Evaluation Guidelines.* 3rd. Edition. Washington, 1974.

20. Deboeck, G.J. *Case Studies of Monitoring and Ongoing Evaluation Systems for Rural Development Projects.* Washington: World Bank, 1976.

21. World Health Organization. *Evaluation of Family Planning in Health Services.* Technical Report Series No. 569. Geneva: 1975.

22. Anderson, D., *Issues in the Monitoring and Evaluation of Rural Development Projects: A Progress Report.* Washington: World Bank, 1976.

23. Suchman, E., *Evaluation Research.* New York: Russel Sage Foundation, 1967.

24. United Nations. *Monitoring and Evaluation Systems for Assessing Developmental Impact at the Local Level,* New York: ESA/SDHA/ Misc. 17., 1976.

25. Stromberg, J.S. Community involvement in solving local health problems in Ghana. *Inquiry,* 12, supplement:146-155, 1975.

26. Nugroho, G., A community development approach to raising health standards in Central Java, Indonesia. In: K.W.Newell (ed.).

Health by the People. pp. 91-111. Geneva: World
Health Organization, 1975.

27.   International Secretariat for Volunteer Services. *The Mobili-*
      zation of Response Structures from the Grassroots to-
      wards Health Services: Report of a Workshop, Manila,
      Philippines, July 8-11, 1974. Manila, Philippines:
      ISVS Asian Regional Office, 1974.

28.   World Health Organization. Regional Office for Africa.
      Primary Health Care: Report of the WHO Regional
      Expert Committee on Primary Health Care. pp. 52-67.
      AFRO Technical Report Series No. 3. Brazzaville, Congo,
      1977.

COMMENTS

R. Galán Morera, *Superintendente Ministerio de Salud,*
Bogotá, Colombia

INTRODUCTION

Before beginning my commentary, I want to congratulate the author on his excellent presentation of a topic of great interest
and importance for the countries of Latin America. His thoughtful
review of the factors that are now limiting the use of evaluation
studies, and the suggestions he offers throughout his paper, give
the participants food for thought about the present situation.
Perhaps because we are in the midst of it, we have failed to explore
some issues thoroughly enough to propose practical ways of improving the results of the evaluation studies done so far, and of
extending their coverage.

His paper opens with a review of some examples of the use and
non-use of evaluation studies in developing countries though they
are also of value to countries throughout the world. He then
proposes strategies that might assure an optimum level of utilization of those studies, and closes with the proposal for mechanisms
that could disseminate their findings more widely. In this contribution to the discussion, I will follow the same sequence.

EXPERIENCE REPORTED

In the light of the experiences reviewed, there can be no
doubt that the central problem lies in the structural relations
between evaluation work and programs of action. These two links
in the same chain have been separated, and the linkage or connection between the *evaluators* on the one hand and the *users*
(whether the latter are called politicians, technicians or

administrators) on the other hand, has been impeded by the kind
of work they each do and the different spheres of action in which
they move.

Everyone knows how decision-makers, intent on their own purposes, always want to be supplied with data and information so
fast that they drive the researcher to dispair at being unable to
deliver that information fast enough. The control machinery he
uses to ensure research quality and validity delay his purpose
and, in many cases, by the time the findings are known at last,
events have moved on and the "historical moment" is no longer of
any interest.

The experiences reported by Stromberg in Southeast Asia and
Africa furnish two good examples of changes in government policies
and situations occuring in the course of the evaluation study
which limit and deprive it of its initial interest. On the other
hand, it is also important that evaluation studies be responsive
to the needs and problems of their prospective users so that their
findings may be put to immediate use as in West Africa.

In my own country, Colombia, we have observed that fact-find-
ing studies often are not used because they were designed without
any regard for the requirements and needs of the decision-makers.
In an attempt to solve this problem, the following strategies have
been prescribed:

a.   that they (the decision-makers or users) be the ones to
      set the objectives in conjunction with the research
      group; and

b.   that, it is hoped, they will take part in the analysis
      of the results and, if this is not feasible, that they
      specify the desired frame of reference and general
      orientation of the analysis.

It is worth recalling here that the more active the participation in any effort, the stronger the commitment to and interest
in its implementation will be.

At this point, I would like to consider another aspect: that
of the limited cooperative participation by local groups in international studies. Because those studies are identified with
exclusively "external interests", national and international requirements are not properly reconciled. Clearly, the international interest -- being based on comparability -- sometimes requires more
general information than is wanted at the national level, or at
the regional area or district level in any one country, and thereby
much of its significance is lost. It may be advisable to allow

local groups to go into detail and extend the coverage of their
information so that they can carry out an in-depth analysis that
satisfies their own requirements while fulfilling international
requirements. This will strike an appropriate balance between
the two interests, which are not mutually exclusive but indeed
are complementary.

I have been struck by the other barrier that Stromberg
identified as yet another impediment to the use of evaluation,
namely the use of sophisticated evaluation techniques. I agree
that this is definitely a limiting factor, but I also believe that
(just now when overall evaluation is in fashion, in which structure
process, result, and impact are analyzed altogether) a proper
balance might be sought between simplicity and sophistication carried to the extreme. I expect this meeting to shed some light on
this matter and help to define the level of detail evaluation
studies should seek in the areas of nutrition and health.

Still there is one obvious question which we sometimes make
no effort to answer, namely "who are the users of a given evaluation study?". This question makes more sense when it is shifted
from specific programs, in which users are fairly easy to
identify, to actions in the aggregate, such as the design of an
evaluation model for the national health system. In such a setting, the number of users may be so great and the interests to be
satisfied so diverse that a quite complex research effort would be
needed to identify them.

PROPOSED STRATEGIES

The paper gives a clear, straightforward summary of three
models described by Davis and Salasin (1) and called respectively
"Research, Development and Dissemination", "Problem-Solution", and
"Research-Action".

I am inclined as is Stromberg, to rely on the last of these,
the "Research-Action" model, as a general guide to and basis for
strategy. My reasons for this preference are that the first model
is devoid of any dynamic or of any interactive relations between
the two basic elements examined (i.e., the evaluation process and
the prospective users). The second, though it endeavors to reduce
problems of this kind by starting from the needs of the users as
the diagnostic basis for the planning of sound solutions, sometimes falls short of its aim because the situations analyzed are
often so specific that no generalization can be drawn from them.
Furthermore, the user is not always able to come up with a good
answer to the question "what are your needs or requirements at a
given time?".

The "Research-Action" model tries to remove the difficulties
of the other two and, as Stromberg says, is based on a dynamic
process that focus on the predefined activities and aspects to be
evaluated and, thus, brings the evaluation much closer to the
requirements of the users. Furthermore, this model appears best
suited to our situation and needs when we consider that fact-find-
ing evaluation not only identifies critical points, but ties in
with the actual performance of integral health care services.
Thus acquiring a dynamic of its own, it provides the regular feedback which is needed for decision-making based on direct experience.

The performance of this model depends to a large degree on two
principal factors. The first is the establishment of educational
requirements and the training of all the staff involved in the
process in order not only to make communication easier within the
multidisciplinary team but to furnish standard and appropriate
analytical tools and techniques that will help make operations more
successful. Two types of training should be encouraged here: one
that could be offered at the undergraduate level and another as
refresher instruction just before the start of the evaluation study.

The second factor is the actual content of the evaluation.
Although here there is no consensus, it is clear that several components or variables must be considered. A conceptual epidemiological model is useful to define possible outcomes and indicators
needed. The components follow a sequential order related both to
the planning and implementation of the program, and to the evaluation process itself. These five components are:

Environmental Variables

This component expresses not only the characteristics and
magnitude of nutrition and health problems but also the environmental conditioning factors involved, since they are clearly multiply
determined. These variables reflect the existing demand to be
satisfied by program activities. This component is a basic point
of reference for the evaluation of the final effects (impact or
outcome) of the program on the individual and the community. It
includes, among others, the existing prevalence of nutritional
diseases and health problems related to them, (e.g., measles, whooping cough, diarrheal diseases, etc.) as well as demographic data
and socio-economic characteristics of the target groups.

Structure

The structure component includes all the resources and the

organizational structures made available by the program to the
target population (existing and new resources). Human, physical
and financial resources are all included here. Similarly, the
community resources for the program should not be forgotten. Within the organizational structure are included the levels of complexity which are closely related to the decision-making levels.
They include three kinds of interrelationships: intra-institutional,
intra-sectoral and inter-sectoral. The latter has a special relevance for the necessary inter-sectoral coordination of food and
nutrition programs.

Process

The third component specifically refers to the different types
of technical and administrative activities which comprise the
services provided by the program to the population. They are
implemented through different kinds of service units according to
the types of nutrition and health-related interventions involved.
The process components also include the level of community participation and the mechanisms of supervision. Knowledge of how closely
the process approximates that planned is essential to make corrective adjustments in the program. In the analysis of this component, both quality and costs of the corresponding activities should
be considered.

Results

This component indicates the output of the program in terms of
achieved coverage of different target groups. It includes also an
indication of *per capita* concentration of services as well as percent untilization of service units.

Impact or Final Effect

The last component refers to the final outcome of the program.
The analysis of this component will give a measure of the real effectiveness of the program. The final effect must be related to
the ultimate objectives of the program in terms of decreased morbidity and mortality due to malnutrition or nutrition-related diseases, real improvement of the diet (control of food intake gap)
and specific protection against some communicable diseases.

The evaluation of cost-effectiveness of the program as a whole
is also included within the total evaluation process. It is a
measure of the financial cost of achieving the favorable changes
obtained.

REQUIREMENTS FOR EVALUATION

Although some of them are obvious, a number of prerequisites for a sound evaluation process may be agreed upon:

a. A clear picture of the environmental factors (baseline situation) is essential as a basis for program planning and evaluation;

b. The objectives of change and respective measurable targets for impact must be clearly defined before the start of the program. This will allow the final evaluation of effects. In addition, a set of indicators and measures of those changes must be developed;

c. The operational targets (including process and results) also must be defined in relation to all technical and administrative aspects of the program. Concrete and objective indicators and measures must also be established for them;

d. An information system must be developed for continuing evaluation of the program. It should include simplified pre-coded forms, cards and periodic reports in order to facilitate collection and analysis of data;

e. Finally, it must be recognized from the beginning that the description of the findings is itself not the end of the process. The evaluation should include also an analysis and explanation of the findings as well as the prediction of future behavior. The evaluation process should then go further and consider both normative and methodological aspects. This is because the real objective of the evaluation is not knowledge *per se* of the outcome of the program but rather the creation of a sound basis for future reorientation of the program in order to maximize its effects and minimize its costs.

ROLE OF THE COMMUNITY

So far my comments have dealt essentially with two elements, namely, the "evaluators" and the "users". I have left until now another element which Stromberg mentions in his paper but which I want to emphasize once again: the active and organized part that the community must take in the final or evaluative stage of the planning process. This is the third link in the chain I referred to at the beginning, namely, the community itself as both the means and the end of all health measures.

There can, in my view, be no doubt of the capacity to evaluate
any program. However, giving the community a part to play improves
not only the evaluation process but also the results that program
staff expect from it. These benefits could be greater yet if
these strategies sprang from the thinking of the community itself.

I hope these remarks will help stimulate discussion on this
important topic and contribute to the emergence of a conceptual
and methodological basis that at the level of our countries can
help make better use of the information furnished by evaluation
studies.

REFERENCES

1.   Davis, H. R., and S. E. Salasin. The utilization of evalua-
        tion. In: E. L. Struening, and M. Guttentag (eds.).
        Handbook of Evaluation Research. pp. 621-666. London:
        Sage Publications, 1975.

PRACTICE AND PROBLEMS OF EVALUATION:

A CONFERENCE SYNTHESIS

Henry W. Riecken
University of Pennsylvania
Philadelphia, Pennsylvania

The task of the "relator" is to identify some of the major threads of the papers, the critiques and the oral discussion and to try to weave from them a more or less coherent summary of what this conference was all about. I have tried to prepare a mixture of summary and personal reaction to some of the issues that have arisen. This turned out to be a task that resembles what a friend of mine calls "suturing clouds", for the discussion in these four days has been extremely wide ranging. About a dozen points stand out, however, and will serve well enough as a framework for these concluding comments.

DIVERGENT APPROACHES TO EVALUATION

One general observation may serve to justify further some of my subsequent comments. I believe that everybody here would agree that there are enormous differences in viewpoints, in backgrounds, in experience and in purpose on the part of participants in this meeting. For example, we have come from different disciplines that have socialized us in different ways, so that physicians look at problems in a somewhat different fashion from economists, or from sociologists, political scientists, or planners. These differences in viewpoint cause us to have different concerns in the matter of evaluating social programs, and to emphasize different aspects of the problem. Political scientists think in terms of power and are quite sensitive to that dimension, while psychologists may treat political power as an annoying intrusion upon an experimental design. Disciplines differ in the way they handle data. In my experience economists generally prefer to work with data that has already been collected by someone else, whereas sociologists and

psychologists are suspicious of all archival data and would rather
go out and get their own. Anthropologists generally believe there
is no substitute for direct contact with a human informant, but de-
mographers hardly ever question people directly.

We all approach the problem of program evaluation from slightly
different perspectives. Furthermore, we have different points of
engagement with the social system and that leads to differences in
point of view between the academic or theoretical orientation and
that of the active planner, program manager, or policy maker in a
national agency. We have people here whose chief point of engagement, so to speak, is in applied social research, the conduct of
field studies and data analysis, others who are concerned primarily
with program planning, and still others whose orientation is to
national or agency policy.

Moreover, we have a variety of topics on our minds -- a large
number of different images in our heads -- as we talk about evaluation. Sometimes "program" evokes the image of vaccinating against
smallpox, sometimes that of distributing contraceptives or giving
dietary supplements, making cash payments to the poor based on
earned income, persuading peasants to change crops or cropping methods, or motivating mothers to use maternal and child health services. Such a variety of concrete images of the program to be evaluated must contribute to our sense of sometimes talking at cross
purposes or talking past one another.

We have also discussed a variety of purposes for evaluation:
evaluation for the development of national policy; evaluation for
making budgetary decisions at the agency level; evaluation for program development; evaluation for management of specific interventions. These different purposes surely influence how we express
our thoughts as we talk to each other.

The existence of these various differences leads me to conclude
that we badly need a common language for talking about program evaluation. It might have been difficult to construct a glossary of
terms like the one in this volume prior to the conference, but it
might have helped to narrow some of the communication gaps (1).
I do not mean simply a specialized Spanish-English dictionary,
although the bilingual aspect is important. My concern goes to the
matter of a commonly accepted terminology in either language. The
English speakers at the conference were not always in agreement
about the usage of some terms. Early on in the conference, for
example, the term "causal modeling" was introduced and became established as a descriptor for one type of evaluation. It is a term
that I am not accustomed to use. I think of "causal analysis" or
"path analysis" or perhaps "causal attribution", all of which are
more or less similar terms. I think about modeling as the making
of a representation of a situation or a process but not necessarily

incorporating causation. This is an example of the need for a
glossary of terms.

Among all the various differences, perhaps one has predominated,
and that is the tension between the academicians or theoreticians
on the one hand and the practitioners on the other. I happen to
think it is a useful tension. It has not been disruptive or acri-
monious at this conference. It has not been in the least unpleasant,
but each side has attempted to remind the other from time to time
of its own major concerns. If I may simplify, vastly oversimplify,
these concerns, it would be that the academicians want to get it
right and the practitioners want to get it written. Both sides
want it both ways, of course, but tend to choose differently between correctness and completion when they cannot have both. This
is an understandable difference, because practitioners have different needs from theoreticians, but these sometimes conflicting
purposes often must be compromised.

One more preliminary comment. I think there has been some
confusion in our thinking about complexity, cost, comprehensibility
and completion. Some comments have implied that complex is equivalent to costly, incomprehensible and never completed, whereas on the
other hand, simplicity is equivalent to cheap, easy to understand
and quickly done. I do not think that is true. There can be quite
complex designs that are, in fact, executed -- that is, they are
completed -- and their results communicated -- that is, made comprehensible. Whether they are costly or not depends on a large
number of factors, some having to do with size or scope, but not
necessarily related to the complexity of the evaluation. It is too
simplistic to say that complexity is hard to understand, takes a
long time, and costs a lot of money while simplicity is easy to
understand, done quickly and is cheaper. When an evaluation is
cheap and quick, it is often also not very good. My experience
with evaluation is that there are few bargains, and usually you
get no more than you pay for.

With those introductory remarks out of the way, let me proceed
to the first of my major points.

EVALUATION METHODS

Our discussions have identified three different modes of proceeding in an evaluation; three methods which may be characterized
briefly as experimental, statistical and expert judgment. The
statistical approach can use either specially collected data or
existing data, which may come from archival records, from agency
operating records, from censuses or from any source of regularly
collected information. The point I want to emphasize is that each

of these methods has certain advantages and certain disadvantages,
so that the choice of an appropriate method is not simple. It may
help to clarify that choice and to make it more rational if we look
a bit more deeply into what these various strategies of evaluation
imply.

     In doing so I want to concentrate on data generation or data
collection, not on data analysis. The latter involves very largely
technical statistical questions that generally can be settled best
by technicians.

     Before I go further with my comments on experimental and sta-
tistical approaches, I should say that I do not approach this question from a totally neutral standpoint. My name is on a book called
Social Experimentation and I have been a strong believer in the
experimental model for evaluation for a good many years, not to say
decades (2). I think you should know that bias and be aware that
I do not speak from a totally detached point of view.

     Robinson Hollister, in his paper, commented well and fully on
the limitations of the experimental approach, particularly in terms
of time, costs, and complexity (3). However, it seems to me that
the experimental paradigm generally has greater precision and higher
internal validity than the other methods. *Internal* validity refers
to the capacity to distinguish between the treatment variable --
that is, the intervention program -- and whatever happens to be
going on otherwise: exogenous variables, secular change, the flow
of events, etc. In other words, *internal* validity refers to the
ability of the analyst to separate the effective cause of the observed outcome from background "noise" of simultaneous but irrelevant events. In contrast, *external* validity refers to what has
here often been called "generalizability" -- that is, the extent
to which the evidence from a particular set of observations can be
said to hold for a larger range of people, communities, events, etc.
Experiments may have more limited generalizability, depending on
how the experimental group is chosen.

     Now, this assertion leads to a conclusion that ought to be in-
cluded in your calculations when you think about which evaluation
method to use. As a working rule, if you need high internal validity, if you need to know cause, then the experimental method is the
method of choice. If you need to rule out plausible rival hypotheses
or alternative explanations of impact, then it seems to me that you
are pretty well forced to an experimental approach. On the other
hand, if all you need to know is whether there has been an effect,
that is, for example, whether there is less third-degree malnutrition now than there was earlier -- then you do not need an experiment. There would be no sense in paying for one. Consider what
information is needed and make the decision about the type of evaluation on that basis.

There is at least one other condition in which an experiment is almost unavoidable. This is the condition of a wholly novel, completely new intervention -- something that is completely outside previous experience. In this condition, there are no archival data, there are no records from any agency, there is no evidence in existence that would help you to understand the probable effects of this novel intervention. Let me give an example drawn from recent United States experience. The United States now has several proposals for a national health insurance program. Although health insurance is widely written in the United States, none of the current plans have very high co-insurance provisions. Co-insurance refers to that part of the cost which must be paid by the insured person rather than by the insurer. Most health insurance plans in the U. S. have something like 20 percent co-insurance -- that is, the insurer pays 80 percent and the policyholder (patient) pays 20 percent of the cost of an episode of treatment. There is no experience with, say, 40 or 50 percent co-insurance or higher rates. In order to test the effect of high co-insurance rates on utilization of health services, it is necessary to establish a new situation. Call it an experiment, call it a trial program, whatever. It is necessary to create the situation in which the behavior to be observed *can* occur.

The limitations of the "statistical" method, either from specially collected data or from existing data, have also been commented upon during the conference, emphasizing "selectivity bias" -- that is, when there has been no random assignment, the participants may be selected on the basis of special motivation or some other characteristic that may seriously distort the response to the program. The question of non-availability of data (i.e., certain kinds of information that cannot be obtained from existing records) has been mentioned as a limitation of "statistical" studies, as well as the question of simultaneity -- that is to say, the co-existence of a behavioral variable interrelated to the independent variable. Finally, the whole question of exogenous variables troubles non-experimental designs, especially those which do not incorporate a control or comparison group.

On the other hand, the statistical approach to evaluation can have high external validity as long as the sample is representative of the population to which one wants to generalize. The statistical approach usually falls short in internal validity or causal attribution. It is very difficult to tease out from macroeconomical or macrosociological data the relationship between any particular limited intervention and the change in the social indicator of interest. It is much harder to make the desired causal inference. The necessary causal attribution and, hence, the method usually has lower internal validity.

Very little was said during the conference about the use of expert judgment. That method was referred to in only one session

and, I thought, almost in a sort of despairing way. The comment
was to the effect that since the more elaborate technologies had
been criticized so heavily, perhaps the safest recourse was to return to intuition and to expert judgment. I would personally resist that very strongly. Expert judgment *seems* simpler though it
is actually more complex. It suffers from more limitations than
almost any of the other methods, largely because expert judgment
is so difficult to replicate. It is very difficult to know what
the expert's process of analysis has been and, therefore, difficult
to know whether the analysis has been carried out correctly or not.
There is no assurance that a different expert would reach the same
judgment, and no way to tell who was more correct.

Thus, it seems to me that the precision of expert judgment is
poor, the internal validity is poor, and the generalizability is
questionable; it is indeed cheap, it is indeed quick, and I think
you get what you pay for.

Mushkin, during the discussion of her paper, introduced another
notion which had not really occurred to me as evaluation but I think
it is worth consideration. I would like to call it "situation
assessment". She pointed out that with some back-of-the-envelope
calculations based on a few numbers from education records and the
census, it was possible to calculate how much of children's nutritional needs were being met by a particular school lunch program.
She calculated that the school lunch program in the United States
met something like four percent of the estimated nutritional needs
of children. Hence, it seemed clear that the program could not
have much of an impact on nutritional status and that more elaborate data analyses might not be necessary. This would be a kind of
evaluation of a program in a rather special sense. It could be a
very useful technique for judging whether an intervention could
possibly have the kind of impact that it is intended to have --
that is, whether it is "in the ball park". It ordinarily would be
very quick and very cheap and it sometimes would tell you that the
intervention is so weak or small that it could not accomplish its
purpose -- that you have to go back to the drawing board and start
thinking the whole thing through again. On the other hand, situation assessment will not tell you much about change. Maybe four
percent is a vast improvement over what the situation was before
the school lunch program was introduced; and it does not tell you
very much about differential impact within families -- maybe that
four percent is concentrated in those who suffered from the greatest
nutritional deficiency and so it is a good program. Lots of other
questions would need to be asked along those lines, but still situation assessment is often a useful, quick technique for arriving at
a first approximation to impact, and it may direct attention to
important questions about an intervention.

Permit me one further general observation about method. In
practice, the choice among methods is not nearly so stark nor so
simple as it has been made out here. It is ordinarily necessary to
use both so-called "soft" methods and so-called "hard" methods if
you want to get a decent answer to an intelligent question. It is
always prudent to begin any evaluation as if you knew nothing whatsoever about the program or the situation in which it was being
conducted -- as if you were a man from Mars to whom everything
had to be explained. The reason for that prudence is that the
knowledge of specific real-life situations that exists at high levels in bureaucracy or in academia is often very slim. Sitting in
an office in Washington or Bogota (or in University City especially),
one can have all sorts of images of what life is like in the *barrios*
and they can all be wrong. They can be wrong in many dimensions so
that it is always prudent to go directly to the real-life local
situation and examine it as an experienced anthropologist, socio-
logist, social psychologist, or other social scientist would -- go
and look just to see what is there. When I was in the public opinion measuring business, we used to do preliminary studies before
designing the questionnaire. We called it "scouting" the situation.
That meant we would go to a village or to a part of a city, wherever
the survey was to be done, and spend a bit of time just talking to
people we would meet on the street, in bars, in restaurants, in the
public library, anywhere we could pick up a conversation. It did
not take a month or even a week but just a couple of days to find
out what was on people's minds and what was not -- what they would
and would not talk about readily, what they were unaware of, un-
concerned about, uninformed about. From that, it was possible to
construct a questionnaire. I propose that the first step in all
evaluations is "scouting" or direct observation of the program in
action, direct interaction with the participants.

The second step is developing a model of the process with which
the evaluation is concerned. Here we enter into some very danger-
ous semantic territory because the term "model" in the social
science literature is used with almost as much looseness and free-
dom as the term "parameter". I will use both terms in the subsequent discussion. I think it is only fair to warn you that what
I mean by parameter or by model is not necessarily what anybody
else means by these terms. Let me try to make clear my own meaning.
A statistician friend, Lincoln Moses, says that, in his experience,
the word "parameter" is so loosely used that it means "any fixed or
variable quantity to which I wish to refer". I will, therefore, use
"parameter" to mean a specific factor in a "model".

Now, "model" in the sense that I am using it is a simplified
version of reality. It is a stripped-down, bare-bones representation of some social, economic, psychological or physiological process; a representation that retains only the essential features of
the process -- the ones that are essential to understanding what

the process is into which the program is going to intervene. There
may be more than one process that is of interest and, hence, more
than one model. And models can be more or less complex.

For the sake of illustration, let me start with a very simple
model. Suppose that we are interested in a nutrition program. We
might well want to have a model of the household distribution of
nutrients. That is, before designing a program, we want to know
what is the current state of affairs among the population. In order
to know who's getting how much food, we examine activities in the
household, perhaps through a survey of households. We also must account for the relative share of nutrient or food that each member
of an average (modal) household receives. We will find that father
is getting a particular share (probably a rather large share) of the
nutrient input while mother is getting a smaller amount. Next to
mother is Aunt Mary who does a little embroidery and sells it in the
market... she gets slightly less than mother. On the other side,
Uncle Joe, who plays in a mariachi band, brings home cash income; he
also has a big appetite and eats a lot. The oldest son gets more
than the next two male children. The girls don't do quite so well.
They get smaller rations, and we notice in our survey that there are
fewer surviving females. Some of the food goes to the chickens and
some is used for the feeding of the pig. Some is just wasted, stolen
eaten by pests or otherwise excluded from human consumption.

This model is not a "causal" model, but it's a very useful model of distribution which helps us to ask appropriate questions about
how and why nutrients are distributed within the household. At least
it helps us to avoid false assumptions about that distribution.

The model can be made a little more dynamic (and more complicated) by including in the activities of household members which
contribute to the provision of nutrient -- that is, how their labor
contributes to the provision of food, as well as how their labor
relates to their caloric needs. Now the model begins to suggest rationale, or "causes" for the existing pattern of distribution. Father works hard as an agricultural laborer (high calorie demand)
but does not earn much money. Uncle Joe, on the other hand, is relatively highly paid and can lay claim to a large part of the nutrient supply because he is a big contributor to the budget. On the
other hand, his work does not require as many calories, and Uncle
Joe is perhaps overweight. The caloric need and productivity can
be calculated for mother, who labors in the garden, and for other
members of the household.

From this sort of model, we begin to understand the familial
patterns of work and eating, an understanding that is a necessary
preliminary to designing an intervention and to evaluating the

impact of the intervention. To repeat, this model is not a "causal" model. It does not incorporate factors that might produce change in consumption patterns, or factors that, historically, produced the current situation. It describes an ongoing process that is in some approximate equilibrium, without saying how that equilibrium came about or what forces sustain the equilibrium level of consumption of nutrients by individuals in the household. (Those are the two possible meanings of "cause" in this context). The understanding of causation, which may be speculative at the time of designing the intervention, will ordinarily become clearer from the analysis of program impact. To be sure, this understanding will depend in part upon what kinds of questions are asked in the impact evaluation.

In principle, any social, economic, physiological, etc. process can be modelled if data are available, and the building of a model will help in understanding the process. A health planner, for example, may be interested in the distribution of enteric disease in a community, especially if a proposal has been made to take some environmental sanitation measure such as providing clean potable water or improving methods of waste disposal. Before deciding what particular measures to institute, the planner would be well advised to survey a sample of households in the community and construct a model that depicted the distribution of diarrheal disease. The model might well show the prevalence of diarrhea among family members, just as the nutrition model showed distribution of caloric intake. The enteric disease model would probably show that prevalence was greater among children than adults, and the younger the child the larger the number of days of illness. The model might also represent the relation between average household prevalence and, say, distance from its commonly used water supply; or proportion of water intake from various sources of varying cleanliness. The model would incorporate those features of family and community that the model builder wanted to take into account in analyzing the situation before taking the next step.

This brings us to step number three in the evaluation process, namely, constructing a conceptual framework and deciding with which "eventual outcomes" the program planner and the impact analyst should be concerned. The "eventual outcomes" which Chernichovsky suggested might underlie a national nutrition policy are an appropriate illustration (4). He identified three: survival, morbidity, and productivity. This is a plausible set of eventual outcomes, though not necessarily the only set. Another analyst or program planner might approach the problem with a different set of eventual outcomes or might add to this list. From those eventual outcomes one then derives the principal dimensions of the problem, its "parameters" if you like it, about which it is necessary to have evidence.

Then, and it seems to me only then, after this procedure (which is laborious to describe but not hard to do) has been completed, is it time to think about what sort of evaluation *method* to employ. I agree with the conferees who said "let's not concentrate too much on methods and let's not let method dictate our choice of problem". The problem must determine the method. One must first go through the analytic steps I have identified before it is at all important or appropriate to decide on the method of evaluation. The heart of the matter is the problem, not the method.

RELATIONSHIP OF EVALUATION TO PROGRAM OPERATION AND PLANNING

My second point concerns a matter that came up several times during this meeting and on which there seemed to be some difference of opinion. It is the question of how the evaluation group should be related to the program operating agency -- how much distance or closeness should there be between them? What are the gains or penalties from a close or a distant relationship?

Two quite distinct situations may exist, it seems to me. One is the situation in which the intervention program has been planned and has been in operation for some period of time before the evaluation takes place. This situation is perhaps the most common, and it leads to such questions as: Who should do the evaluation? When should the evaluation be done? What will be the relationship between the evaluator and program operation? etc. The other situation, clearly distinct, is that in which evaluation is but one phase in program development. It is clearly recognized as a phase of program development and may be described as a "pilot program", "demonstration", "trial" or "randomized experiment". Such evaluation effort proceeds concurrently with the development of the program. It is of a piece with that whole effort; it is not added later. The two situations are quite distinct in terms of their incentive structure -- by that I mean the way in which the people involved are motivated to behave and in terms of the likely outcomes that evaluation will have.

In the first kind of situation, the action team is undoubtedly committed to the program by the time the evaluator gets there. They have been through the pain of developing the program, they have been through the birth pangs and growing pains, they know what a terrible struggle it has been to get something going in the field and they are pretty sure that what they have is a very good thing. It is doing good things for the people that it's intended to serve. The program staff may know its faults pretty well and they may perceive some of the unintended consequences that it's having. They may be sensitive to some of its problems, but mainly they are committed to it. In that situation evaluation can very well be a threat because almost all interventions fall short of the expectations of their inventors. Our reach always exceeds our grasp and no program ever does as well as those who sponsor it hope it will do. So it is not surprising that evaluation is a threat and it is not surprising that evaluation is resisted, that data are held back (data that would discredit the program), data are made hard to get, and there is often an unpleasant adversarial relationship between the evaluators and the program operators.

In the other situation in which the program is developed from the outset as a trial and its form is explicitly tentative, there is less danger of premature commitment to a single form or to a single version of the program. Sometimes this is exploited by having two or more versions of a particular intervention that are placed in comparison with each other. This sometimes can lead to rivalry but it is unlikely to lead to the kind of dedicated commitment to a program that the first situation does.

So, these two situations produce quite different problems as far as the strategy of evaluation is concerned. In our discussion of program evaluation we have not always distinguished one kind from the other and I think some of the questions -- Where should the evaluator come from? How should he be related to the program operation? What should his skills and talents be, and so on -- all are related to, or are at least conditioned by, the thought of the structural relationship of evaluation to program operation.

Furthermore, these two situations have different implications for implementation of the recommendations arising from evaluation. Implementation may well depend, as we have heard, upon having addressed the questions that the operating agency wants to answer rather than some other question, and giving answers that allow the agency to take some action to do something about it -- that is, focusing on what I like to call "manipulable" variables. Thirdly, successful implementation may well depend on involving the program operators in the design of the evaluation as well as in the data collection and analysis. It is easy to see how these two different situations lead to very different relationships in these three domains that will have a bearing on implementing evaluation.

What should we conclude about the relative merit of "outside" versus "inside" evaluation? Are there advantages and disadvantages to each? I think there certainly are. The outside evaluator is more likely to be insulated from undue influence by the program operators -- that is, to maintain his objectivity, his detachment, and perhaps to be fair and unbiased. At the same time, such a person has less familiarity with the program, is not quite so likely

to be sensitive to the questions that the agency wants to have
answered, and, indeed, may not put his answers in terms that they can
do anything about. On the other hand, the inside evaluator, while
he has the advantage of familiarity and closeness to the questions
of the operating agency, may well tend to collude with the program
operators to defend it and may be more biased. The suggestion was
made that outside evaluation is perhaps preferable in the case of
what is called summative evaluation where the decision is a "go/no
go" decision. It's a decision to continue the program or to cut it
off, fund it for another year or phase it out. Inside evaluation
may be more suitable for formative evaluation, that is, for data
collected to shape the program as it goes along and events develop.
This seems to me a very plausible position. Furthermore, I would
like to express my strong view that programs will benefit more from
formative evaluation, in which the evaluative activity is used as
an integral part of program development, rather than from summative
evaluation which seems to come *ex cathedra* and pronounces summary
judgment upon a program that may have been underway for a long time
and perhaps should have been examined earlier before it became set
in its ways.

Somewhat the same reasoning applies to the question of the
timing of an evaluation. The drawbacks of waiting too long to evaluate versus starting too soon were well articulated by Conference
participants. If one waits too long, the program has become "established" -- that is, its procedures and customs have begun to
become rigid; the program staff have developed attachments to the
"right way" to carry it out; and the target audience, the clients
of the program, have adapted to it. No one is very eager to change.
On the other hand, if one starts an evaluation too soon, some conferees argued, the program will not have had time to demonstrate
its effects, it will still be in a developmental phase, and its
staff will be trying to work out unforeseen operating problems.
Premature evaluation will almost always conclude that the program
is not effective and will dampen staff morale, discourage sponsors
and lead to abandonment -- wrongly, in many cases.

It is hard to disagree with the conclusion that any evaluation
(or anything else, for that matter) should occur neither too early
nor too late, but how are we to determine what is the "right time"?
I suggest that no satisfactory general answer can be given in terms
of weeks, months or years; and that it will be hard to judge when
a program has begun to jell but has not become rigid. Instead of
trying to pick *the* right time for a summative evaluation, we should
try to introduce the notion of evaluation and the expectation of
evaluation right at the beginning of program planning. Evaluation
should appear as a natural and ordinary concomitant of program development, not as a "day of reckoning" or as an indication that all

is not going well. If evaluation appears early, in a collaborative
stance, that also increases the likelihood that its results will be
used.

Elsewhere I've suggested that there may be a third way out of
this. It's been explored very little but it's worth, I think,
some thought. The "third way" is to vest the responsibility for
developing and testing interventions in the hands of a special agency -- an agency that is not given responsibility for program operation. My reasoning on this matter is that the trouble with both
outside and inside evaluation is that the incentive structure is
wrong. The incentive structure is set up to reward a successful
program, successful intervention. In order to have successful evaluation, that is,objective, fair and adequate evaluation, rewards
ought to be structured in such a way that the research activity
itself pays off rather than the success of the program. This was
tried very briefly and I think inconclusively in the United States
in the latter part of the Johnson Administration in the form of the
Program Plans and Evaluation section of the Office of Economic Opportunity. This section of OEO did not develop or sponsor specific
anti-poverty measures, but rather tested proposals that others made
for combating poverty. It sponsored the New Jersey Negative Income Tax experiment and several experiments to evaluate educational
interventions, for example, and might have gone on to other types
of anti-poverty experimentation had not its existence been terminated
early in the Nixon administration.

In some sense, putting the evaluation of programs in the hands
of an independent agency is justified by the same logic that puts
the evaluation of drugs in the hands of the Food and Drug Administration in the United States, or the evaluation of certain kinds of
technical products in the National Bureau of Standards. The rewards
are not for making a better antibiotic or a better automobile bat-
tery but for testing antibiotics and batteries to judge their adequacy. I suggest this as an alternative locus for evaluation
projects and evaluation procedures.

IMPACT EVALUATION AND PROCESS EVALUATION

We've repreatedly had our attention called to shortfalls in the
delivery of an intervention or to misuse of the intervention supplied. That is, poor people in the United States use food stamps
to buy expensive but fattening pastry instead of nutritious meats
and vegetables, let's say. Or people in less developed countries
sell their powdered milk in order to buy transistor radios or liquor
or whatever it is they want. There are two points to be made. One
is that any evaluation needs some sort of process monitoring to

make sure that the interventions are appropriately delivered; or
when they're not properly delivered to know how they were delivered
so that the variable intensity of treatment can be taken into account in the analyses. Otherwise, it's not a fair test of the intervention, since the extent of impact is almost surely influenced
by treatment intensity.

The second point is perhaps more important. When an evaluator
observes some **sort** of shortfall in delivery of treatment, it should
be an occasion not for blaming the participant, or blaming the program administration, or blaming the politician, but for asking one-
self the question "Why did that happen?". Think of Alexander Flem-
ing. Suppose he had said, as he looked at his petrie dishes that
fateful day in 1927, "Damn that mold! It ruined all my bacteria".
Instead, he asked why. It is incumbent upon evaluators to ask: Why
don't the health workers distribute all the pills? Why don't some
families use the clinic? Why are the powdered milk supplements sold
rather than consumed?, and so on. You can learn a lot about the
basic problem as well as about the intervention by asking that kind
of question.

EVALUATION FOR WHOM?

A fourth point that caught my attention was initially raised as
a question: Who should decide what is to be evaluated? Who should
design the evaluation? Who should benefit from it? Who should decide what aspects of the intervention are to be evaluated? I suppose that conventionally the sponsor of the intervention program,
the ministry or the agency, has a major interest and it presumably
needs the information in order to make some decisions. Proverbially,
he who pays the piper calls the tune, which seems to give the ministry the right to set the terms of evaluation. But, looking at the
matter in terms of equity, it has been proposed that other parties
also have a legitimate interest in the evaluation of the intervention, specifically the target audience. They are the persons who
are most likely to be affected by the intervention, whether it is
well designed or poorly designed, whether it is effective or defective, and that they should have a right to participate in any attempt to assess its impact (and side effects).

One can look at this suggestion in two lights. It may be considered an outgrowth of the new consumerism, the democratic egali-
tarian ideology that holds that people should have a wider opportunity for self-determination and they shouldn't be victimized by the
bureaucracy; they shouldn't be made to participate in madcap ventures
against their will, against their better judgment, and against their
experience. This really is a political idea. It is a revision of
the traditional notion, at least in the U.S., that the bureaucracy
is controlled by the elected representatives who are in turn

controlled by the people and that, when this long chain operates in its intended fashion, ineffective programs and unjust laws are eliminated. The challenging view says no, the chain doesn't work well but one can shortcut the process by going directly to the people who are participating in an intervention. The target audience has a right to say what the effects on them are or have been.

Without either endorsing or disputing this position, it is possible to look at the suggested strategy in another light and to conclude that it would be prudent to involve the target audience for quite another reason, namely: the quality of the evaluation will be better. People who have been the objects of treatment can tell an evaluator more and different things about the treatment than either those who are providing it or those who designed it. Participants' experience will help the evaluator to find things that he might otherwise miss, including unintended consequences, side effects, shortfalls of delivery or perversions of treatment, and so on. It is in the self-interest of the program operator (and evaluator) to involve the participants in the design of the evaluation regardless of his position on equity, social justice and the role of bureaucracy.

It was also suggested during one of our discussions that a prudent program developer would consider using some variant of Delphi Technique to forecast the probable effects of the intervention before installing it. Concretely this suggestion assumes that experts would be employed in the Delphi process and I think that's an interesting idea. But, consistently with what I've said above, I think also the target audience might well be involved in making the Delphic forecasts.

BASIC RESEARCH

It is clear from the prepared papers, critiques and spontaneous discussion that there is a considerable amount of fundamental ignorance about important aspects of health and nutrition. We have heard, for example, that there is only one scientifically demonstrated measure of nutritional status (growth) and that it is a fairly gross measure which is responsive to changes in nutrition but may not be selectively responsive -- that is, it may respond to other changes as well. At the same time there has been comment bordering upon incredulity that no measure of morbidity is consistently related to nutritional status. Likewise, some conferees find it hard to believe that there is no relationship between nutritional status and mortality -- or, at least, longevity.

Similarly, we seem to know perilously little about the biology of nutrition in relation to the psychology of cognitive impairment.

We do not know how long the effects of severe but time-limited malnutrition may last, or whether these effects are reversible or ir-
reversible. We are not sure what the effect of mild to moderate
malnutrition is upon mental functioning, intellectual achievement
or performance.

There also seems to be some uncertainty about the relationship of nutrition and income, beyond the fact that it is positive,
so that the income elasticity of expenditures for diet is not well
established.

If we cannot measure response to nutritional changes unequivocally, it is hard to know how to evaluate most nutritional interventions; and, if we are not sure how biological and psychological
factors are related, it is hard to know what kind of intervention
to design. If we do not know something about differential responsiveness in the population, it is hard to know how to target an
intervention for maximum impact.

The missing knowledge can often be supplied best through basic
research, perhaps undertaken separately from program evaluation but
certainly guided in its purpose by the practical questions that program developers must answer. It is not always necessary to conduct
basic research and evaluation studies separately, however, and
there may be gains to both from putting the two purposes together.
What I want to emphasize, however, is the importance of getting more
knowledge about fundamental problems and unanswered questions that
underlie many health and nutrition programs.

COSTS OF EVALUATION

There was a great deal of interest at this Conference, as there
always is, in how expensive evaluation is; and there was even an
expression of the view that no resources ought to be "diverted" from
program operations to evaluation research.

It is hard to say anything definitive, or even anything intelligent, about costs because, I believe, we don't know what things
cost in this business. We do not have a decent cost accounting system for evaluation, for social experiments, or for applied social
research of any kind. In the absence of such a system, I am reluctant to come to any conclusion about the comparative costs of experiments, statistical analyses of archival data, sample survey
studies and so on. It seems pretty clear that the larger the scope
of the evaluation and the longer the period of observation, the more
costly it will be and, other things being equal, the more useful
information it will provide.

There may be some ways to cut costs but I don't know any widely
applicable general rules. I am also suspicious of "obvious" inferences here. Recall Hollister's point about archival data (3). Just
because a file of information exists doesn't mean that it will be
cheap to use; the costs involved in cleaning, editing, reordering
or reforming an archive may exceed the cost of new data collection,
Hollister believes. Under some circumstances, I'm sure he is right.

A related point has to do with assigning a fixed portion of
the program budget for evaluation purposes. This has sometimes been
done in the legislation for social improvement programs and, in the
U.S., has varied from 1 percent to more then 5 percent. Any percentage is arbitrary and no particular number makes sense across
the range of possible program expenditures. Imagine, for example,
an intervention that is cheap to administer, like a tax imposed
upon certain employees. The marginal cost of collecting the new
tax might be less than $100,000 while the effects of the tax upon
employment practices might be great. It would not be reasonable to
prescribe 5 percent or to limit the cost of evaluation to $5,000.
At the opposite extreme, it seems clear that the costs of a national
health insurance program in the United States will run into the bil-
lions annually but it might not be necessary to spend more than a
few million on a one-time experiment whose answers may help to avoid
the costly mistakes of Medicare.

Just as it is difficult to cost account evaluation research,
there is no commonly agreed upon method for cost accounting social
intervention programs. Accordingly, there is no satisfactory approach to the cost effectiveness of intervention, no commonly accepted way of measuring the efficiency of program expenditures.

Lastly, one comment on the "diversion" of program resources to
evaluation. It is hard to imagine that an adequately conducted evaluation could ever incur greater costs than a program that did not
achieve its intended impact. The cost of finding out whether program funds are being expended without effect is a cheap cost indeed.

Certainly, there seem to be sound reasons for proceeding cau-
tiously with innovative programs. It is prudent to try such programs on a small scale, under somewhat controlled conditions, in
order to learn: a) whether the intervention has the desired effect
at all; b) what the unforeseen problems and complications of its
administration are; c) what unintended and unwanted effects the
intervention has; and d) how much more the program actually costs
to operate that its designers thought.

At several points in our discussion here, some conferees expressed the opinion that impact evaluation, and especially experi-

mentation, took too long to be helpful. By the time an evaluation
study has been completed, some said, the problem has disappeared
or has changed so much that the results are unuseable. This comment might be interpreted as a plea for less delay in analyzing
results and preparing reports. I cannot disagree with the opinion
that many studies come in grossly behind schedule.

But it might also be interpreted as an opinion that our response to social problems and social issues must be more rapid and
that experimental trials are a needless deferral of action. Here
I would disagree, if only on the ground of prudence in the face of
ignorance: we don't know how to solve many social problems, so
let us be cautious in trying out new ideas. But also I would disagree with the view that social problems quickly disappear or quickly change in fundamental ways. It was pointed out here that two
major issues in the United States -- the welfare system and national health insurance -- have been on the verge of change for almost
a decade. In both cases, numerous analysts and commentators derided
the idea of experimentation on the ground that the legislation would
have been enacted before the results were in. In both cases they
have been wrong. As Pastore remarked during the discussion "Programs come and go but issues have a way of enduring".

To be sure, some aspects of an issue or a problem may change
quickly, but these are likely to be surface features. Part of the
strategy of evaluation is to choose for investigation those features of a social problem that are not merely superficial, but are
more fundamental. Not only will such features be more enduring so
that studies will not be inappropriately late, but they will be
the more important aspects of a problem, more worthwhile addressing
for the purposes of change.

TECHNICAL ISSUES

A number of technical questions were raised and discussed,
most eagerly I thought, by the academic social scientists at the
meeting. Several contributors made constructive suggestions about
explaining randomization to participants and to program operators,
overcoming resistance to randomization and maintaining the integrity of random assignment. Some mentioned contemporary innovations
in statistical methods for dealing with departures from randomization and for comparing non-equivalent groups, but also stressed the
need for further development of such methods. Another issue was
the development of measuring instruments, including data series to
serve as indicators as well as questionnaires, tests and intervening procedures. Much of this area of discussion emphasized validity
and usability -- i.e. the appropriateness of a particular procedure,

the necessity for "tailor-making" measuring instruments to fit both
the specific problem and the specific population or linguistic-
cultural situation in which it was to be used. I think it would be
unprofitable to rehash these points here, and I would simply emphasize the desirability of securing adequate technical assistance,
which is available for dealing with those issues in the specific
context of a concrete evaluation problem.

A significant technical issue is data processing and, especially, the establishment and maintenance of data storage files from
which information can be quickly, cheaply and accurately retrieved.
This problem is especially important in longitudinal studies with
repeated observations of the same individual, and in studies that
make multiple observations of the same person or unit. For example,
if evaluation of a health program requires observing height, weight,
presence or absence of disease, heart rate and blood pressure on
three annual physical examinations, it is essential that the records
of each individual be complete on each occasion, that they do not
become confused with the records of other individuals with similar
names, for instance, and that a particular datum is not mistakenly
entered in the wrong column of the record card. So stated, the
problem seems simple to solve but when many thousands, or hundreds
of thousands of such entries have to be stored on computer tape in
such a way as to make it easy to compare height changes between
control and experimental groups accurately, it turns out not to be
easy to solve. Let me reiterate Hollister's good advice: do not
try out novel systems of data storage in large scale studies (3).
They will always have unanticipated difficulties that will cost
lots more money.

Social scientists know more about some of these technical issues than we do about some of the more profound questions (cf. Basic
Research, above) and have written extensively on them. It is perhaps unfortunate that we do not always agree upon tactics in a concrete situation, and that we are more fond of giving wise advice
that we are of taking it. Nevertheless, there are some general
principles about measurement and some specific techniques that are
widely applicable and accessible through trained professionals.

One question that has been implicitly if not explicitly asked
is: how much of the technology of evaluation, as developed in the
U.S., is transferable to Latin America (supposing that someone
might want to use it there)? It is with some trepidation that I
give my answer, since I have not personally directed or executed
an evaluation study in Latin America and things always look simpler
before you try them.

In principle, all of the technology of evaluation is transferable with what I would take to be the ordinary and necessary adap-

tations to circumstances -- adaptations that we take for granted
when we shift language, culture, geography, etc.; adaptations of
form, not usually of substance. Certainly there is evidence of
application of portions of the technology in Latin America. Social
experiments have been carried out in Guatemala, Colombia, El Sal-
vador and elsewhere. Sample surveys are not uncommon. Census data
and other archival records are regularly collected in usable form.
Computing capacity is available, though I am unclear about its ubiq-
uity or cost. (Computing programs and machine compatibility are
problems in the U.S. too).

Are there special problems of an administrative, bureaucratic
or political character that make the transfer of evaluation technology difficult or impossible? I have not learned of any such
obstacles at this meeting. The one paper that touched upon this
range of issues did not make the case that the *methods* were non-
transferable, but only that the process of introducing and managing
intervention was differently located in the socio-political system.
This means, to me, that generating interest in program evaluation
and getting its recommendations accepted and implemented may take
on different dimensions in Latin America than in the U.S., but it
does not deny the transferability of technique.

HUMAN RESOURCES AND THE INSTITUTIONALIZATION OF EVALUATION

How does evaluation become more than merely a passing fancy
and how can a body of professionals be developed? This matter has
been mentioned but not prominently in our discussion, but I think
it's a matter that requires some very careful reflection and extensive discussion, particularly in terms of the Latin American
situation. Although I don't pretend to know Latin America well,
I want to make a couple of comments about the situation in the
United States in the spirit of letting you know that things aren't
all that good north of the border either. At one point I worked
with a committee concerned with evaluating social experiments. We
concluded that there were not many organizations who were capable
of conducting adequate evaluation operations and that many of those
which do conduct evaluations are not strong. Secondly, we concluded
that individuals with appropriate training and experience were not
in abundant supply.

These conclusions were reached three or four years ago, and
the labor market in the social sciences has been changing rapidly
in the United States at least. Some modification of that conclusion might be justified as of 1978 but don't think it will be vastly
different from what I just said: there are not many competent individuals or organizations.

Organizations that do evaluations need a variety of talents --
they need persons with skills in study design, questionnaire construction, statistical analysis, data processing, interviewer supervision and training. Most of these skills are not taught to can-
didates for degrees in the average North American university. If
they're learned at all, they're learned on the job, learned through
apprenticeship. Indeed, that may be the only way to teach them
because they are all applied skills and can be learned primarily
through application. In order to develop such people, such talents,
organizations need a continuous work flow. That is, the organization must be able to hire inexperienced, untrained individuals
(who have demonstrated substantial personal ability as graduate
students) who are looking for an opportunity to learn a craft that
is not taught at universities (with few exceptions). These trainees
must learn on the job and there must be enough jobs to provide
training opportunities. Evaluation studies offer an exceptional
opportunity to develop the sort of skill that they wish to acquire.

Perhaps the same conditions obtain in Latin America. Certainly, it appears from the discussion here that the organizational
and institutional base for education in Latin America needs to be
strengthened. How might this be accomplished? How might a capacity for conducting evaluation studies be developed? How might a
consultative or advisory service be provided and training ground
be fashioned for professionals who wish to move from established
disciplines to the newer and less developed field of assessing program impact? It is only in the last 15 years or so that governments and private citizens have begun to ask for an accounting of
social interventions. Until then, the advocates of an intervention
had only to demonstrate good faith and pure hearts -- good intentions and a plausible program. Now the concerned governments are
beginning to ask whether the intervention is useful, effective,
helpful. Does it do what it proposes? This attitude, this quiet
challenge, will not, I propose, abate or disappear. If anything,
it will grow stronger and more insistent as the efforts to ameliorate social problems mount, while problems yield reluctantly, if
at all.

Should there be established a Latin American Institution for,
say, the conduct of evaluations, for consultation on evaluation,
for training personnel and developing the capacity for evaluation
in institutional form? Should it be an international (e.g. Pan-
American) institution? Should it promote collaboration among existing institutions? Should it serve as a technical development center or an archive of evaluations or a bibliographic aide?

These are questions that Latin American colleagues should address and they will deal more deftly with the intricacies than I can.

But I venture to suggest some attributes such an evaluation institute might have:

a.   A staff that could provide the professional and technical
     services needed for evaluation, and which kept itself in
     trim by conducting evaluation studies themselves -- on
     request, by bidding on jobs, etc.; or by providing tech-
     nical consultation on specific services (e.g. design,
     sampling, data processing) to program operating agencies.
     The staff might also act as broker to identify help and
     resources for its clients to engage directly;

b.   An advanced level training program for social scientists,
     physicians, public health workers, etc. at the profes-
     sional level; and training for technicians in data pro-
     cessing, survey management and the like. These might be
     short to medium term programs (3 to 18 months) depending
     on training objectives. Like many "internship" programs,
     trainees would be expected to return to countries/agencies
     from which they had come.

It is almost universal experience that an idea, a style of inquiry, a movement in thought and action will wax if it is given a
name, a formal status and an organizational identity. If impact
evaluation of intervention programs is a promising and useful thrust,
it will be the more so by being embodied in an institutional form.

SELF-SUSTAINING INTERVENTIONS

As one participant pointed out, many interventions are not bold
enough, they're not powerful enough to have much impact on the problems they address. Some are too conventional and some are unimagi-
native, but most of them fail to meet what I will call Herrera's
criterion, namely: that the most important outcome of an intervention program ought to be that the intervention as such can wither,
can be withdrawn, can disappear without having the target population
slip back to where it was before the intervention (5). In other
words, the behavior or the state of affairs that the intervention
seeks to influence should become self-sustaining as a result of the
intervention. It should not be necessary to carry on an intervention program *ad infinitum* -- it should result in a change that is
self-sustaining.

IS EVALUATION A DISTINCT AND UNIQUE PROCEDURE?

My final point addresses the question of whether it is reasonable to talk about evaluation as if it were a unique method or a

singular technique. Is there a distinctive body of knowledge, theory or practice that can be unequivocally defined as "evaluation"?

     It was frequently pointed out here that the techniques of eval-
uation are not clearly different or distinct from conventional social scientific research. In fact, all of the techniques for collecting and analyzing data for evaluation purposes are drawn directly
from one of the conventional scientific disciplines, usually those
of the social sciences.

     Furthermore, it is important to dispel the notion that there
is *an* evaluation methodology, broadly applicable, that can simply
be taken off the shelf and used to assess the impact of any program. The truth is quite otherwise. There is no single evaluation
methodology (and, above all, no single "simple and inexpensive"
technique). Rather, there are multiple techniques. Often these
are alternative techniques that are equally plausible and useful
in a particular situation. This last phrase is the key to the puz-
zle -- "in a particular situation". The methodology of evaluation
is not rigid but flexible. Good practice consists of choosing from
a wide range of possibilities the most appropriate techniques for
the particular situation, for the concrete task at hand and for the
particular constraints that surround it: cost, time, level or precision needed, availability of data, and other resource limitations.
The skillful evaluator is able to combine appropriate techniques,
adjust to unforeseen difficulties, and exploit unanticipated opportunities. A well designed evaluation is indeed "tailored" to the
program itself.

     What is distinctive about evaluation then? Is it just another
kind of social research? Not quite. The distinctive feature of
evaluation is that it is social research embedded in a context of
power and policy. That means at least two things: evaluation must
focus upon issues of policy and program operation -- it must be
relevant; and, second, if it is well done, the evaluation will suggest changes that threaten some established portion of the power
structure which exists around the program being evaluated. In concrete terms, evaluation is social science research applied to public policy problems and to the operation of ameliorative social
(or economic, medical, etc.) programs. And evaluation is social
science research that inevitably takes on the character of a political act (in the English language sense of "political"), whether
or not the evaluator wishes it.

     As a consequence of all of these attributes, evaluation does
have a distinctive character but not a simple physiognomy. Its
character derives from the demand to use the tools of social science
to gather relevant and useful information about a public policy and

to analyze and interpret that information so as to influence the use of political power. Thus, evaluation has the character of an applied science carried out in a political context. But evaluation is a type of applied social research, not a singular set of techniques, but a special combination put together for each singular occasion.

So we see that evaluation is not a panacea, nor yet a new miracle treatment for sick programs or debilitated policies. It is, however, a rational sensible way of using existing technical resources to help improve the ways in which we intervene to ameliorate social problems.

REFERENCES

1. Hennigan, K. M., B. R. Flay, and R. A. Haag. Clarification of concepts and terms commonly used in evaluative research. In: R. E. Klein, M. S. Read, and H. W. Riecken, (eds.). *The Practice of Impact Evaluation*. New York: Plenum Publishing Corporation, 1979.
2. Riecken, H. W., and R. F. Boruch. *Social Experimentation. A Method for Planning and Evaluating Social Interventions*. New York: Academic Press, 1974.
3. Hollister, R. G. Comments on: Recent United States experiences in evaluation research with implications for Latin America, by T. D. Cook, and E. G. McAnany. In: R. E. Klein, M. S. Read, and H. W. Riecken, (eds.). *The Practice of Impact Evaluation*. New York: Plenum Publishing Corporation, 1979.
4. Chernichovsky, D. The economic theory of the household and impact measurement of nutrition and related health programs. In: R. E. Klein, M. S. Read, and H. W. Riecken, (eds.). *The Practice of Impact Evaluation*. New York: Plenum Publishing Corporation, 1979.
5. Herrera, G. Comments on: Special issues for the measurement of program impact in developing countries, by J. W. Townsend, W. T. Farrell, and R. E. Klein. In: R. E. Klein, M. S. Read, and H. W. Riecken, (eds.). *The Practice of Impact Evaluation*. New York: Plenum Publishing Corporation, 1979.

CLARIFICATION OF CONCEPTS AND TERMS COMMONLY USED

IN EVALUATIVE RESEARCH

Karen M. Hennigan*
Brian R. Flay**
    Northwestern University
    Evanston, Illinois

and

Richard A. Haag
ACTION
Washington, D. C.

TABLE OF CONTENTS

*   Karen M. Hennigan is now at University of Southern California.
** Brian R. Flay is now at University of Waterloo, Ontario, Canada.

II.   WHAT IS BEING EVALUATED?

      A.   Program, Project, and Treatment

      B.   Conceptual and Empirical Models

III. RESEARCH DESIGN

      A.   Experimental Design

      B.   Quasi-Experimental Design

      C.   Nonexperimental Design

      D.   Design Issues

           1.   When are measurements taken?
           2.   Who is measured

IV. MEASUREMENT

      A.   What is Measurement?

      B.   Which Variables are Measured?

           1.   Treatment variables
           2.   Outcome variables
           3.   Nontreatment variables
           4.   Variables in empirical models

      C.   How are Variables Measured?

           1.   Operationalizing constructs
           2.   Measurement instruments
           3.   Methods of gathering measurements

      D.   Attributes of Good Measures

           1.   Validity
           2.   Reliability
           3.   Measurement error
           4.   Reactivity and response bias

V.   DESCRIBING THE RELATIONSHIP
      BETWEEN VARIABLES

A.   Statistics

B.   Data Analysis

   1.   Making causal inferences
   2.   Data analysis procedures
   3.   Statistical Significance

C.   The Validity of Causal Inference

   1.   Some threats to internal validity in
         experiments
   2.   Some threats to internal validity in
         non-experiments and some quasi-
         experiments
   3.   External validity

VI.   REFERENCES FOR MORE INFORMATION

VII. INDEX TO CHAPTER

I.   WHAT IS EVALUATIVE RESEARCH?

I.A. Differentiating Evaluation, Evaluative Research,
            and Basic Research

     It is useful to distinguish between evaluation in general and
evaluative research in particular. In the broadest sense, *evaluation* is the process of generating information about the operations
and impact of implemented programs or policies. When a particular
program is being evaluated this general process is often called *program evaluation*. *Evaluative research* is the application of scientific, empirical research methods to program evaluation leading to
logically defensible, causal statements about the effectiveness of
a program. Thus, evaluative research can be considered a subset of
the more general process of evaluation.

     Judgments resulting from evaluative research are empirically
based and aim to be replicable, whereas judgments from evaluations
in general may include assertions made with little or no objective
evidence to back them up. Therefore, gathering experts' opinions
about the merits of a particular project is a form of evaluation --
called *expert judgment*, but not a form of evaluative research. Even
a systematic procedure of gathering experts' opinions that results
in their reaching a consensus, such as in the *Delphi Technique*,

should not be considered evaluative research, for its results are based on experts' estimates of the likelihood of certain outcomes rather than on measures of the actual outcomes.

Evaluation activities which do not involve the application of scientific research methods (such as expert judgment and the Delphi Technique) are sometimes conducted as adjuncts of or preliminary to evaluative research. Two other forms of general evaluation that can complement or precede evaluative research that were discussed in this book are situation assessment and administrative history.

Situation assessment, suggested by Mushkin, refers to a procedure for making a quick estimation of the magnitude of the service offered to a target population relative to some standard or to some estimate of the magnitude of the problem. For example, if a project gives daily food supplements to women with infants, the percentage of mothers' daily nutritional needs that these supplements represent can be estimated (assuming daily nutritional needs are known). If this percentage turns out to be quite low, this simple assessment is enough by itself to suggest that the project will not have an impact. Riecken discusses the strengths and weaknesses of this and the expert judgment approach, either of which could provide an initial assessment of the worth of a program before full-scale evaluative research is undertaken.

An *administrative history* typically is a case study (a description of one particular case, one particular project). It includes a narrative summary of how the project was implemented over time, what key administrators did and why. It may include a blow-by-blow description of the staff and recipients' activities from an administrator's point of view. An administrative history may provide valuable information about the implementation and operations of a project.

For the most part, this book is concerned with evaluative research in particular rather than evaluation in general. While this distinction between evaluative research (empirically-based and scientifically defensible evaluation) and evaluation in general (including subjective, often opinion-based evaluation) is quite important, many writers use the terms evaluation, *evaluation research,* and evaluative research interchangeably, taking for granted that readers notice the extent of scientific rigor of the evaluation activity being discussed. Which term writers in this book actually use, then, is not so important. This book is primarily concerned with evaluation that leads to empirical, scientifically defensible, causal statements about the effectiveness of nutrition and other health-related programs or policies.

Evaluative research should also be distinguished from basic research. *Basic research* is often a prerequisite to evaluative research. For example, basic research would be needed to identify what kind of nutrition supplements, consumed in what quantities over what periods of time are likely to meet the dietary deficits prevalent in a certain locale. After basic research has established that a certain nutrition supplement is physiologically effective, a program might be designed to distribute the supplement, and the effectiveness of the implemented program might be evaluated. Program evaluative research would investigate the effectiveness of distributing this nutrition supplement in a *field setting* -- that is, a naturally occurring situation. Program evaluative research is always conducted in a field setting, for its purpose is to assess empirically the implementation and impact of a program or policy as it actually operates in a community, state, or country.

This book mentions basic research on health and nutrition in several places but evaluative research is its major focus and the terms and concepts clarified here reflect this focus.

I.B. Two Dominant Approaches to Evaluative Research

Two dominant methodological approaches to evaluative research appear in this book -- the experimental approach and the statistical control approach. The two approaches differ primarily in how they *control* for the influence of nontreatment variables on outcome variables. Both approaches seek to disentangle the effects of treatment and nontreatment variables on outcome variables. For example, was it the nutrition supplements that were given to children at a school that caused a change in their health (as measured by height, weight and morbidity) or were the observed changes in health due to the normal processes of growth and maturation or seasonal fluctuations in prevalence of disease-causing agents? Both approaches seek to determine whether the treatment delivered by the project being evaluated has a real impact on the outcomes of interest, over and above any influence of nontreatment factors, but the two approaches use different methods to accomplish this.

I.B.1. The experimental approach. The *experimental approach* or the experimental control approach is characterized by two practices. First, measures of outcome variables are compared across two or more groups of persons who have received different amounts of the treatment (usually some vs. none) that is delivered by the project being evaluated. The groups that are compared are called *comparison groups*. Second, the comparison groups are formed by *random assignment* (see Section III.A). The purpose of random assignment is to create comparison groups that are randomly equiva-

lent -- that is equivalent on the average in every way except that
one group will receive the treatment being evaluated and the other
group will not. In this way all the nontreatment variables are
said to be *experimentally controlled* (see Section III.A). Only
the treatment variables being evaluated distinguish one comparison
group from another. Therefore, if differences between comparison
groups appear in the outcome variables after the treatment has been
delivered, and if the groups were initially equivalent in every
way (including on all nontreatment variables), then researchers
can conclude that the observed differences between the groups were
caused by the treatment rather than by nontreatment factors.

The experimental approach is typically *prospective* in that it
involves asking what outcomes a project will produce. Thus, prospective studies begin before all outcomes are known and they typically involve designing measures around the expected effects of
the particular treatment and outcomes being studied. Prospective
experimental research not only involves the generation of new data,
but, by specifying in advance what is to be considered evidence of
program success, it avoids capitalizing on accidental outcomes.

I.B.2. The statistical control approach. While the experimental approach to evaluative research is characterized by the
creation of randomly equivalent comparison groups, the *statistical
control approach* is characterized by the use of statistical adjustments to control for the influence of nontreatment variables (see
Section III.C). When it is impractical or impossible to create
randomly equivalent comparison groups, but the treatment, nontreatment, and outcome variables can be measured for individuals who
have received different amounts of exposure to the treatment,
there the evaluator can analyze the statistical relationships between relevant variables under various assumptions about the causal order of the variables. Further, the evaluator can make statistical adjustments for the nontreatment variables in order to estimate the independent relationship between the treatment and outcome variables.   In other words, the statistical control approach
makes use of what is known and can be assumed about the relationship between variables and the observed correlations to make statistical adjustments that remove the influence of nontreatment
variables on outcome variables so that the independent relationship between the treatment variables and outcome variables can
be estimated. While we will call this the statistical control
approach, others call it the *nonexperimental approach* (since it
typically uses nonexperimental research designs) or the *econometric approach* (since it uses many of the methods developed by
economists and sociologists to study economic variables).

The statistical control approach to evaluative research typically is *retrospective* in the sense that it involves examining

the outcomes that a project has already produced. Retrospective studies can be begun after the project has been completed and can focus on outcomes that have already been observed. Thus, retrospective studies can use data from project records. The object of the study is to determine to what extent the project was responsible for the observed outcomes.

While the differences described above -- experimental vs. statistical control, prospective vs. retrospective research -- differentiate the experimental and statistical control approach, some evaluative research studies do not use exclusively one approach or the other. For example, experimental evaluators often use statistical adjustments to control for nontreatment variables that cannot be randomized conveniently.

I.C. Kinds of Evaluative Research

Not only may evaluators adopt different methodological approaches, but their evaluations may be directed toward different ends -- that is, they may be aimed at answering different sets of questions. A key distinction of this sort is often made between formative and summative evaluation.

I.C.1. A key distinction. *Formative evaluation* is intended to provide information to those who are responsible for developing programs about the project's operation and implementation -- information that can be used to improve the management and probable impact of the project. In contrast, the goal of *summative evaluation* is to determine how well the treatment delivered by a project achieved its objectives, and what side effects the project may have had. The primary concern of summative evaluation is to determine the nature of the project's impact -- that is, to describe what particular outcomes the project caused. Formative evaluative research, on the other hand, is typically conducted when a new project is first being implemented in order to maximize the efficiency of its operation and the consistency between its operation in practice and its planned operation. Summative research typically begins to collect data after an initial shakedown period since its focus is on assessing the impact of the project as it operates in practice.

A distinction similar to the distinction between formative and summative evaluation is made between process and impact evaluation. *Process evaluation* is often used, like formative evaluation, to denote the examination of factors that may facilitate or inhibit the project's impact on its targets rather than the actual outcomes *per se*. In this sense process evaluation is primarily concerned with the implementation process -- that is, with the organ-

ization and operations of a project. This focus is also called
implementation evaluation. In contrast, *impact evaluation* is like
summative evaluation in that it focuses on assessing the impact of
the project being evaluated. The label "process evaluation" can
also be used to denote an emphasis on studying process variables
or mediating variables (e.g., the ways that cultural mores may
affect acceptance or use of an innovative procedure). In this
sense both summative and formative evaluation can involve process
evaluation (e.g., the process by which a project has an impact or
the process by which a project's treatment is received).

Most of the chapters in this book devote more attention to
summative than to formative evaluative research concerns, or they
emphasize a combination of the two, often termed *comprehensive e-
valuation.* Though comprehensive evaluation is advocated in most
instances, there are some conditions under which either formative
or summative evaluative research activities are stressed. For example, a formative evaluation might be given greater priority if
there is reason to suspect that a treatment is not operating as
planned, or a summative evaluation might be given greater priority
if there is already ample evidence that the treatment has been implemented and delivered according to plan.

I.C.2. Other distinctions.   There are numerous adjectives
that have been used to identify a particular emphasis or procedure
in evaluation. Writers in this volume, for example, have used the
terms: secondary evaluation, administrative evaluation, multiconstituency evaluation and cost-effectiveness to highlight a particular evaluation approach or method. But these terms are not
mutually exclusive, nor are they distinct from formative and summative evaluation. Rather, they are used to draw attention to a
particular procedure or approach that may or may not be a part of
formative or summative evaluative research.

Administrative evaluation, advocated by Ugalde and Emrey, is
primarily directed toward evaluating the impact of cultural, political, and administrative factors on the implementation and usage
of project services. This approach to evaluation grows out of
their argument that the political and administration-based implementation problems are more limiting to social improvement in Latin
America than lack of treatment impact *per se*. Hence, administrative evaluation focuses on measuring and testing relationships between an intervention and the political and administrative factors
that affect its selection, acceptance, implementation and subsequent utilization or distribution while placing less emphasis on
measuring treatment impact.

Administrative evaluation is not the same as administrative
history (see Section I.A.). Administrative evaluation is orient-

ed toward a set of questions that may be answered by evaluative research. Administrative history, on the other hand, has been identified as general evaluation procedure -- a chronology of the history of a program from an administrative point of view.

Multiconstituency evaluation, advocated by Cook and McAnany, typically involves asking both formative and summative questions. It is distinguished from other kinds of evaluation by the way the set of evaluation questions (or research hypotheses) are generated and selected for study. A multiconstituency evaluation seeks to answer a broad range of questions chosen to represent the interests of each of the different consitituencies involved in a social, health or nutrition program. For example, it would seek to answer questions of importance from the recipients' and the community's perspective, and from the project staff's, project developers' and project sponsors' point of view, as well as the general public's point of view.

Secondary evaluation or secondary analysis refers to the re-analysis of previously analyzed evaluative research data by a second group of researchers. These researchers may check the original finding by repeating the analysis; or they may ask different questions of the data, or analyze the data in different ways. Their results may confirm, contradict, or go beyond the original researchers' conclusions.

Cost-effectiveness refers to the procedure of contrasting the cost of a treatment or different ways of delivering a treatment with the effectiveness of the treatment in achieving particular outcomes.

II. WHAT IS BEING EVALUATED?

II.A. Program, Project and Treatment

The term *intervention* is used most often by writers in this volume to denote some aspect of the entity which is being evaluated. Intervention is to be distinguished from the next most commonly used term, "program". Program can refer to several interventions at several geographic locations all aimed at reaching a general common goal like improving public health. Or, program can refer to a single intervention at a single geographic location aimed at achieving a specific goal, like preventing smallpox. To avoid confusion, Cook and McAnany suggest the word *project* be used to refer to the latter, a single intervention, and *program* be used to refer to the former, multiple interventions aimed at achieving a general goal. The U.S. Peace Corps, then, is an example of a program, and it includes hundreds of specific projects.

On the other hand, "intervention" is sometimes used to denote a project (e.g., providing a nutrition supplement at a single site may be called an intervention) and other times used to denote the goods or services the project is delivering -- that is, the project *treatment*. Every project offers some treatment and it is the treatment that is supposed to effect some improvement in some aspect of the recipient's status (e.g., nutritional, health, educational). To avoid confusion here, we will use the words program, project, and treatment to denote the three levels at which the entity being evaluated can be described. Programs contain multiple projects, projects deliver one or more treatments. The convention of distinguishing these three levels by these three terms is not universally followed and these terms are sometimes used in different ways by other authors.

A project may offer multiple treatments, a *global treatment package* consisting of multiple components (e.g., nutrition supplements and medical care) or it may consist of a single component (e.g., nutritional supplements only). If a treatment has multiple components that are carefully planned to complement one another in order to increase their combined effectiveness, it may be called an *integrated treatment*. In addition, a treatment may be a *well-defined treatment* (e.g., smallpox vaccinations) or an *unfocused treatment* (e.g., the addition of a nurse to the staff of a local clinic).

In this book, projects have been variously labeled, experimental or controlled, demonstration or pilot, and phantom. Describing a project as an *experimental* or *controlled intervention* indicates as explained above, that the project is implemented in such a way that the effect of the treatment on outcomes, could be distinguished from the possible influence of nontreatment variables. In particular, if the project is described as experimental, this ability to distinguish between treatment and nontreatment influences has been achieved by randomly assigning persons to groups that did or did not receive the treatment. For controlled interventions, the ability to distinguish may have been achieved by random assignment to treatment and no-treatment groups, or it may have been achieved by other means.

Projects described as *demonstrations* or *pilot projects* typically are of a relatively small scale and are "experimental" only in the sense that they are untested. These may or may not be implemented in an experimental ways, i.e., with random assignment to treatment and control groups.

When a project is described as a *phantom intervention*, the writer is suggesting that the project was not implemented as planned, i.e., either it was not delivered at all or it was not delivered to the target persons. For example, when the planned vaccina-

tions in a smallpox eradication project were given in a neighboring
wealthy community rather than in the targeted poor community, or the
nutrition supplements meant for nursing mothers were actually consumed by others in the family, a phantom intervention has occurred.

The *implementation* of a project requires the *delivery of an
intervention*, or more accurately the *delivery of a treatment*. Implementation is of concern to evaluators since it is necessary to
evaluate the impact of a treatment as it actually operates not as
it was planned to operate. Similarly, the *utilization* of a treatment is of concern. Most projects have designated *target populations* or persons whom the treatment is planned to help. Evaluators
must determine whether the targets are actually using the project's
services. When those in the target population who receive a treatment are self-selected rather than randomly assigned, the persons
who do take advantage of a project's services are almost always
systematically different in some way (e.g., in terms of their level
of need, income, motivation to work with the project staff, etc.)
from those who do not take advantage of its services. This self-
selection blurs the effect of treatment by confounding it with the
personal characteristics of persons who sought or did not seek treatment.

II.B. Conceptual and Empirical Models

In one sense the entity being evaluated is a conceptual model,
or a theory that certain aspects of the project treatment will lead
to particular outcomes. Every project embodies an underlying *conceptual model*, an explicit or implicit theory about the relationship between treatments and outcomes it is supposed to cause. For
example, a project planned to deliver a particular nutritional supplement to malnourished and illiterate children may be based on a
model (or theory) which specifies the ways different aspects of the
treatment should affect the health and intellectual status of malnourished children. In a simple case, for example, the model may
specify that when malnourished children consume x amount of a
particular supplement y times a week over z months, then a specified improvement in health status will result, and subsequently
their intellectual status will improve. This simple model is a
model of linkages between treatment variables and outcome variables.
If a project is implemented for a given range of x, y, and z values,
an investigation of the impact of the treatment on health status
and intellect tests this model.

Both the experimental and the statistical control approach to
evaluative research are, in this sense, testing some conceptual
model. An explicit theoretical approach develops the conceptual
model into an *empirically-based model* that may include multiple treat-

ment and outcome variables as well as nontreatment variables. From
this approach, the object of the evaluative research exercise is to
build an empirical model comprehensive enough to explain most of the
variation in the outcome variables, to order the causal relationships in this model, and to estimate empirically the values of *parameters* such as the x, y, and z in the example above. This approach, sometimes called *causal modeling* depends on adequate statistical control (see Section III.C.) in the data analysis style (see
Section V.B.).

III.   RESEARCH DESIGN

The *design* of evaluative research is the blueprint for the research -- it is the research plan. The key to understanding different kinds of designs is to identify the nature of comparison and
the nature of control employed. An evaluation may use an experimental, quasi-experimental or nonexperimental research design. Each
of these differs primarily in terms of what is compared and the
method and extent to which the influence of nontreatment factors
is controlled.

III.A.   Experimental Design

As noted earlier, *experimental design* calls for comparing the
outcomes of two or more *randomly equivalent comparison groups*. One
or more of the comparison groups does not receive the treatment
(called a *no-treatment group, no-treatment control group,* or simply
a *control group*) or receives some treatment other than the intervention treatment (called an *alternative treatment group,* or an *alternative treatment control group*). Another one or more of the
groups does receive some amount of the treatment (called a *treatment group, project group,* or sometimes *experimental group*). Experimental designs call for the *random assignment* of persons or
groups of persons to either a treatment group or control group.
This means that a pool of eligible persons or groups of persons are
identified and a random procedure (e.g., the flip of a coin) is
used to divide the pool into treatment and control groups.

A variety of procedures may be used for random assignment in
field situations (see for example 1, 2) but they all result in form-
ing randomly equivalent comparison groups. The assumption is then
made that the comparison groups are alike on all dimensions except
the treatment variables that are being evaluated. Consider, for
example, that treatment and control groups for a mother's nutritional supplement project are formed by random assignment, then (by the
laws of probability, given that the number of women is large enough)
each group of women will have about the same average age, height,

weight, prior health status, number of previous births, number of living children, and so on. This is important since we know that in addition to the nutritional supplements given, nontreatment factors like these can influence the subsequent health status of newborns. These nontreatment factors that can influence the outcomes an evaluator is studying are called *confounding* factors or variables. By randomly assigning mothers to receive or not receive the treatment (nutritional supplements) the possible confounding effect of these nontreatment factors on the outcomes of interest (newborn health) is *experimentally controlled* by approximately equating the treatment and control groups on these variables from the start. In other words, the object of random assignment is to form comparison groups that are approximately the same (on the average) in every way except that treatment groups receive the project's treatment and control groups do not receive the treatment. The similarity between groups extends to confounding and to apparently irrelevant factors as well. Theoretically, then, if treatment groups are later found to have healthier newborns, the evaluators can safely infer that the treatment the project delivered (nutritional supplement) is responsible for this outcome.

Typically, experimental designs call for the measurement of outcome variables before the project treatment is delivered to any group and measurement of treatment variables (e.g., frequency of treatment, kind of treatment). Finally, outcome variables are measured once again after the project treatment has been received and has had time to be effective.

III.B. Quasi-experimental Design

A *quasi-experimental design* also typically involves comparisons between treatment groups and control groups (either no-treatment or alternative treatment groups). However, unlike with experimental designs, these groups are not formed by random assignment. Instead, *nonequivalent comparison groups* are formed using one of a number of specific alternatives to randomized assignment that have been identified (see 1, 2, 3). These alternatives guide evaluators in choosing comparison groups in certain nonrandom ways, and in measuring suspected outcome variables at certain times, that will produce some degree of control over the influence of confounding variables.

Two strong quasi-experimental designs discussed in this book are *interrupted time series designs* and *regression discontinuity designs*. These designs are discussed in detail elsewhere (1,2) and cannot be fully described here. Briefly, however, an interrupted time series design involves taking repeated measurements of an outcome variable before and after a specific project is introduced. If the project has an effect, there will be an interruption in the

regular data pattern observed over time, and the interruption will
coincide with the point at which the project began operation (or
was in operation long enough for an effect to be expected). Briefly, a regression discontinuity design is useful when persons are
given or not given project services according to whether they are
above or below a cut-off point on a quantified continuum of merit
or need. If the project does affect the group that receives the
treatment, a discontinuity or interruption should appear in the regression line relating the merit or need variable and the outcome
variable of interest.

III.C.   Nonexperimental Design

A *nonexperimental design* typically does not involve comparing
designated treatment and control groups. Instead, nonexperimental
designs call for the researcher to examine the statistical relationships or correlations between treatment variables (e.g., kinds of
treatment, frequency of treatment) and outcome variables (e.g.,
health status on newborns, infant mortality) as well as a variety
of nontreatment variables (e.g., age of mothers) in a large number
of persons or groups of persons (some or all of whom have received
some treatment). Instead of achieving control by comparing randomly equivalent groups or special kinds of nonequivalent comparison
groups, control is achieved by statistical means. These nonexperimental studies are sometimes called *natural experiments*. Calling
them experiments is a misnomer in some senses since, technically,
the word "experiment" is reserved for studies that randomly distribute the treatment to some persons in the target population and
not to others. The emphasis, then, is on the word "natural". These
studies are natural in the sense that the researchers do not intervene in the process by which some persons in the target population
receive treatment and others do not.

Nonexperimental studies depend on *statistical control* rather
than experimental control to disentangle the influence of treatment
variables from the influence of nontreatment variables on the outcome variables. Here is a single example of how statistical control
is used. Consider again the example of a nutritional supplement
project for nursing mothers in a certain village. A nonexperimental
study would measure the treatment variables (e.g., how much of the
supplements which mothers consumed), nontreatment variables (e.g.,
infant's health) after the project had been in operation for some
time. Then researchers would conduct statistical analyses to determine the correlations between all these measured variables. Suppose that the researchers found (a) that infants whose mothers consumed more of the nutritional supplements were healthier than infants whose mothers consumed less (or more) of the supplements (a
positive correlation between infant's health and mother's consump-

tion of nutritional supplements); (b) that infants with younger mothers were healthier than infants with older mothers (a negative correlation between infant's health and mother's age); and (c) that younger mothers consumed more nutritional supplements than older mothers (a negative correltation between mother's age and consumption of nutritional supplements). Researchers need to determine whether some infants were healthier than others because of the nutrition supplements provided to their mothers, or simply because their mothers were younger. To do this researchers must be able to make some assumptions and test certain empirical relationships.

To begin with, the researchers can assume that the nutritional supplements did not cause the age of the mothers, rather the age of the mothers was in some way responsible for the amount of nutritional supplements consumed (i.e., younger mothers chose to or were more able to take advantage of the nutritional supplements offered). By making this assumption, the researchers rule out the possibility that the nutrition supplements alone were responsible for the differences in infant health. Next, they need to determine whether the supplements contributed at all to infant health, or whether the differences in infant health were totally due to the age of the mother.

To determine which of these explanations is true, the researchers rule out the possibility that the nutrition supplements alone were responsible for the differences in infant health. Next, they need to determine whether the supplements contributed at all to infant health, or whether the differences in infant health were totally due to the age of the mother.

To determine which of these explanations is true, the researchers examine the statistical relationship between the consumption of supplements and infant health with the influence of mother's age eliminated statistically by "partial correlation" method (i.e., the relationship between the consumption of supplements and the health of infants not counting their joint correlation with mother's age). If they find no relationship between these variables (once mother's age is controlled in this way), then, the researchers would be inclined to accept the second explanation as being closest to the truth.

This is an oversimplified example, in part because it involves only three variables, in part because the statistical methods that would be applied are more complex than this example suggests. But it does demonstrate the necessity of making assumptions about causal order where possible, and gathering empirical clues about the causal order of the other relationships studied. Note that accurate statistical control depends on accurate measurement and accurate assumptions.

The process described above used to analyze data in nonexperimental studies is often called *causal modeling*. Causal modeling calls for the measurement of treatment variables, outcome variables, and a host of nontreatment variables (since the influence of each nontreatment variable on the outcome variables must be distinguished from the influence of treatment variables on outcome variables).

In practice, evaluative research designs sometimes call for a mixture of experimental and statistical controls. Notice that experimental design primarily indicates how comparison groups should be formed and when measures should be taken, while nonexperimental designs call for accurate measurement of all nontreatment as well as treatment and outcome variables, and often requires a causal modeling approach to data analysis.

III.D. Design Issues

III.D.1 When are measurements taken? Evaluative research designs, particularly experimental designs, often call for pre-treatment measurements called *pretests*, or *baseline measures*, as well as post-treatment measurements called *posttests*. Baseline measures gauge the level of the problem for all persons in the study (e.g., persons in the experimental and control groups) before the project begins. In general, the more points in time at which measurements are taken before and after the project begins, the more confidently the outcomes of a project may be determined. In experimental designs, measures over time contribute to an understanding of the persistence of outcomes and possibly the sequence of outcomes from the most immediate to those that develop more slowly. In quasi-experimental designs, measures of nonequivalent comparison groups over time contribute to an understanding of the magnitude and nature of the nonequivalence between comparison groups as well as an understanding of outcomes. The more knowledge the researchers have about the nonequivalence of comparison groups, the more confidently they can separate the influence of those factors from the influence of the treatment on the outcomes measured.

In general, any time the same persons are measured on a set of variables at several points in time, the data is called *longitudinal data*. On the other hand, when a number of persons are measured on a set of variables at one point in time, the data is called *cross-sectional data*. Longitudinal data can involve pretests and posttests or multiple posttests. Experimental designs almost always involve some longitudinal measurement that can be used to determine whether a person's status on outcome variables changed. Two kinds of longitudinal measurement sometimes used in nonexperimental or quasi-experimental research are panel data and time series data.

Panel data is cross-sectional data taken at two points in time on the same persons. An advantage of panel studies is that they include measures of *lagged correlations* and *cross-lagged correlations* as well as *synchronous correlations*. The correlation between one variable as measured at time A and the same variable at time B is a lagged correlation. The correlation of one variable with a second variable at time A is a synchronous correlation. The correlation of one variable at time A with a second variable at time B is a cross-lagged correlation. Using lagged and cross-lagged correlations is advantageous because comparing correlations at different points in time aids in making assumptions about the order of causal relationships.

A *time series* is a special kind of longitudinal data. It involves measures of the same variables at multiple points in time for the same measurement unit (e.g., a person, a group, a community).

Most nonexperimental evaluative research uses data collected on a cross-section of people at one point in time. A cross-sectional sample typically includes persons who have received different amounts of the treatment being evaluated. There are many different ways this cross-section of people can be selected (see Section III. D.2.).

III.D.2. Who is measured? Every project that is to be evaluated has a *target group* or *target population* which is defined by the characteristics of the persons the project is trying to reach. The defining characteristics may be geographic, or related to need, or age, or virtually anything. For example, a nutrition supplement project might be aimed at mothers of newborns who live within walking distance of a new clinic, or it might be targeted at all school age children who attend a village school. In the first case, even though all the mothers of newborns within walking distance of the clinic may be in the target population, they will not all actually take advantage of the treatment the project offers. In the second case, all the children in the target population may participate if the treatment is delivered to each of them at school. The point is simply that the target population or target group for a project may not be the same as the group who actually receives the treatment. Only a small part of the target population may actually receive treatment. Ideally, treatment and control comparison groups both come from the target population.

An evaluative research design may call for measures from the entire target population, or if the target population is very large it may call for measures from a *sample* (a portion) of the target group. The target population is the *universe* from which samples are drawn. There are a number of ways to select a sample from some defined population or universe. A sample can be randomly selected, or purposely selected in a nonrandom way, or self-selected through volunteering.

Random selection of a sample involves selecting a particular number of persons at random from a larger group to be in a sample. The purpose of *random sampling* is to create a smaller group that is *representative* of the population sampled from, in this case, the target group. In other words, the smaller group or sample should contain about the same proportion of men and women, rich and poor, healthy and sick, and so on, as the target population contains. Random selection of a sample is not the same as *random assignment* to comparison groups although similar methods are used to achieve randomness. Recall that the purpose of random assignment is to divide a large group (not necessarily the entire target group) into two or more randomly equivalent comparison groups. The comparison groups may or may not be representative of the total target population. On the other hand, the purpose of random sampling is to select a smaller group that is representative of the larger group (target population) from which it was selected. After random assignment, the researcher has two (or more) groups that are randomly equivalent to each other, whereas after random selection of a sample, the researcher has one group that is representative of the total target population.

Nonrandom samples are sometimes selected, but it should be remembered that they are typically not representative of the target population. One form of nonrandom sampling is *purposive sampling for heterogeneity*. Researchers may select a sample that contains instances of all the different kinds of persons or kinds of treatment-related problems in the target population rather than choosing a strictly representative sample which also includes instances of all the different people or problems, but in the same proportion that they are present in the target population. The former is a purposive sample selected for heterogeneity, while the latter is a representative sample.

A sample is sometimes *stratified* across certain variables, for example, a sample of treatment recipients may be stratified across income. This means that recipients from each of several designated income levels are chosen for the sample. While stratification may lead to nonrandom samples if persons with designated income levels are purposely chosen, on the other hand, the samples may be randomly selected from designated income levels. In other words, a sample may be randomly selected within each income level but stratified (nonrandom) across designated income levels.

Another form of nonrandom sample is a *volunteer sample*. A volunteer sample is a *self-selected sample*. For example, a project distributing a new crop fertilizer might provide the fertilizer to any farmer in the village who wished to try it. The treatment group for this project would be a volunteer (or self-selected) sample of farmers from the village. Self-selected samples are almost never representative and are usually *biased* in unclear or unknown ways. Therefore, it is usually not legitimate to generalize from self-selected samples to the population from which they come.

While sampling most often involves selecting persons to be studied, it can also involve selecting projects from a defined population of projects (i.e., a program) or selecting any units from a defined population of those units.

IV MEASUREMENT

IV.A What is Measurement?

Measurement is an attempt to specify the type and/or level of certain objects, properties, or behaviors on some qualitative or quantitative scale. There are four levels of measurement. At the least precise level is nominal or categorical measurement, in which objects, properties, or behaviors are simply classified into groups that are qualitatively different. Grouping people according to their political party, or whether they are farmers or non-farmers, are examples of nominal measurement.

Ordinal measurement, in which objects or properties are ordered in a quantitative dimension is a level of measurement with more precision than nominal measurement. *Rank ordering* people from least healthy to most healthy is an example of ordinal measurement. Assigning people a level on some ordered quantitative scale is also ordinal measurement. For example, people might be classified as more healthy or less healthy than a particular standard level. When there are only two levels of an ordinal measure it is said to be *dichotomous*. When there are three or more levels of an ordinal (or interval or ratio) measure, it is said to be *continuous*. Ordinal measurement is often used in evaluative research.

The difference between the highest score and the next highest score on an ordinal scale may not be the same as the distance between any other two contiguous scores on the scale. For example, the difference between the healthiest person in a group and the second healthiest is not necessarily the same as the difference between the second and the third or the third and fourth healthiest. Interval measurement is involved when consecutive scores on a scale are the same distance apart. Temperature measured by degrees Centigrade or Fahrenheit is measured by an interval scale -- the difference between one consecutive degree and another is the same regardless of how high or how low the temperature might be. Interval scales are only occasionally used in evaluative research.

Interval scales do not permit the formation of ratios because they have arbitrary zero points. Zero degrees of temperature Centigrade does not indicate the absence of temperature, so that even though the number 4 is twice as big as the number 2, 4° of temperature does not represent twice as much as 2°. If a scale allows the formation of ratios then ratio measurement is involved. Length, mass, and time are ordinarily measured with a ratio scale. (Temperature can also be measured with a ratio scale when it is recorded in degrees Kelvin).

All four levels of measurement can be used in evaluative research. Though there is a preference for the more precise levels, it is often only possible to measure the variable of interest on an ordinal scale.

IV.B.   Which Variables are Measured?

While the research design indicates who is to be measured and when, it is the conceptual model of hypotheses about the project treatment that determines which variables are measured. In evaluative research, these variables fall into three broad categories: (1) treatment variables; (2) outcome variables; and (3) nontreatment variables.

IV.B.1.   Treatment variables. Alternative labels that denote variables that fall in this category are *inputs* or *input variables, intervention variables, project variables,* and *program variables.* The focus here is on variables that indicate answers to questions such as: What kinds of services did a project provide to whom? How much of which services did which project recipients actually use? Over what period of time did recipients receive services? How well were the project services or treatments delivered? What skills did the dispensers possess? In short, treatment variables describe the nature and extent of the project as implemented, who received its services, and what the qualifications of the project's staff were.

The treatment variables are also called the *independent variables.* They are intended to operationally represent the project and its treatment as it was implemented. Taking these variables as given, researchers look for changes in outcome variables that are caused by, or are dependent on, the project treatment, as represented by the treatment variables. Independent variables are often *controllable* or *manipulable variables* in the sense that they can be purposely set at particular levels. For instance, the grams of nutritional supplements distributed to each project client can be controlled or set by an administrator. If clients are asked to consume the supplement while they are at the project site, the grams of nutritional supplements actually consumed by each client may also be controlled.

IV.B.2. <u>Outcome variables</u>. The measured *effects, outcomes,* or *impact* of a treatment of project are the *outcome variables,* or *impact variables.* The outcomes of a treatment are dependent on the level of the treatment and so they are also called *dependent variables.*

The effects of a treatment may accumulate over time. For example, shortly after a nutrition project is started, weights and other anthropometric indices may increase but IQ scores may not be effected. Given time, however, IQ scores may improve and ultimately the impact of such a project may be to stimulate desires for higher education or more challenging jobs. Thus, writers often distinguish between *immediate* and *ultimate outcomes, initial* and *eventual outcomes, proximal* and *distal outcomes,* or even *outcomes* and *impacts.* When these distinctions are made, it is assumed that there is a *chain of cause and effect,* whereby the occurrence of an immediate, initial or proximal outcome (e.g., increased weight/anthropometric indices) is followed by an ultimate, eventual, or distal outcome or impact (e.g., increased IQ scores).

Sometimes even more distal outcomes are later observed or measured. For example, the children of adults in a reading project may demonstrate improved reading skills. Or many people with improved reading skills might become unemployed because they would like more challenging jobs which are not available. Such effects are known as *unintended outcomes* or side effects. As demonstrated above side effects may be desirable or undesirable.

IV.B.3. <u>Nontreatment variables</u>. We define as "nontreatment variables" any variables that are neither treatment (independent) variables nor outcome (dependent) variables. While treatment variables describe project inputs and outcome variables describe project outcomes or impact, *nontreatment variables* represent conditions other than the treatment that may influence the effects of the treatment. Context variables, confounding variables, mediating variables, and control variables are names for different roles that a nontreatment variable may play in the research.

Context variables simply describe the social situation or context in which the program being evaluated is taking place. Examples of context variables include the educational status or economic status of the recipients, or political forces operating in the community. For example, a nutrition supplement might be administered only to people of low educational attainment. The effects of such a program cannot be generalized to people of higher educational attainment.

When a nontreatment variable is present at one level for the control group and a different level for the treatment group it is impossible to say whether any outcomes are due to the treatment or this other variable. Such variables are known as *confounding variables* because their effects on outcomes cannot be separated from the effects of the treatment (i.e., they may "confound" the results). When a nontreatment variable is known or assumed to influence, moderate, or mediate the effects of a treatment on an outcome, it is known as a *mediating variable* (or *moderating, intervening, intermediate,* or *intermediary variable* or *conditioning factor*). For example, if nutrition supplements are administered to children of both high and low socio-economic status but effects are found only for children of low socio-economic status, then socio-economic status mediates the effect of nutrition supplements and is called a mediating variable. Alternatively, it may be that all children respond to nutrition supplements but lower class children respond to a greater degree than higher class children. If this is known before a study, and the effects of socio-economic status are statistically controlled when the effects of the treatment are being assessed, then social class may be known as a *control variable*.

It is evident that the four roles of nontreatment variables described above are not always mutually exclusive. Sometimes one variable such as social class status may be cast in the role of a context variable, sometimes as a control variable, and even sometimes as an outcome or dependent variable. Any division into types of variable is only a heuristic device, and we have indicated some distinctions often but not always, made between types of non-treatment variables.

IV.B.4. Variables in empirical models. Just as nontreatment variables may be labeled differently according to the role they play in the research and data analysis, variables in empirical models (see Section II.B.) are also labeled according to their role. The variables in a model are called exogenous or endogenous. *Exogenous variables* are variables that are assumed not to be caused by any of the variables in the model. Exogenous variables are taken as given, the researcher makes no attempt to explain their cause. In this sense, they are independent of the other variables in the model. They play the role of causal variables and not effects. The variables in a model that are studied as effects, the variables whose cause the researcher is trying to identify, are called *endogenous variables*. Endogeneous variables may be mutually dependent on each other as well as dependent on exogeneous variables.

IV.C. How are Variables Measured?

IV.C.1. Operationalizing constructs. Researchers use the word *variable* in two senses. It can mean a conceptual variable or abstract concept such as health, mathematical reasoning ability, or intelligence, or it can refer to concrete questions or observations like a medical examination, a white blood cell count, twenty questions on a mathematical reasoning test, or an IQ test. Conceptual variables are called *constructs*. Concrete (measurable) variables are called *operational variables*. Though researchers often think and write in terms of constructs, these conceptual variables typically cannot be directly measured. So constructs are *operationalized* or *operationally defined* by selecting one or more concrete, measurable variables that capture the meaning of the construct. *Measures*, then, are operational variables. *Indicators* or *indices* refer to operational variables that reflect or estimate the underlying designated construct.

IV.C.2. Measurement instruments. Scales, tests, questionnaires and interviews are all measurement instruments. Continuous variables are measured on *scales*. For example, a recipient's satisfaction with the treatment can be measured on a continuum from very satisfied to not at all satisfied. This can be accomplished using the simplest kind of scale that requires the recipient to answer one question that places his or her feelings on the continuum, or it may be accomplished by combining the recipient's responses to several questions (e.g., about different aspects of the treatment). One kind of simple scale format is a *semantic differential*. It provides the respondent with opposite adjective pairs as end points on a continuum (e.g., satisfied_ _ _dissatisfied), and requires that the respondent indicate where his feelings lie on the continuum, usually with five or seven points in between (e.g., satisfied _ x _ _ _ dissatisfied). Asking respondents to *rank order* a set of responses or events from least to most important, satisfying or healthy (etc.) is another kind of scale. Sometimes a set of questions are asked or a set of observations are taken and researchers use this information to form an *index* that places each individual on some continuum (e.g., health index). Sometimes quite complex methods are used to determine a single scale score from several items of information. Established sets of questions, particularly those that scale a person's abilities,knowledge or achievements are often called *tests*.

Questionnaires and *interviews* typically ask about (aim to measure) several different variables. They involve a list of questions that may be answered in a structured or in a flexible format using either *closed-ended* or *open-ended* questions. Closed-ended questions have precoded response options. This means the respondent or interviewer merely has to check or circle the most appropriate response. Open-ended questions on the other hand, allow respondents to give answers in their own words. Their responses may later be subjected to *content analysis* in which the researcher develops categories of answers and classifies each respondent's answers according to these categories.

In many countries important economic, social, and health characteristics of the population are routinely monitored. This means that many *indicators* of the economic status (economic indicators), social well-being (social indicators), or health status (health indicators) of the population are available to evaluation researchers. Examples of indicators of health include death rate, age at death, infant mortality rate, morbidity rate, etc. Sometimes social or economic indicators are used as *proxy measures* of health status because they are known to be correlated with more direct measures of health status. Proxy measures are used when more direct measures of the construct of interest are unavailable or cannot be taken.

The usefulness of indicators often depends on the *unit of measurement,* or the *level of aggregation* of the information. The measurement unit may be individuals, classrooms, households, communities, or even countries. The unit of measurement for the gross national product, for example, is the country if this indicator is based on country-wide production statistics. On the other hand, the unit of measurement for a country's female marriage ratio is the individual. The marriage ratio for women in the U.S., for example, would be based on determining whether each individual woman in the U.S. was married or not, then taking the ratio of married to unmarried women. Both of the examples just given are *aggregated* to the country level. The first example, gross national product, could not be *disaggregated* if the original data was collected at the national level. However, if the original data was collected at a state or regional level, disaggregation to these levels would be possible so long as those records were kept. The second example, marriage ratio, might be disaggregated to the state level, or city level, by taking the ratio of married to unmarried women within each state or community. While it is possible in theory to disaggregate an indicator such as the marriage ratio, it may not be possible in practice. Often the individual level data that is needed to form the indicator is destroyed or unrecoverable and only the aggregated indicator is available for use.

IV.C.3. Methods of gathering measurements. There are a number of major methods that a researcher may use to gather measurements, each of which may incorporate a variety of techniques such as the administration of formal tests, direct physical measurement, and other kinds of systematic observation. Some of the basic tools are archives, observation, surveys, interviews, and questionnaires.

Some projects routinely record information about their clients, their staff, and their interactions. These project *archives* of information are sometimes useful to evaluators. Archives of country and local, economic and social or health indicators, may also be consulted by evaluators. Since the information in archives is usually collected primarily for other purposes (project administration, government administration), it may be distorted in ways compatible with its purpose but not with evaluative research. Before using

such data, evaluators familiarize themselves with the process by
which the information is archived, so that they are aware of its
probable completeness and accuracy. Often, researchers will choose
to supplement *archival data* that is available with data they gather
themselves by making systematic observations or conducting surveys
or interviews.

Observation involves researchers observing certain events or
behaviors, or taking direct physical or chemical measures, and recording the data in a systematic way. Usually more than one observ-
er or more than one observation of the same event is required to increase the reliability of the recorded information. To make the observation less obvious and to minimize possible disruption of the
normal routine, researchers sometimes become participants in the
project event themselves and make observations as participants.
This is called *participant observation*.

Surveys involve asking persons, via a questionnaire or an interview, to respond to groups of questions, check lists, inventories or
items on tests that are designed to measure certain constructs. *Interviews* basically involve asking persons to respond to an oral questionnaire. When administering surveys or interviews, it is advantageous to use a set of *standard procedures*. This reduces the variability in answers due to extraneous factors such as different word-
ings, settings, etc.

The development of *interview schedules* and survey questionnaires,
tests or scales is sometimes called *instrumentation*. The first step
in instrumentation is to determine how the constructs of interest
can be operationalized. Questions and items are then developed according to the operational definitions. At a final stage of instrumentation researchers may test their instruments on a group of persons who are very similar to, or are a small sample of, the target
population to follow the planned measuring procedures and answer
the planned questions. This *pilot testing* (or *pretesting*) stage
usually results in several reviews of the procedures and questions.
It is important in maximizing the attributes of good measures.

IV.D. Attributes of Good Measures

IV.D.1. Validity. The most important characteristic of a
measure is its *validity*. Operational measures are said to have
construct validity to the extent that they truly represent the intended constructs. While an empirical coefficient of validity is
not typically calculated, instruments can be *validated* in several
ways. First, measures can have face validity, in that those who
are familiar with the project and its operations agree that the
measures are reasonable operationalizations of the constructs of
interest. Second, if measures are valid, then there should be

congruity among alternative measures of the same construct; that is, they should be highly correlated. This is called convergent validity. On the other hand, measures of different constructs should not be highly correlated. This is called divergent validity. Measures with high validity are *specific* in that they reflect variations in the target construct but do not reflect variations in other constructs. The validity of measures can sometimes be checked by comparing the measures with behavioral criteria or archival records of an event. For example, the validity of mothers' reports of their children's ages might be checked by locating old hospital and clinic records that list the birth dates. This approach to assessing validity is also known as the *multicriteria* approach in that multiple criteria are used.

A further aspect of validity, familiar to epidemiologists, is the ability of a measure, a test or a screening procedure to classify people or their attributes correctly according to some criterion. There are two ways in which a test can be wrong. It can "detect" an attribute that the individual does not possess (false positive); or it can fail to detect the attribute when the person does in fact have it (false negative). The *sensitivity* of a measure or procedure is the extent to which individuals who truly manifest an attribute are so classified by the procedure. The more sensitive a screening test is the smaller the number of *false negatives* it produces, with the perfectly sensitive test yielding no false negatives. The converse of sensitivity is *specificity*, which is the ability to identify correctly those who do *not* have the attribute -- hence to minimize the number of false positives. Specificity and sensitivity are not necessarily complementary: a sensitive procedure may also be specific, but it may not be. Some tests are both sensitive and specific while others are neither and hence are useless. In choosing a test for a specific purpose in an evaluation, it may be necessary to accept poor specificity in order to have adequate sensitivity (or vice versa, depending on which property is more important for the evaluative purpose).

Finally, when a measure is being used to classify people or their attributes according to some criterion, it may be possible to adjust the *cutting point* (or *cut-off score*) so as to maximize either specificity or sensitivity. The *cutting point* is the value of the variable at which an individual is assigned to the "has attribute" category. For example, a cutting point for classifying a child as malnourished might be chosen as the 5th percentile on the Boston weight/age norms or as the 25th percentile. Obviously the former cut-off score would produce fewer false positives (i.e.fewer children classified as malnourished who were in fact not malnourished but only slight of build; hence, it would be more specific than a cut off at the 25th percentile). On the other hand, a 25th percentile cutting point would yield a much larger number of children

classified as "malnourished" and would be more sensitive since it
would misclassify fewer genuinely malnourished ones. In this particular example, greater specificity is achieved at the cost of less
sensitivity and vice versa.

IV.D.2. Reliability. A second important characteristic of
measures is *reliability*. Reliable measures yield stable, consistent
measures of a construct. If measures are reliable, then one gets
almost the same measurement each time the same person is measured.
Height and weight, for example, can be measured quite reliably
while the percentage of fat in the body or the tone of muscles are
measured less reliably. The more reliable the measurement, the
more capable it is of detecting changes in the construct. Even an
unreliable scale can detect a 10-pound weight gain in a child, but
a very reliable one is needed to establish a gain of one ounce.

Empirical coefficients of reliability can be calculated for
measures when *redundancy* is built into the measurement process. For
example, if five questions are asked about a person's understanding
of the principles of home sanitation, the correlations among each
person's answers to these five questions will reflect the internal
consistency or *constancy* of the knowledge-of-home-sanitation index
formed by these questions. The internal consistency among several
items designed to measure a single construct is the basis of one
method of empirically estimating measurement reliability. Other
methods include giving the same test or set of questions to the
same persons twice (test-retest reliability method) or comparing a
person's responses on half of a test with those on the other half
(split-half reliability method).

Elaborate procedures have been developed to maximize the reliability and comparability of measures taken by tests designed to
measure constructs such as intelligence, aptitude, and achievement.
Such tests are often *standardized tests* which means not only that
they are administered according to a set of standard procedures,
but also that the scoring of the tests is based on the performance
of a representative sample of the population they are intended for.
Further, many tests (whether standardized tests or not) report results in terms of *standard scores* which facilitate comprehension,
comparison between tests (or alternate forms of the same test) and
with established norms.

IV.D.3. Measurement error. No matter how carefully measures
are taken, there will almost always be some *error in measurement*.
If a person's height were measured four times on the same day and
the height recorded to the nearest millimeter, the four estimates
would probably vary slightly. The more reliable the measurement,
the less error in measurement. Less reliable measures include a
larger component of error. Most of the analysis techniques that re-

searchers use assume *random errors of measurement* -- that is, that
a measure just as often errs by overestimation as by underestimation.
Systematic error in measurement, sometimes called *measurement bias*,
is quite different. Whenever a test result is systematically larger than the true value (or systematically smaller), the measure is
said to be biased. For example, when a measuring instrument is
wrongly calibrated, it may always overestimate the quality it is
measuring.

IV.D.4. Reactivity and response bias. A third important characteristic of measurement is *reactivity*. Researchers want to minimize reactivity in measurement. Measurement is said to be reactive
to the extent that the act of measuring itself influences the responses measured. Persons may act differently if they know an
evaluator is making observations. Or, persons may not answer according to the way they actually think or act, but according to the way
they think they ought to think and act, or the way they think the
researcher would like them to think or act. These last examples of
reactivity are examples of a *response bias*. Respondents' answers
to questions are sometimes affected by the image they want to present of themselves or the image they think the researcher is looking for. Researchers attempt to word questions and design measurement procedures in ways that minimize response bias.

One way to avoid reactivity in measurement is to avoid staging
an event or asking questions just for the purposes of measurement
as is the case with surveys or interviews. Measures that avoid
reactivity in this way are called *unobtrusive measures*. Gathering
data in naturally occurring situations like measuring physical
traces that are indicative of certain activities (e.g., counting
empty containers to estimate food consumption) or making observations as one of the participants (participant observation) in a
situation are two examples of unobtrusive measures. Gathering data
from archival records that are routinely collected anyway, is a
third source of data for unobtrusive measures.

V. DESCRIBING THE RELATIONSHIP BETWEEN VARIABLES

V.A. Statistics

A major object of data analysis is to describe accurately the
relationship between variables. When two variables are *statistically related* in a systematic way, they are said to be *correlated, associated,* or *linked*. This means that when one variable changes, the
other variable can be expected to change also. When two are related in this way each is said to be a *correlate* of the other.

The degree of relationship between variables is indicated by the *correlation coefficient* which can range from +1.00 through to -1.00. When two variables are significantly correlated the correlation coefficient is significantly (see statistical significance in Section V.B.3.) different from zero. When there is a *positive correlation* between variables an increase in one will be accompanied by an increase in the other. When there is a *negative correlation* between variables an increase in one will be accompanied by a decrease in the other. For example, weight gain is positively correlated with caloric intake and negatively correlated with energy expended on work or exercise.

In addition to the relationship between two variables, researchers are often interested in the average value of a variable, or some other measure of "central tendency". The average may be either a *mean* or a *median* (middle), depending on the nature of the data. Both give an indication of the most common or most likely value of the variable for a given group of persons. A third basic statistic, the *range, variance, standard deviation* or *coefficient of variation,* is a measure of the dispersion or scatter of values around central tendency; it describes the *variability* among observations.

Some characteristics have more variability than others. For example, in any given rural community the heights of adult males will vary much less than their incomes. The range of heights might be from 165 to 180 cm. with an average height of about 175 cm. The range (15 cm.) is less than one-tenth as large as the average. In contrast, cash income might well vary from one thousand to as much as ten thousand pesos with a median income of, say, 2000 pesos. For income, the variability is much greater, for the range (9000 pesos) is more than four times as large as the average.

The mean, median, and variance can be calculated for any continous variable measured for a particular group of persons.

The variance associated with the outcomes measured in evaluative studies is quite important because the object of data analysis is to explain as much of this variation as possible, and in particular to estimate the portion of the variance that was caused by the treatment. This is done by estimating the size of several identified components of variance (e.g., that due to specific treatment factors, and non-treatment factors). In general there are systematic and random components of the variance. The systematic or deterministic variance is the portion that is contributed by identifiable factors. The random or stochastic variance arises from errors in measurement. This component is also known as *disturbance, noise,* or *error variance,* or just *error,* or, since it is typically estimated by what is left when the deterministic variability is taken out, it is sometimes called the *residual variance* or *residual error.*

V.B.   Data Analysis

V.B.1. Making causal inferences. In the data analysis stage,
evaluative researchers are ultimately concerned with the nature of
the relationship between treatment and outcome variables -- is there
a causal relationship? Making this judgment is called making a *causal inference*, or a *causal attribution* or determining that there is
a *causal link* between two variables. There are three conditions
that must be considered in order to determine whether a relationship is causal.

The first requirement for making a causal inference is to establish that the two variables of interest are systematically related. One variable cannot be a cause of the other unless the two variables are correlated in some way. However, being correlated is
not enough to establish that there is a causal relationship between
the two variables, for correlations are *bi-directional*. The correlation coefficient does not suggest which variable may have preceded the other (e.g., did A cause B or did B cause A?). Logically,
a cause must precede its effect. So a second requirement for making
a causal inference is that the *direction of causality* must be clear.
It must be clear that the presumed causal variable preceded the presumed effect. In the case of evaluative research, the researcher
needs to demonstrate that the treatment (presumed cause) precedes
an observed improvement in the outcomes of interest (presumed effect) rather than the other way around. For example, if researchers find a positive correlation between the number of visits to a
local clinic and a measure of health (e.g., morbidity), they must
determine whether making visits to the clinic preceded better health
(and therefore may have caused better health via the treatment delivered) or whether better health preceded visits to the clinic
(and may have caused visits to the clinic in the sense that only the
healthier people were able to reach, or were interested in going to
the clinic).

The third requirement for making causal inferences is to rule
out the possibility that some third variable or variables caused
both of the variables of interest. In particular, evaluative researchers need to establish that nontreatment variables were not
the sole cause of all observed improvements.

In all research, the first requirement for making a causal inference -- that the two variables in question are systematically
related -- is determined by statistical calculations. Various procedures may be used, but they all involve estimates of correlation
and estimates of variance. The second requirement -- that the direction of causality be established -- is achieved in different
ways. In experimental research, the order of variables is known.

Differences on treatment variables are created across comparison
groups that initially are randomly equivalent on outcome variables
and on nontreatment variables. If some time later, a difference
between comparison groups on the outcome variables is observed, the
researchers know that the difference on outcome variables was preceded by a difference on treatment variables. In nonexperimental
research, however, the order of variables is not known, particularly
in research that uses data that was all collected at one point in
time. This produces the problem of *simultaneity*. When all the
measures in a study are taken simultaneously, the direction of causality between variables is not known with certainty. In many instances, however, researchers can make assumptions about the causal
order, relying on common sense, other data, and partial correlations or other statistical procedures to provide clues.

The third requirement for making causal inferences -- to rule
out the possibility that some third variable (e.g., a nontreatment
variable) is the cause of both of the variables in question -- is
also achieved differently in experimental and nonexperimental research. In experimental studies the influence of nontreatment variables is controlled experimentally. *Experimental control* is explained in Section III.A. In nonexperimental studies, the influence
of nontreatment variables is controlled statistically, in the data
analysis stage. *Statistical control* is explained in Section III.C.

V.B.2. Data analysis procedures. Several specialized procedures have been developed to suit the particular data analysis needs
of a research design. In the data analysis stage, experimental researchers are primarily concerned with establishing whether there
is a statistically significant correlation between treatment and
outcome variables. The other two requirements for making causal
inferences are met before the data analysis stage in experimental
studies. Experimental data is typically analyzed using some kind
of *analysis of variance* procedures. A discussion of these procedures is beyond the scope of this chapter, but interested readers
may consult (4, 5) both of which are good basic textbooks on the
analysis of experimental data.

In nonexperimental research, all three requirements for making
causal inferences must be met in the data analysis stage. Consequently, there are several different approaches to data analysis
that are commonly used including *multiple regression,* or *path analysis* or causal modeling using regression, *structural equations*, or
simultaneous equations. For a discussion of these procedures, interested readers are referred to such basic texts (6, 7, 8).

Of course, many evaluative research studies including those
with quasi-experimental research designs, use combinations of techniques that are typical in experimental research and techniques

that are typical in nonexperimental research.

   V.B.3. Statistical significance.   When researchers find that
a treatment probably did cause an outcome (i.e., the requirements
for making a causal inference are met), they have found a *treatment effect* or simply, an *effect*. To aid them in their search for
treatment effects, researchers typically hypothesize that certain
variables cause certain outcomes (*causal hypotheses*). Conceptual
models involve a set of causal hypotheses. It is in the data analysis stage that researchers test each of their causal hypotheses
and determine which are effects. However, since there is error in
measurement and variables themselves sometimes have considerable
variability, researchers are careful to determine the likelihood
that any apparent treatment effect is real and not simply due to
chance variations in the variable. For this reason data analysis
procedures include *tests of significance* that compare the estimated
magnitude of a treatment effect to the amount of variability in the
data. By convention, researchers call an observed effect *statistically significant* when this test suggests that an effect of the
magnitude observed would occur strictly by chance less than five
out of 100 times. An estimate of the probability that an effect
occurred by chance alone is called the *confidence level* or the *significance level*.

   When the detected effect is not a real one, the finding is
called a *false positive*. When a test fails to detect an effect
where the treatment actually does cause improvements in outcomes,
the finding is called a *false negative*. If the measures taken have
construct validity (see Section IV.D1.), the researchers may estimate
the likelihood of *spurious negative findings* (false negatives) by
calculating the *statistical power* of the particular data analysis
they used to detect an effect for a given set of variables.

   In a general sense, statistical power can be thought of as an
estimate of the capacity of a particular statistical analysis to detect effects of various sizes. Statistical significance can be
thought of as an estimate of how likely it is that an observed effect is not simply due to chance.

   It should be noted that statistical significance does not necessarily imply *social significance*. When the number of people measured is great, a small effect may be detected as statistically significant (i.e., very likely to be a true effect). However, it may
be too small to make a practical difference in peoples' lives or
to be the basis of a policy decision.

V.C. The Validity of Causal Inference

   A major concern of researchers is the validity of causal inference. This type of validity, called *internal validity*, should

be distinguished from construct validity, discussed in Section IV.
D.1., and external validity discussed in Section V.C.3. Internal
validity is concerned with whether or not there was a cause and effect relationship between the independent or treatment variable as
operationalized. Researchers must be wary of common *threats to internal validity* or *plausible rival hypotheses* that could explain
observed effects (see 1, 3).

V.C.1. Some threats to internal validity in experiments. Random assignment for group comparability rules out most threats to internal validity. However, three threats mentioned in this volume
that random assignment does not rule out are attrition, resentful
demoralization of controls, and compensatory rivalry.

It is almost inevitable that some people will drop out of the
treatment and control comparison groups that were randomly formed
at the start of the research. If more persons or different kinds
of persons drop out of one group than another, the researchers are
faced with a problem called *systematic* or *differential attrition*.
This is a problem because an observed difference between a treatment
and a no-treatment group at the end of the research may be due to
attrition rather than the effectiveness of the project. It could be
due to the fact that the persons who dropped out of the treatment
group were worse off in the beginning than those who completed the
project. Or, it may be due to the fact that all the persons for
whom the treatment was ineffective dropped out before the post-
project measurements of outcomes were taken. In any case, experimental researchers must carefully monitor attrition in order to decide
whether this plausible alternative explanation for differences found
between comparison groups can or cannot be ruled out.

Other problems experimental researchers may encounter have been
called the *resentful demoralization of controls* and *compensatory
rivalry*. If the persons who are in a control group are aware of the
fact that persons in a project group are receiving some treatment
that they are not receiving, these persons in a control group may
resent this difference. This resentment or demoralization may lead
persons in control groups to behave in ways they would not have otherwise. For example, they may actively seek to obtain the experimental treatment or an equivalent treatment and may be wholly or partially successful. Such an occurrence can change a no-treatment control group -- a group that feels resentment. Awareness of the difference in treatment received may lead to rivalry on the part of
members of a control group in the sense that they may try to outper-
form the treated group on outcome measures -- e.g., to feed their
children better, improve their houses or the cultivation of their
crops. Their increased motivation, again makes a no-treatment control group more like an alternative treatment group. These problems
are most likely to arise when control and treatment groups are in

close contact or communication, and when the project is aimed at affecting some outcome that is within voluntary control. Evaluation
researchers must always consider the possibility of such influences
on the control group and decide to what extent they may have affected
the nature of differences between the treated and control groups.

V.C.2. Some threats to internal validity in non-experiments
and some quasi-experiments. Important threats to the internal
validity of nonexperimental and quasi-experimental designs have been
identified and discussed in detail elsewhere (1, 3). Only those
threats mentioned in this book will be described here.

One of the primary threats to internal validity in non-experimental research is the problem of *simultaneity* (see Section V.B.1).
Whenever all of the variables of interest are measured at one point
in time the causal order (i.e., which is the cause and which is the
effect) is not known. Another important threat to internal validity
in nonexperimental research is *omitted variable bias*. Since the
influence of nontreatment variables must be statistically controlled, each nontreatment variable that may affect the outcomes must
be measured in order for its influence to be controlled.

Selection bias is a third threat to internal validity in non-
experimental and some quasi-experimental research. In experimental
research comparison groups are assumed to be equivalent at the start,
because they are randomly assigned, but in quasi-experimental designs and in the statistical control approach to evaluative research, comparisons are made between admittedly nonequivalent
groups. Unless the receipt of a treatment is randomly assigned,
there are bound to be differences between the persons who do and
do not receive the treatment. Treatment may go to the neediest,
the first to come in, the most highly motivated, the youngest, the
oldest, the poorest, the richest and so on. When persons are selected to receive a treatment in a nonrandom way (especially if it
is self-selection) a selection bias is introduced in determining
the effectiveness of the treatment being evaluated. If there is
later found a difference between persons who received the project
treatment and those who did not, this may be due to the effectiveness of the treatment or to the ways that persons who were in the
project were already different from persons not in the project.
For example, children enrolled in a reading project may have been
better educated to begin with than children who were not in the
project. Or the mothers involved in a nutritional supplement project may have been initially less well nourished than mothers who
were not involved in the project. Such pre-project differences on
the outcomes that a project is designed to affect, are called *pretest differences*.

Since these pretest differences confound the meaning of any
post-project differences, researchers have sometimes tried to use

statistical adjustments to eliminate the influence of pretest differences on the analysis of posttest differences. Unfortunately, it
has been shown that the influence of pretest differences cannot be
completely removed by such means; instead, these adjustments typically introduce an *underadjustment bias*.

Sometimes nonexperimental researchers try to avoid the problems
caused by pretest differences by *matching* characteristics of persons
in a treatment group with the characteristics of persons who did not
receive the treatment in order to select a matched no-treatment control group. For example, suppose that a nutrition project is set
up in a community where the children are severely malnourished. In
order to determine the effectiveness of the nutrition project, researchers want to select a no-treatment control group but feel morally obligated to feed all the children in the "experimental" community. So they search surrounding communities (where malnutrition
in general is not as severe as in the project community) in order to
identify children who are just as severely malnourished as children
in the project. While this matching procedure eliminates pretest
differences in malnutrition between the project and control group,
it introduces other problems in interpreting the posttest results.

The principal problem this sort of matching introduces has to
do with *statistical regression*. All measures have some amount of
random error. If a person is measured several times on the same
variable, a distribution of different scores will be obtained. When
the errors in measurement are random, the measures are just as likely to be too high as too low. This means that the middle score,
the mean, is the best estimate of the person's true score on that
variable. If a person scores unusually high at one point in time,
it is likely that the next time the person is measured on that variable his score will be lower, closer to what would be the mean of
his distribution of scores if he had been measured on the variable
several times. In short, persons who score unusually high at one
point can be expected to score lower and persons who score unusually
low at one point in time can be expected to score higher. This is
called *regression toward the mean*.

When a group of persons are measured, one can expect just as
many persons to be measured too high as too low. So when this
group is measured again, the average or mean score for the group can
be expected to remain the same even though those in the group who
scored unusually high the first time will tend to score lower and
those who scored unusually low the first time will tend to score
higher. When, on the other hand, a group is composed of persons
who were selected because of their high scores, one can expect that
a greater number of persons in that group have scores that are too
high than scores that are too low. So when this group is measured
again, one would expect the average or mean score for the group will

be lower since many persons whose scores were unusually high the first time will tend to score lower. Therefore, if evaluators compared children from a very poor community which has a nutrition project with children from other communities selected because their malnutrition scores were as high as the project children's malnutrition scores, one would expect the next time the children in both groups were measured that the control group of children would score lower on malnutrition than the project group scores simply because of statistical regression. This is called a *regression effect*.

V.C.3. External validity. A third major type of validity is called external validity. A treatment effect has external validity when it is believed to *generalize* to other settings, other people, other places, at other times. For example, if a nutritional supplement project was successful at a clinic in a city, would it be as successful at an outpost serving a rural area? Whether or not a treatment effect is generalizable depends on the extent to which the procedures used, the setting, and the characteristics of the target population served by the project being evaluated are representative of those to be used elsewhere. That is, external validity depends on the correspondence between the sample (of procedures, people, or projects) studied and the population to which generalization is desired.

It is sometimes difficult to maximize both the internal validity and the external validity of research at the same time. When sacrifices have to be made, the experimental approach to evaluative research sacrifices some external validity in favor of maximizing internal validity, while the statistical control approach sacrifices some internal validity in favor of maximizing external validity.

ACKNOWLEDGEMENT

The authors would like to thank Henry W. Riecken and Thomas D. Cook for their very helpful comments and criticisms on drafts of this chapter.

VI.   REFERENCES

1.   Cook, T. D., and D. T. Campbell. The design and conduct of
        quasi-experiments for field settings. In: M. D. Dunnette
        (ed.). *Handbook of Organizational and Industrial Psychol-
        ogy*. Skokie, Illinois: Rand-McNally, 1976.
2.   Riecken, H. W., and R. F. Boruch (eds.). *Social Experimenta-
        tion: A Method for Planning and Evaluating Social Inter-
        vention*. New York, Academic Press, 1974.

3.   Campbell, D. T., and J. C. Stanley. *Experimental and Quasi-experimental Designs for Research*. Chicago: Rand McNally, 1966.
4.   Winer, B. J. *Statistical Principles in Experimental Design*. McGraw-Hill, 1971.
5.   Keppel, G. *Design and Analysis: A Researcher's Handbook*. Englewood Cliffs: Prentice Hall, Inc., 1973.
6.   Blalock, H. M., Jr. (ed.). *Causal Models in the Social Sciences*. Chicago: Aldine, Atherton, 1971.
7.   Bock, R. D. *Multivariate Statistical Methods in Behavioral Research*. New York: McGraw-Hill, 1975.
8.   Goldberger, A. S. and O. D. Duncan. *Structural Equation Models in the Social Sciences*. New York: Serninan Press, 1973.

For additional reading about the basics of evaluative research see:

Anderson, S. B.; S. Ball; R. T. Murphey & Associates. *Encyclopedia of Educational Evaluation*. Jossey-Bass, 1975.
Suchman, E. A. *Evaluative Research*. New York: Russell Sage Foundation, 1967.
Weiss, Carol. *Evaluation Research*. Prentice Hall, 1972.
Shortell, S. M., and W. C. Richardson. *Health Program Evaluation*. St. Louis: C. V. Mosby, 1978.

VII.   INDEX TO CHAPTER

The preceding chapter was written to aid the uninitiated reader by attempting to clarify the meaning of evaluative research terms and concepts that are used throughout this book. To facilitate its usefulness, the terms being clarified are in *italics* in the text, and a separate index for this chapter has been prepared. You may turn immediately to the section clarifying a particular term or concept by finding the appropriate section number after the term in the alphabetical list below.

While this chapter does include many of the most basic terms and concepts in evaluative research, several important terms are not discussed. This chapter is not meant to be comprehensive; rather it is organized around clarifying the meaning of basic evaluative research terms and concepts that were used by authors in this book.

PARTICIPANTS

Giovanni Acciarri
Universidad del Valle
Apartado Aéreo 2188
Cali, Colombia

Nelson Amaro
Banco de la Vivienda Popular
22 Avenida 31-56, Zona 12
Colonia Santa Elisa
Guatemala, Guatemala

Jaime Arroyo
Programa de Salud Familiar
Ministerio de Salud
Apartado 2048
Panamá, Panamá

Nicolás Arditto Barletta
Ministerio de Planificación y Política Económica
Apartado 3543, Zona 1
Panamá, Panamá

José María Bengoa
Comisión Nacional de Investigación Científica y Tecnológica
(CONICIT)
Apartado Postal 70617
Caracas, Venezuela

Abby Bloom
Agency for International Development (USAID)
United States Embassy
Panamá, Panamá

Ricardo Bressani
Instituto de Nutrición de Centro América y Panamá (INCAP)
Apartado Postal 1188
Guatemala, Guatemala

James A. Brown, Jr.
Office of Development Planning
Bureau for the Near East
Agency for International Development (USAID)
Department of State
Washington, D. C. 20523

William P. Butz
Economics Department
The Rand Corporation
1700 Main Street
Santa Monica, California 90406

Rubén Cáceres
Ministerio de Salud Pública y Bienestar Social
Asunción, Paraguay

Herbert Caudill
Agency for International Development (USAID)
United States Embassy
Panamá, Panamá

Adolfo Chávez
Instituto Nacional de Nutrición
San Buenaventura y Viaducto Tlalpán
México 22, D. F., México

Dov Chernichovsky
Population and Human Resources Division
The World Bank
1818 "H" Street, N. W.
Washington, D. C. 20433

Thomas D. Cook
Department of Psychology
Northwestern University
Evanston, Illinois   60201

Héctor Correa
Graduate School of Public Health and International Affairs
University of Pittsburgh
Pittsburgh, Pennsylvania   15260

John A. Daly
Office of Health
Agency for International Development (USAID)
Department of State
Washington, D. C. 20523

Joseph H. Davis
Office of Health
Agency for International Development (USAID)
Department of State
Washington, D. C. 20523

Carlos H. Daza
Division of Family Health, Nutrition Section
Pan American Health Organization
525 Twenty-third Street, N. W.
Washington, D. C. 20037

Michael Draper
Evaluation Division
Canadian International Development Agency
122 Bank Street
Ottawa, Canada K1A/0G4

Robert Emrey
Association of University Programs in Health Administration
1 Dupont Circle N.W.
Washington, D. C.

Luis F. Fajardo
Universidad del Valle
Apartado Aéreo 2188
Cali, Colombia

Timothy Farrell
Instituto de Nutrición de Centro América y Panamá (INCAP)
Apartado Postal 1188
Guatemala, Guatemala

Brian R. Flay
Health Studies Department
University of Waterloo
Waterloo, Ontario, Canada

Ricardo Galán Morera
División de Investigación
Ministerio de Salud Pública
Bogotá, Colombia

John Michael Gurney
Caribbean Food and Nutrition Institute (CFNI)
University of the West Indies
P. O. Box 140
Kingston 7, Jamaica

Richard A. Haag
ACTION
Washington, D. C.

Jean-Pierre Habicht
National Center for Health Statistics
Center Building, Room 2-58
3700 East-West Highway
Hyattsville, Maryland 20782

Nair Carmen de Oliveira Hamann
Proyecto Nutricao INAN/Banco Mundial
Brasilia, Brazil

Jerianne Heimendinger
Agency for International Development (USAID)
Department of State
Washington, D. C. 20523

Karen M. Hennigan
Psychology Department
University of Southern California
Los Angeles, California 90024

Guillermo Herrera
Department of Nutrition
Harvard School of Public Health
665 Huntington Avenue
Boston, Massachusetts 02115

Robinson Hollister
Department of Economics
Swarthmore College
Swarthmore, Pennsylvania 19081

Alberto Chen Hurtado
Programa de Desarrollo Rural-Urbano
Organización de Estados Americanos
6 de Diciembre 4585
Quito, Ecuador

Nicholas Imboden
Development Centre
Organization for Economic Cooperation and Development (OECD)
94 Rue Chardon-Lagache
Paris 16, France

José Jordan
Ministerio de Salud Pública
Habana, Cuba

Robert E. Klein
Instituto de Nutrición de Centro América y Panamá (INCAP)
Apartado Postal 1188
Guatemala, Guatemala

J. Michael Lane
Bureau of Smallpox Eradication
Center for Disease Control
Atlanta, Georgia 30333

Kenneth Leslie
Caribbean Food and Nutrition Institute (CFNI)
P. O. Box 140
Kingston 7, Jamaica

Flavio Machicado
Organización de las Naciones Unidas para la Agricultura (FAO)
Apartado Postal 1424
Santo Domingo, República Dominicana

Patrick J. H. Marnane
Division of International Health Programs
American Public Health Association
1015 Eighteenth Street, N. W.
Washington, D. C. 20036

Leonardo J. Mata
Instituto de Investigación en Salud
Universidad de Costa Rica
Ciudad Universitaria "Rodrigo Facio"
San José, Costa Rica

Emile McAnany
Institute for Communication Research
Stanford University
Palo Alto, California 94304

Selma J. Mushkin
Public Services Laboratory
Georgetown University
3600 "M" Street, N. W.
Washington, D. C. 20007

Cutberto Parillón
Sistema Integrado de Salud de Veraguas
Ministerio de Salud Pública
Panamá, Panamá

José Pastore
Instituto de Pesquisas Econômicas
Universidad de Sao Paulo
Sao Paulo, Brazil

Gretel Pelto
Archeology and Human Ecology Department
University of Connecticut
Box U-176
Storrs, Connecticut 06268

Sebastián Piñera
Comisión Económica para América Latina (ECLA)
Avenida Dag Hammarskjold
Santiago, Chile

Ernesto Pollitt
Department of Nutrition and Food Sciences
Massachusetts Institute of Technology
Cambridge, Massachusetts 02139

Alberto Pradilla
Fundación para la Educación Superior (FES)
Apartado Aéreo 002805, Cod. 144
Cali, Colombia

Robert Pratt
Office of Nutrition
Agency for International Development (USAID)
Department of State
Washington, D. C. 20523

Frank C. Ramsey
National Nutrition Unit
The Queen Elizabeth Hospital
Martindales Road, St. Michael
Barbados, West Indies

Emirto Raudales
Sistema de Análisis y Planificación de la Alimentación y Nutrición
(SAPLAN)
Consejo de Planificación Económica
Tegucigalpa, Honduras

Merrill S. Read
Division of Family Health, Nutrition Section
Pan American Health Organization
525 Twenty-third Street, N. W.
Washington, D. C. 20037

Robert L. Robertson
Mount Holyoake College
South Hadley, Massachusetts

A. Kimball Romney
Department of Anthropology
University of California at Irvine
Irvine, California 92664

Henry W. Riecken
School of Medicine
University of Pennsylvania
36 Hamilton Walk, Room M-151
Philadelphia, Pennsylvania 19104

Roberto Rueda-Williamson
CONTESEN
Calle 70, No. 4-50
Apartado Aéreo 090-400
Bogotá, Colombia

Paul Schultz
Yale Economic Growth Center
Yale Station, Box 1987
New Haven, Connecticut 06520

Susan C. M. Scrimshaw
School of Public Health
University of California at Los Angeles
Los Angeles, California 90024

Giorgio R. Solimano
Institute of Human Nutrition
Columbia University
College of Physicians and Surgeons
511 West 166th Street
New York, New York 10032

C. Richard Stark
Pregnancy and Infancy Branch
National Institute of Child Health and Human Development
Bethesda, Maryland 20014

Jerome Stromberg
Division of Strengthening of Health Services
World Health Organization
1211 Geneva 27, Switzerland

John W. Townsend
Instituto de Nutrición de Centro América y Panamá (INCAP)
Apartado Postal 1188
Guatemala, Guatemala

Antonio Ugalde
Department of Sociology
University of Texas
Austin, Texas 78712

Beverly Winikoff
Rockefeller Foundation
1133 Avenue of the Americas
New York, New York 10036

INDEX